MINIMALLY INVASIVE GYNECOLOGY SERIES

Myomectomy

GENERAL SERIES EDITORS

Eric J. Bieber, MD
Assistant Professor
Director of Reproductive Endoscopy
Department of Obstetrics and Gynecology
The University of Chicago
Chicago, Illinois

Franklin D. Loffer, MD
Gynecological Associates, Ltd.
Phoenix, Arizona

FORTHCOMING IN THE SERIES:

Management of Ectopic Pregnancy
edited by R. Leach
and S. Ory

MINIMALLY INVASIVE GYNECOLOGY SERIES

Myomectomy

edited by

Eric J. Bieber, MD
Assistant Professor
Director of Reproductive Endoscopy
Department of Obstetrics and Gynecology
The University of Chicago
Chicago, Illinois

Victoria M. Maclin, MD
Assistant Professor
Chief, Section of Reproductive Endocrinology and Infertility
University of Nebraska Medical Center
Omaha, Nebraska

Blackwell
Science

Editorial Offices:
350 Main Street, Malden, MA 02148-5018, USA
Osney Mead, Oxford OX2 0EL, England
25 John Street, London WC1N 2BL, England
23 Ainslie Place, Edinburgh EH3 6AJ, Scotland
54 University Street, Carlton, Victoria 3053, Australia

Other Editorial Offices:
Blackwell Wissenschafts-Verlag GmbH
Kurfürstendamm 57
10707 Berlin, Germany

Blackwell Science KK
MG Kodenmacho Building
7–10 Kodenmacho Nihombashi
Chuo-ku, Tokyo 104, Japan

DISTRIBUTORS

USA
Blackwell Science, Inc.
Commerce Place
350 Main Street
Malden, Massachusetts 02148
(Telephone orders: 800-215-1000 or 781-388-8250; fax orders: 781-388-8270)

Canada
Copp Clark, Ltd.
200 Adelaide St West, 3rd Floor
Toronto, Ontario
Canada, M5H 1W7
(Telephone orders: 416-597-1616 or 800-815-9417; fax orders: 416-597-1617)

Australia
Blackwell Science Pty, Ltd.
54 University Street
Carlton, Victoria 3053
(Telephone orders: 03-9347-0300;
fax orders: 03-9349-3016)

Outside North America and Australia
Blackwell Science, Ltd.
c/o Marston Book Services, Ltd.
P.O. Box 269
Abingdon
Oxon OX14 4YN
England
(Telephone orders: 44-01235-465500;
fax orders: 44-01235-465555)

Notice: The indications and dosages of all drugs in this book have been recommended in the medical literature and conform to the practices of the general medical community. The medications described do not necessarily have specific approval by the U.S. Food and Drug Administration for use in the diseases and dosages for which they are recommended. The package insert for each drug should be consulted for use and dosage as approved by the FDA. Because standards for usage change, it is advisable to keep abreast of revised recommendations, particularly those concerning new drugs.

First published 1998
Acquisitions: Chris Davis
Production: Kevin Sullivan
Manufacturing: Lisa Flanagan
Typeset by Best-set Typesetter Ltd., Hong Kong
Printed and bound by Edwards Brothers
Printed in the United States of America
98 99 00 01 5 4 3 2 1
The Blackwell Science logo is a trade mark of Blackwell Science Ltd, registered at the United Kingdom Trade Marks Registry

Library of Congress Cataloging-In-Publication Data

Myomectomy / [edited by] Eric J. Bieber, Victoria M. Maclin.
p cm.
Includes bibliographical references and index.
ISBN 0-86542-381-4
1. Myomectomy. 2. Uterine fibroids—Surgery. 3. Smooth muscles—Tumors—Surgery. 4. Infertility. Female—Surgery. I. Bieber, Eric J. II. Maclin, Victoria M.
[DNLM: 1. Uterine Neoplasms—Surgery. 2. Myoma—Surgery. WP 458 M997 1998]
RG301.M96 1998
616.99′366059—dc21
DNLM/DLC
for Library of Congress 98-21524
CIP

Contents

Contributors

Marvin D. Almquist, MD
Department of Obstetrics and Gynecology
Good Samaritan Hospital
Cincinnati, Ohio

Michael S. Baggish, MD
Professor of Obstetrics and Gynecology
University of Cincinnati
Chairman, Department of Obstetrics and Gynecology
Good Samaritan Hospital
Cincinnati, Ohio

Michael P. Diamond, MD
Professor and Director
Division of Reproductive Endocrinology and Infertility
Department of Obstetrics and Gynecology
Wayne State University School of Medicine
Detroit, Michigan

Dee E. Fenner, MD
Assistant Professor
Department of Obstetrics and Gynecology
Rush-Presbyterian-St. Luke's Medical Center
Chicago, Illinois

Samir N. Hajj, MD
Head of Gynecology
Department of Obstetrics and Gynecology
Pritzker School of Medicine
Head of Gynecology
Department of Obstetrics and Gynecology
University of Chicago
Chicago, Illinois

Lisa A. Hasty, MD
Clinical Assistant Professor
Division of Reproductive Endocrinology and Infertility
Department of Obstetrics and Gynecology
Emory University School of Medicine
Atlanta, Georgia

Lawrence C. Layman, MD
Chief, Section of Reproductive Endocrinology and Infertility
Department of Obstetrics and Gynecology
The University of Chicago
Chicago, Illinois

Richard E. Leach, MD
Assistant Professor
Division of Reproductive Endocrinology
Department of Obstetrics and Gynecology
Wayne State University School of Medicine
Detroit, Michigan

Beth A. Plunkett, MD
Resident, Obstetrics and Gynecology
Northwestern University Medical School
Home Officer, Obstetrics and Gynecology
McGaw Medical Center of Northwestern University
Chicago, Illinois

Elizabeth Puscheck, MD, FACOG
Assistant Professor
Department of Obstetrics and Gynecology
Northwestern University Medical School
Chicago, Illinois

Valerie Montgomery Rice, MD
Senior Staff Physician
Division of Reproductive Endocrinology and Infertility
Department of Obstetrics and Gynecology
Henry Ford Center for Reproductive Medicine
Detroit, Michigan

Gloria Richard-Davis, MD
Assistant Professor
Department of Obstetrics and Gynecology
Tulane University Medical Center
New Orleans, Louisiana

Joseph S. Sanfilippo, MD
Chairman, Department of Obstetrics and Gynecology
Allegheny University of Health Science
Pittsburgh, Pennsylvania

Barbara A. Soltes, MD
Assistant Professor
Department of Obstetrics and Gynecology
Clinical Director, Women's Health Research Center
Rush-Presbyterian-St. Luke's Medical Center
Chicago, Illinois

Elizabeth A. Stewart, MD
Assistant Professor of Obstetrics, Gynecology, and Reproductive Biology
Harvard Medical School
Brigham and Women's Hospital
Boston, Massachusetts

Howard C. Topel, MD
Department of Obstetrics and Gynecology
Lutheran General Hospital
Park Ridge, Illinois

Togas Tulandi, MD, FRCS, FACOG
Director, Division of Reproductive Endocrinology/Infertility
Professor of Obstetrics and Gynecology
McGill University
Montreal, Quebec

Rafael F. Valle, MD
Professor, Department of Obstetrics and Gynecology
Northwestern University Medical School
Chicago, Illinois

Jenn-Ming Yang, MD
Department of Obstetrics and Gynecology
Good Samaritan Hospital
Cincinnati, Ohio

Foreword

Howard A. Kelly and Thomas S. Cullen published one of the first texts in this field, *Myomata of the Uteri*, in 1909. In 723 pages, detailed case histories of 1674 women and relevant pathology were carefully discussed. Cullen noted the reduction of mortality to less than 1% with the development of surgical technique. Moreover, advances in antiseptics and anesthesia added to the reduction in morbidity.

Today, rarely do the sequelae associated with enormously large myomas arise because a patient has failed to seek medical advice. However, there continues to be significant symptomatology requiring treatment. Advances in technology and pharmacology have expanded our therapeutic options. *Myomectomy*, edited by Eric J. Bieber and Victoria M. Maclin, summarizes our progress in the diagnosis and treatment of leiomyomas to date. The editors have assembled an outstanding group of authors to address surgical technique, by both endoscopy and laparotomy, as well as vaginal myomectomy. Special chapters on adhesion prevention, medical therapy, and reproductive performance after surgery add to a pertinent, up-to-date review for practicing physicians.

Myomectomy continues the exemplary tradition of Kelly and Cullen by thoroughly addressing the current diagnosis and treatment of leiomyomata uteri. This text is a valuable addition to the medical literature and will serve as a comprehensive resource for practicing gynecologists, both in the United States and abroad.

John A. Rock, MD
James Robert McCord Professor and Chairman
Department of Gynecology and Obstetrics
Emory University School of Medicine
Atlanta, Georgia

Preface

Approximately 25% to 30% of women in their reproductive years develop uterine leiomyomas, 80% of which are asymptomatic (1,2). Asymptomatic leiomyomas almost never require operative intervention unless they are believed to be a contributing factor to infertility. In general, indications for surgical treatment of uterine leiomyomas include menorrhagia, pelvic pain and pressure, a rapidly growing leiomyoma, and infertility.

Hysterectomies outnumber myomectomies 10 to 1 in the surgical treatment of uterine leiomyomas (3). This statistic may be due in part to the perceived incidence of recurrence after myomectomy, which has been reported to range from 10% to 50% (4–6). Buttram and Reiter reported a 15% average recurrence rate in over 3000 myomectomies. Acian and Quereda used life-table analysis to report a 10-year recurrence and reoperation rate of 38% and 18%, respectively. Fedele and colleagues reported a 5-year cumulative probability of recurrence of 51%. Interestingly, most recurrences were asymptomatic. The increased incidence of hysterectomy versus myomectomy in the treatment of uterine leiomyomas has also been attributed to the notion that there is a higher morbidity rate associated with myomectomy. Contrary to this perception, a recent retrospective study by Iverson et al (1) revealed that myomectomy compared favorably to hysterectomy, with a decreased risk for visceral injury and infection. Therefore, myomectomy is a reasonable option for women who wish to preserve their uterus.

Uterine preservation is a desired outcome for many women, regardless of desire for future reproduction. This issue is addressed in Chapter 11, "Myomectomy in the Nonreproductive Woman." For those of us who appreciate the positive role that myomectomy plays in the treatment of women with symptomatic and asymptomatic leiomyomas, this book should prove to be a helpful guide. We have attempted to take a comprehensive look at the epidemiology, pathophysiology, diagnosis, and treatment of uterine leiomyomas. The contributing authors were selected because of their knowledge and practical experience. The various approaches to myomectomy are presented with detailed advice pertaining to patient selection and operative technique.

The contributing authors were instructed to write chapters that could stand alone, as we realize that most readers do not read medical textbooks from cover to cover. Because of this, some inevitable redundancy and crossover exist in the text. In addition, the reader may note differing opinions in various chapters. Rather than attempting to homogenize the views of the contributors, we have kept the heterogeneity of opinions in the belief that this reflects the true nature of medicine and surgery.

We are hopeful that the information contained within will help advance the knowledge of the reader and increase the practitioner's confidence in myomectomy as a useful alternative to hysterectomy for the treatment of uterine leiomyomas. For patients with asymptomatic leiomyomas requiring myomectomy for treatment of infertility, we hope that this text enables the practitioner to approach the procedure in a manner that minimizes adhesion formation and optimizes reproductive potential.

E.J.B.
V.M.M.

REFERENCES

1. Iverson RE, Chelmow D, Strohbehn K, et al. Relative morbidity of abdominal hysterectomy and myomectomy for management of uterine leiomyomas. Obstet Gynecol 1996;88:415–419.
2. Parker WH. Myomectomy: laparoscopy or laparotomy. Clin Obstet Gynecol 1995;38:392–400.
3. National Center for Health Statistics. Hysterectomies in the United States, 1965–1984. Vital and Health Statistics, Series 13, No. 92. Publication 88-1753. Bethesda, MD: Public Health Service, 1987.
4. Buttram VC, Reiter RC. Uterine leiomyomata: etiology, symptomatology, and management. Fertil Steril 1981;36:433–445.
5. Fedele L, Parazzini F, Luchini L, et al. Recurrence of fibroids after myomectomy: a transvaginal ultrasonographic study. Hum Reprod 1995;10:1795–1796.
6. Acien P, Quereda R. Abdominal myomectomy: results of a simple operative technique. Fertil Steril 1996;65:41–51.

Acknowledgments

I would like to thank my staff, especially Therese Reczek and Lisa Missal, for invaluable help in the preparation of the manuscript. I would also like to express my gratitude toward my wife, Edie Bieber, and my two sons for tolerating the time away from their lives. Finally, I would like to thank my father and mother, George and Audrey, for embodying the search for truth and knowledge.

E.J.B.

I would like to express special appreciation to my family, especially to my children.

V.M.M.

We would both like to thank the many individuals who made this text possible, including the staff at Blackwell Science, and the many mentors who have shaped our careers and are too numerous to name here.

E.J.B.
V.M.M.

CHAPTER

1

Fibroids: Basic Information

Dee E. Fenner

Uterine leiomyomas are the most common uterine neoplasms. They are benign proliferations of smooth-muscle cells and fibrous connective tissue that arise from the uterine smooth muscle. They are noted clinically in 20% to 30% of women greater than 30 years of age and are found in up to 75% of hysterectomy specimens when they are searched for systematically (1). Leiomyomas are the most common indication for hysterectomy in the United States, accounting for approximately 30% of all procedures in two large collaborative trials (2,3). Based on the total number of hysterectomies performed in the United States annually, it would be expected that each year approximately 165,000 to 175,000 hysterectomies are performed for leiomyomas. This results in a direct cost for inpatient care alone in excess of $1 billion (4).

Most uterine leiomyomas are detected in reproductive-aged women, are uncommon in adolescents, and are clinically detected less frequently in postmenopausal women. Leiomyomas are more common in black than in white women.

Uterine leiomyomas may be single or multiple and range in size from 1 to 2 mm to greater than 20 cm in diameter. They may be located within the uterine wall, may be intramural, or may protrude into the endometrial cavity as submucosal fibroids. Fibroids may lie under the serosal surface of the uterus or grow from a stalk as a pedunculated fibroid. Pedunculated subserosal tumors that outgrow their uterine blood supply and obtain a secondary blood supply from another organ such as the omentum are termed *parasitic leiomyomas*. Rarely, a condition known as disseminated peritoneal leiomyomatosis (DPL) is encountered unexpectedly at the time of cesarean section or laparotomy. DPL appears as multiple, small, granular white or tan nodules on the pelvic and abdominal peritoneum and on the surfaces of the uterus, adnexa, intestine, and omentum. The nodules are distributed randomly and most of them are less than 1 cm in diameter. Generally this is a benign condition but must be differentiated from metastatic leiomyoma sarcoma. Most often this condition is seen with pregnancy, estrogenizing granulosa tumor, or oral contraceptive use. Once the hormonal stimulus is removed, the tumors regress and excision is not needed (5,6).

EPIDEMIOLOGY OF UTERINE LEIOMYOMAS

Risk factors associated with the development of uterine leiomyomas have been reported in a few retrospective analyses. These clinical reports have relied on physical examination to select a control group. Work by Cramer and Patal (1) has shown that the incidence of uterine fibroids may be grossly underestimated when physical examination or routine pathologic evaluation is relied on for determination of the presence or absence of leiomyomas. Therefore, while these studies are valuable, their validity is questionable.

The first study, conducted at the Oxford Family Planning Association in Oxford, England, and reported by Ross et al (7), used hysterectomy specimens for the study group as compared to age-matched controls determined by clinical examination. At the time of surgery, 535 women were evaluated. Case control analysis showed that reproductive experiences were closely linked to the development of fibroids. Risk of fibroids decreased consistently with increasing number of term pregnancies. Women with five term pregnancies had only a quarter of the risk of nulliparous women. Risk also decreased consistently with increasing duration of oral contraceptive use, as the risk of fibroids was reduced by 31% in women who had used oral contraceptives for at least 10 years. Cigarette smoking was also associated with a decrease in fibroids. Smokers of 20 cigarettes a day had roughly two-thirds the risk of nonsmokers.

A study conducted in Milan by Parazzini et al (8) evaluated subjects with pathologically confirmed leiomyomas versus controls. The control group was comprised of women admitted for acute medical problems. Specifically excluded were women admitted for gynecologic, hormonal, or neoplastic disease or those with a past history of hysterectomy. Comparison was made between 275 women with histologically confirmed fibroids and 722 control subjects. Questions were asked about menstrual and reproductive histories, education, and lifetime use of oral contraceptives and other hormonal treatments. The risk of uterine fibroids was found to be reduced in parous women relative to nulliparous ones, with a relative risk of 0.6. Postmenopausal women had a relative risk of 0.1 when compared with premenopausal women of the same age. Women with fibroids tended to have an earlier age at menarche, to be more educated, and to use intrauterine devices and oral contraceptives more frequently, although these findings were not statistically significant. Current smoking but not past smoking lowered the fibroid risk by about 40%. No association was found with body mass index, history of spontaneous or induced abortions, or age at first birth.

Both the Oxford and Milan study showed an increasing risk of leiomyomas with age, with a peak in the fifth decade of life. Both studies agreed on the decreased risk of leiomyomas with parity. Women with five births had only 25% the risk of nulliparous patients in the Oxford study and a relative risk of 0.6 in the Milan study (Table 1.1).

A study of a larger group of women with uterine leiomyomas that uses women whose uteri have been removed and serially sectioned as control subjects is desirable to confirm the Oxford and Milan data. The relationship of parity, timing, and number of pregnancies and the risk of leiomyomas needs to be further studied. These associations leave open the question of the extent to which leiomyomas may cause infertility as opposed to how infertility may promote the development of leiomy-

TABLE 1.1

Reduced risk of leiomyomas

	RELATIVE RISK
Any term pregnancy vs. nulliparous	0.60
Greater than 5 pregnancies vs. nulliparous	0.25
OCP use greater than 10 yr	0.70
Smoking	0.66
Postmenopausal vs. reproductive-aged women	0.10

OCP, oral contraceptive pills.
Source: Ross RK, Pike MC, Vessey MP, et al. Risk factors for uterine fibroids: reduced risk associated with oral contraceptives. Br Med J 1986;293:359–362; and Parazzini F, La Vecchia C, Negri E, et al. Epidemiologic characteristics of women with uterine fibroids: a case-control study. Obstet Gynecol 1988;72:853–857.

omas (9). Cramer et al suggest that to some extent the association with infertility may reflect menstrual irregularities impeding parity and at the same time promoting the development of leiomyomas. They evaluated uterine specimens of 22 women undergoing hysterectomies for various causes who were sectioned at 2-mm intervals to establish the absence or presence of leiomyomas. They compared 22 women to 8 controls with false-positive clinical diagnosis of fibroids. While this study is small, they noted a trend supporting the negative association of leiomyomas with smoking. Cramer's group specifically evaluated the hypothesis that abnormal uterine bleeding might be a risk factor in the development of uterine leiomyomas. However, due to the sample size they did not find statistical significance ($p > .2$) in the relationship of abnormal bleeding in patients with myoma versus controls, although they did see a trend.

A larger prospective study is warranted to evaluate the hypothesis of abnormal uterine bleeding or unopposed estrogen action having a role on the growth of uterine leiomyomas. It may provide a possible explanation for the negative correlation of myomas with cigarette smoking, which is thought to lower circulating estradiol levels. While estrogen may be an important promoter of growth in uterine leiomyomas there is no evidence that hormones or other growth factors cause the chromosomal abnormalities that are now being documented in the etiology of uterine leiomyomas.

ETIOLOGY

Townsend and coworkers (10) discovered that cells that compose a single leiomyoma are of identical glucose 6-phosphate dehydrogenase electrophoretic type, even though the cell type of different tumors from within the same uterus may vary. These data suggest that leiomyomas are of a unicellular origin, arising from a single neoplastic smooth-muscle cell.

Cytogenetic analysis has consistently demonstrated abnormalities, including translocations and deletions involving several chromosomes. Four cytogenetically abnormal subgroups have been described: tumors with aberrations involving the short arm of chromosome 6, tumors with deletion in the long arm of chromosome 7, tumors with trisomy 12, and tumors with 12q (14–15) changes. In the remaining cytogenetically abnormal uterine leiomyomas, various nonrecurrent abnormalities have been found. Precise mapping of chromosomal breakpoints of recurrent tumor-specific translocations followed by molecular analysis of deoxyribonucleic acid (DNA) regions immediately flanking such breakpoints has proved to be a successful approach to identifying and isolating genes involved in tumor development (11). It has been suggested that genes interrupted by these translocations or deletions play a role in the formation of leiomyomas similar to the role played by the t(2;13) translocation in alveolar rhabdomyosarcoma and in the t(11;22) translocation in Ewing's sarcoma (12). Why these nonrandom chromosomal abnormalities occur and at such a high frequency is yet undetermined.

Estrogen has long been implicated as a growth factor for leiomyomas due to their appearance after menarche, growth during pregnancy, and postmenopausal regression (13). In addition, the long-term administration of gonadotropin-releasing hormone (GnRH) agonist, which causes a hypoestrogenic state, has been documented to reduce myoma volume. Wilson et al (14) reported a significantly higher concentration of estrogen receptors in leiomyomas than in normal myometrium in the same uterus. However, Puuka et al (15), Pollow et al (16), and Tamaya et al (17) were unable to demonstrate a difference between the estrogen receptor concentrations of leiomyomas and normal myometrium. Pollow et al also demonstrated a significantly lower conversion of estradiol into estrone in the leiomyoma than in myometrium (16). Their findings suggest that increases in local estradiol concentration may play a role in the pathogenesis of leiomyomas.

Cramer et al in 1985 (18) evaluated the effect of alpha-estradiol and beta-estradiol on the growth of normal myometrium and leiomyoma cells from the same patients. This in vitro study showed that leiomyoma cells had significantly less growth than normal myometrium. The authors proposed the possibility that this heterogeneity in hormonal growth stimulation may be an important factor in the wide variation of growth potential of uterine leiomyomas and that the difference in leiomyoma growth may be a distinctive property of the host hormonal milieu, rather than a distinctive property of the tumor tissue.

The effects of estrogen on myoma growth may be related to estrogen-mediated responses of other receptors and growth factors. There is increasing evidence that estrogen stimulates the production of progesterone receptors [Adams et al (19)], epidermal growth factor [Yeh et al (20)], and insulin-like growth factor–I [Guidice et al (21)]. Andersen et al (22) demonstrated that the expression of estrogen-regulated genes appears to be greater in myomas than in normal myometrium, and therefore may be important in myoma growth.

Pollow et al (16) reported that the concentration of progesterone receptors in leiomyoma was significantly lower than that of surrounding myometrium. Wilson et al (14), however, noted an increase in progesterone receptors in leiomyomas when compared to normal myometrium, although individual variations were noted between samples. Soules and McCarty (23) found the levels of both cytoplasmic estrogen and progesterone receptors in leiomyomas to demonstrate the same quantitative and qualitative changes throughout the menstrual cycle, apparently in response to variations in circulating estrogen and progesterone. Yet several studies have suggested that progesterone may inhibit the growth of leiomyomas. Goldziener et al (24) were able to demonstrate that large doses of medroxyprogesterone acetate, 25 mg given daily to patients 14 to 21 days before hysterectomy, evoked intense degenerative changes in leiomyomas. Smaller doses (2 mg) of norethindrone daily, for 1 to 3 months prior to surgery, however, had no effect.

The concentrations of receptor proteins in target tissue are controlled in part by the endogenous steroid hormones. Estrogen increases the concentrations of both estradiol receptors and progesterone receptors. Progesterone on the other hand decreases the concentration of both receptors (25).

Rein et al (26) recently reviewed the role of progesterone in the pathogenesis of uterine myomas. They noted two studies by Tiltman (27) and Kawaguchi et al (28) that showed increased mitotic activity in myomas removed during the luteal phase or after treatment with medroxyprogesterone. These studies, along with data showing that medroxyprogesterone when given along with a GnRH agonist prevents myoma shrinkage, support their theory of the importance of progesterone in myoma growth (29,30). They further hypothesize that since the rate of mitosis strongly influences the propagation of somatic mutations, progesterone may contribute to myoma formation by increasing the likelihood of somatic mutations.

Peptide growth factors may be important in the regulation of leiomyoma growth. Induction of DNA synthesis by epidermal growth factors in leiomyoma and matched myometrial cell cultures was found to be similar by Fayed et al (31). However, the number of epidermal growth factor receptor sites in leiomyoma cells is significantly lower than in matched myometrial cell cultures. Insulin binding was similar in both normal myometrium and leiomyoma cells. Protein synthesis was stimulated in both tissues when epidermal growth factor or insulin was added to the cells, but when epidermal growth factor and platelet-derived growth factor were both added a significant growth occurred in the leiomyoma cells and not the normal myometrium.

Further investigation to determine what factors initiate somatic mutations, the relationship of the hormonal environment, and the effect of other growth factors is ongoing. It is hoped that these answers will lead to new treatment options for uterine leiomyomas.

CLINICAL FEATURES

The majority of leiomyomas are asymptomatic, with the prevalence ranging from 10% to 40% depending on the population of women sampled (13).

The most common symptom associated with leiomyomas is abnormal bleeding, which typically presents as menorrhagia. In Buttram and Rerterv's (13) review of the literature, of 1698 cases of myomectomy in which symptoms were recorded, 30% of the patients demonstrated menstrual abnormalities. Review of their own 59 patients with leiomyomas who were undergoing surgery for infertility similarly revealed that 29% of patients experienced menorrhagia. However, it should be noted that these series are based on patient reports rather than actual measurement of menstrual flow.

The etiology of leiomyoma-associated menorrhagia is unknown. Ulceration over submucosal tumors has been postulated. However, it is rarely observed in hysterectomy specimens or during hysteroscopic examinations. Furthermore, the incidence of submucous tumors is too low to explain the incidence of menorrhagia (32).

Miller and Ludovici (33) suggested that anovulation associated with uterine leiomyomas is responsible for menorrhagia. However, no studies have conclusively demonstrated that the incidence of anovulation in women with leiomyomas is higher than that of a control group. The presence of regular ovulatory cycles in most women with leiomyomas precludes the diagnosis of dysfunctional bleeding. Sehgal and Haskins (34) demonstrated that the endometrial surface area of a myomatous uterus can obtain the size of more than 200 sq cm, as compared to 15 sq cm for normal uteri. They were further able to show a correlation between severity of bleeding and increased endometrial surface area. Their hypothesis does not suggest the actual mechanism of bleeding and it does not explain bleeding associated with subserosal myomas, which may not distort the uterine cavity.

Farrer-Brown and associates (35,36) attempted to demonstrate that uterine bleeding was the result of compression of the venous plexi of the adjacent myometrium and endometrium. Their study showed radiographic evidence by which leiomyoma arising in various sites caused congestion and dilation of the adjacent endometrial venous plexi by impinging on the veins of the inner myometrium or on the arcuate radial veins throughout the intramural and subserosal regions of the myometrium. It has also been postulated that the uterus cannot contract because of the fibroids. Again, however, few well-controlled studies that actually measured menstrual flow have been performed to accurately record and correlate menorrhagia with leiomyoma size and location.

Pelvic pain or pressure is less frequently caused by uterine leiomyoma. Rubin and Ford (32) found concomitant pelvic disease, such as tubal inflammation, endometriosis, diverticulosis, or ovarian carcinoma, in patients with uterine leiomyomas who had substantial pelvic pain. Acute pain associated with a low-grade fever and tender uterus may be seen with carneous or red degeneration of leiomyomas or possible torsion of a pedunculated fibroid; however, these conditions can generally be managed conservatively and are self-limiting. Before surgery is performed for pelvic pain secondary to uterine leiomyomas, a careful and complete work-up should be performed to rule out other etiologies.

Pelvic pressure and impingement of pelvic viscera, specifically the bladder, resulting in suprapubic discomfort, frequency of urination, urinary retention, or overflow incontinence are rare. Constipation or pain with defecation has also been implicated as a result of a posterior fibroid. However, these should be a diagnosis of exclusion and more common etiologies should be evaluated before surgical management of leiomyomas.

Many reproductive disorders, including infertility, recurrent spontaneous abortions, anovulation, and preterm labor, have all been attributed to uterine leiomyomas. Despite an enormous amount of anecdotal and observational literature, there are at present no controlled data to support a causal association between uterine leiomyomas and infertility or poor reproductive outcomes (37).

Buttram and Rerter (13) reported 700 consecutive major surgical procedures performed for infertility, with only 16, or 2.3%, performed for uterine leiomyomas in women who had no other apparent fertility factors. Therefore, infertility secondary to leiomyomas appears rare.

Buttram and Rerter also reported that approximately 40% of women who underwent myomectomies for either infertility or recurrent pregnancy loss subsequently delivered term infants. These results were similar to pregnancy rates observed in untreated normal couples with infertility or habitual abortions associated with leiomyomas. Again, long-term prospective studies with untreated control subjects must be performed to better assess the impact of uterine myomas on reproductive outcomes.

PATHOLOGY

Leiomyomas are spherical, firm, and encapsulated smooth-muscle tumors. The cut surfaces are white to tan colored with a whorled pattern (see Plate 1). The appearance of leiomyoma may be altered by degeneration changes. Submucosal leiomyoma can be ulcerated and hemorrhaging. Hemorrhaging and necrosis are observed in some myomas, particularly in large myomas of women who are pregnant or who are undergoing high-dose progestin therapy. Dark-red areas represent hemorrhage and yellow areas reflect necrosis. The damaged smooth muscle is eventually replaced by firm white or translucent collagenous tissue. Cystic degeneration may also occur and in some leiomyomas becomes extensively calcified (38).

Microscopically, leiomyomas are composed of whorled uniform fascicles of smooth-muscle cells. The spindle-shaped cells have indistinctive borders and an abundant fibrillar, eosinophilic cytoplasm. The nuclei are elongated with blunt or tapered ends and have finely dispersed chromatin and small nuclei. Mitotic figures usually are infrequent.

Leiomyomas generally have fewer than 5 mitotic figures per 10 high-power fields (HPF). Leiomyomas with 5 to 10 mitotic figures per 10 HPF are termed *mitotically active*. They contain no atypical cells and are benign.

Atypical leiomyomas contain atypical cells but still have fewer than 5 mitotic figures per 10 HPF. Again, these are a benign microscopic variant of uterine leiomyomas (38).

Leiomyosarcoma represents about 1.3% of uterine malignancies and about one-third of uterine sarcomas. Fewer than 1% of women thought clinically to have leiomyomas have leiomyosarcomas (38). These are de novo malignancies that do not arise from preexisting fibroids. Women with benign uterine leiomyoma are not at increased risk for leiomyosarcoma. Microscopically, the three main criteria for diagnosis of leiomyosarcoma are hypercellularity, significant nuclear atypia, and frequent mitotic figures (39).

REFERENCES

1. Cramer SF, Patal A. The frequency of uterine leiomyomas. Am J Clin Pathol 1990;94:435–438.
2. Gambone JC, Reiter RC, Lench JB, Moore JG. The impact of a quality assurance process on the frequency and confirmation rate of hysterectomy. Am J Obstet Gynecol 1990;163:545–550.
3. Dicker RC, Greenspan JR, Strauss LT, et al. Complications of abdominal and vaginal hysterectomy among women of reproductive age in the United States. Am J Obstet Gynecol 1982;144:841–848.
4. National Center for Health Statistics. Health. United States, 1990. Hyattsville, MD: Public Health Service, 1991. DHHS publication no. (PHS) 91–1232.
5. Aterman K, Fraser GM, Lea RH. Disseminated peritoneal leiomyomatosis. Virchows Arch [A] 1977;374:13–26.

6. Tavassoli FA, Norris HJ. Peritoneal leiomyomatosis: a clinicopathologic study of 20 cases with ultrastructural observation. Int J Gynecol Pathol 1982;1:59–74.
7. Ross RK, Pike MC, Vessey MP, et al. Risk factors for uterine fibroids: reduced risk associated with oral contraceptives. Br Med J 1986; 293:359–362.
8. Parazzini F, La Vecchia C, Negri E, et al. Epidemiologic characteristics of women with uterine fibroids: a case-control study. Obstet Gynecol 1988; 72:853–857.
9. Cramer SF, Horiszny JA, Leppert P. Epidemiology of uterine leiomyomas. J Reprod Med 1995;40:595–600.
10. Townsend DE, Sparkes RS, Baluda MC, McClelland C. Unicellular histogenesis of uterine leiomyomas as determined by electrophoresis by glucose-6-phosphate dehydrogenase. Am J Obstet Gynecol 1970;107: 1168–1173.
11. Shoenmahers EF, Mols R, Wanshura S, et al. Identification, molecular cloning, and characterization of the chromosome 12 breakpoint cluster region of uterine leiomyomas. Genes, Chromosomes, and Cancer 1994; 11:106–118.
12. Doney MK, Gerken SC, Lynch R, et al. Precise mapping of t(12;14) leiomyoma breakpoint of chromosome 14 between D145298 and D145540. Cancer Lett 1995;96:245–252.
13. Buttram VC, Rerter RC. Uterine leiomyoma: etiology, symptomatology, and management. Fertil Steril 1981;36:433–445.
14. Wilson EA, Yang F, Rees ED. Estradiol and progesterone binding in uterine leiomyomata and in normal uterine tissues. Obstet Gynecol 1980;55:20.
15. Puuka MJ, Lontula KK, Kauppila AJI, et al. Estrogen receptor in human myoma tissue. Mol Cell Endocrinol 1976;6:35.
16. Pollow K, Geilfuss J, Boquoi E, Pollow B. Estrogen and progesterone binding proteins in normal human myometrium and leiomyoma tissue. J Clin Chem Clin Biochem 1978;16:503.
17. Tamaya T, Motoyama T, Ohono Y, et al. Estradiol 17-B progesterone, and 5-alpha-dihydrotestosterone receptors of uterine myometrium and myoma in the human subject. J Steroid Biochem 1979;10:615.
18. Cramer SF, Robertson AL, Ziats NP, Pearson OH. Growth potential of human uterine leiomyomas: some in vitro observations and their implications. Obstet Gynecol 1985;66:36–41.

19. Adams AD, Hild-Petito S, Donnelly K, Fazleabas AT. Regulation of estrogen (E) and progestin (p) receptors (R) in leiomyomas during the cycle and leuprolide acetate treatment. In: Proceedings of the Forty-ninth Annual Meeting of the American Fertility Society, Montreal, Quebec, Canada October 1993. Montreal: American Fertility Society, 1993:11–14.
20. Yeh J, Rein M, Nowak R. Presence of messenger ribonucleic acid for epidermal growth factor (EGF) and EGF receptor demonstrable in monolayer cell cultures of myometria and leiomyomata. Fertil Steril 1991;56: 997–1000.
21. Guidice LC, Irwin JC, Dsupin BA, et al. Insulin-like growth factor (IGF), IGF binding protein (IGFBP), and IGF receptor gene expression and IGFBP synthesis in human uterine leiomyomata. Hum Reprod 1993; 8:1796–1806.
22. Andersen J, Grine E, Eng CLY, et al. Expression of connexin-43 in human myometrium and leiomyoma. Am J Obstet Gynecol 1993;169:1266–1276.
23. Soules MR, McCarty KS. Leiomyomas: steroid receptor content. Am J Obstet Gynecol 1982;143:6–11.
24. Goldzieher JW, Maqueo M, Ricaud L, et al. Induction of degenerative changes in uterine myomas by high-dose progestin therapy. Am J Obstet Gynecol 1966;96:1078.
25. Thi MTL, Banlien EE, Milgrom E. Comparison of the characteristics and of the hormonal control of endometrial and myometrial progesterone receptors. J Endocrinol 1974;66:349.
26. Rein MS, Friedman AJ, Barbieri RL, et al. Cytogenetic abnormalities in uterine leiomyomata. Obstet Gynecol 1991;77:923–926.
27. Tiltman AJ. The effect of progestins on the miotic activity of uterine fibromyomas. Int J Gynecol Pathol 1985;4:89–96.
28. Kawaguchi D, Fujii S, Konishi J, et al. Mitotic activity in uterine leiomyomas during the menstrual cycle. Am J Obstet Gynecol 1989;160:632–641.
29. Friedman AJ, Barbieri RL, Doubilet PM, et al. A randomized double-blind trial of a gonadotropin releasing-hormone agonist (leuprolide) with or without medroxyprogesterone acetate in the treatment of leiomyomata uteri. Fertil Steril 1988;49:404–409.
30. Carr BR, Marshburn PT, Weatherall PT, et al. An evaluation of the effect of gonadotropin-releasing hormone analogs and medroxyprogesterone acetate on uterine leiomyomata volume by magnetic resonance imaging: a prospective, randomized, double blind, placebo-controlled crossover trial. J Clin Endocrinol Metab 1993;76:1217–1223.

31. Fayed YM, Tsibris JCM, Langenberg PW, Robertson AL Jr. Human uterine leiomyoma cells: binding and growth responses to epidermal growth factor, platelet-derived growth factor, and insulin. Lab Invest 1989;60:30–37.
32. Rubin A, Ford JA. Uterine fibromyomata in urban blacks. A preliminary survey of the relationship between symptomatology, blood pressure and haemoglobin levels. S Afr Med J 1974;48:2060–2062.
33. Miller NF, Ludovici PP. Origin and development of uterine fibroids. Am J Obstet Gynecol 1955;70:720.
34. Sehgal N, Haskins AL. The mechanism of uterine bleeding in the presence of fibromyomas. Am J Surg 1960;26:21.
35. Farrer-Brown G, Beilby JOW, Tarbit MH. The vascular patterns in myomatous uteri. J Obstet Gynecol Br Commonw 1970;77:967.
36. Farrer-Brown G, Beilby JOW, Tarbit MH. Venous changes in the endometrium of myomatous uteri. Obstet Gynecol 1971;38:743.
37. Vollenhoven BJ, Lawrence AS, Healy DL. Uterine fibroids: a clinical review. Br J Obstet Gynecol 1990;97:285–298.
38. Blaustein's pathology of the female genital tract. 4th ed. New York: Springer-Verlag, 1994:489–491.
39. Leibsohn S, d'Ablaing G, Mischell DR, Schlaerth JB. Leiomyosarcoma in a series of hysterectomies performed for presumed uterine leiomyomas. Am J Obstet Gynecol 1990;162:968–974.

CHAPTER

2

Preoperative Evaluation Before Myomectomy

Valerie Montgomery Rice
Gloria Richard-Davis

Uterine fibroids or leiomyomas occur in approximately 20% to 50% of women in the reproductive age group, and they are the most common pelvic tumors in women (1–3). The frequency is higher in women in their thirties and forties. Figures from autopsy reports suggest that the frequency may be as high as 75% (4). The incidence is three to nine times higher in black than in white women, suggesting a genetic predisposition in certain individuals (5). The precise etiology of fibroids has not been established.

Symptoms associated with fibroids include abnormal uterine bleeding, particularly menorrhagia and hypermenorrhea, as well as pelvic pressure or pain, bloating, increased urinary frequency, and constipation. Infertility, first-trimester pregnancy losses, placental abruption, pain, premature labor during the second and third trimester, fetal malpresentation, inertia, and dystocia during labor may also be noted. In addition, postpartum hemorrhage and infection may be associated with uterine leiomyomas. However, many women with fibroids are completely asymptomatic (Table 2.1).

As women delay childbearing, physicians will encounter with increasing frequency patients who wish to maintain their fertility in the presence of symptomatic fibroids. The American College of Obstetrics and Gynecology has long recommended hysterectomy when the uterine

TABLE 2.1

Signs and symptoms associated with uterine leiomyomas

SYMPTOMS	SIGNS
Asymptomatic	Abnormal uterine
Bleeding	Menorrhagia
Pelvic pressure/pain	Hypermenorrhea
Urinary frequency	Infertility
Urinary obstruction	Spontaneous abortion
Rectal pressure/constipation	Recurrent pregnancy losses
Increased abdominal girth	
Pregnancy-related symptoms	
Preterm labor	
Pain	
Placental abruption	
Fetal malpresentation	
Labor dystocia/inertia	

size exceeds that of a 12-week gestation (5). Recently, this recommendation, even in women who have completed childbearing, has been challenged with a proposal that symptoms should be the primary determinant of therapeutic intervention (6). Certainly, in women desirous of future fertility, removal of the fibroid (myomectomy) is the procedure of choice. Hysterectomy is, therefore, reserved for women who are not candidates for myomectomy.

HISTORY

An extensive history should be obtained from patients with uterine leiomyomas. Questions should be directed to elicit information relating to symptoms frequently associated with fibroids. Concerns regarding malignant degeneration of tumors can also be addressed in appropriately directed questions. General information regarding the patient's current and past state of health will be helpful in determining management plans. Any previous surgeries, particularly abdominal surgeries, should also be noted at this time.

SYMPTOMATOLOGY

Of patients with uterine leiomyomas, 20% to 50% are symptomatic. The most common symptoms generally associated with these tumors are menorrhagia and/or metrorrhagia and pain. As fibroids increase in size, pelvic pressure may occur in conjunction with urinary frequency or stress incontinence from bladder compression. Most leiomyomas are stable and do not change, or they change slowly. Patients may become symptomatic when fibroids grow or undergo degenerative changes. Previous studies indicate that up to a third of gynecologic admissions and a high proportion of gynecologic surgical procedures have been related to uterine leiomyomas (7,8). The severity of symptoms experienced by a patient with uterine leiomyomas will depend on the number, size, and location of the tumors. Less commonly, lateral growth compresses the ureters, resulting in ureteral obstruction, hydroureter, hydronephrosis, and, on occasion, flank pain. If the uterus is enlarged significantly, examination of the adnexal structure may be impossible. Consequently, it will be difficult to differentiate fibroids from ovarian masses on pelvic examination.

Based on the patient's presenting symptoms, the preoperative evaluation may include pelvic examination and imaging studies to exclude other pelvic pathology (Fig. 2.1).

Menorrhagia

A review of the literature reveals that menorrhagia is present in approximately 30% of patients who undergo myomectomy. There are several theories explaining why menorrhagia occurs secondary to fibroids. It has been suggested that ulceration over submucosal fibroids results in men-

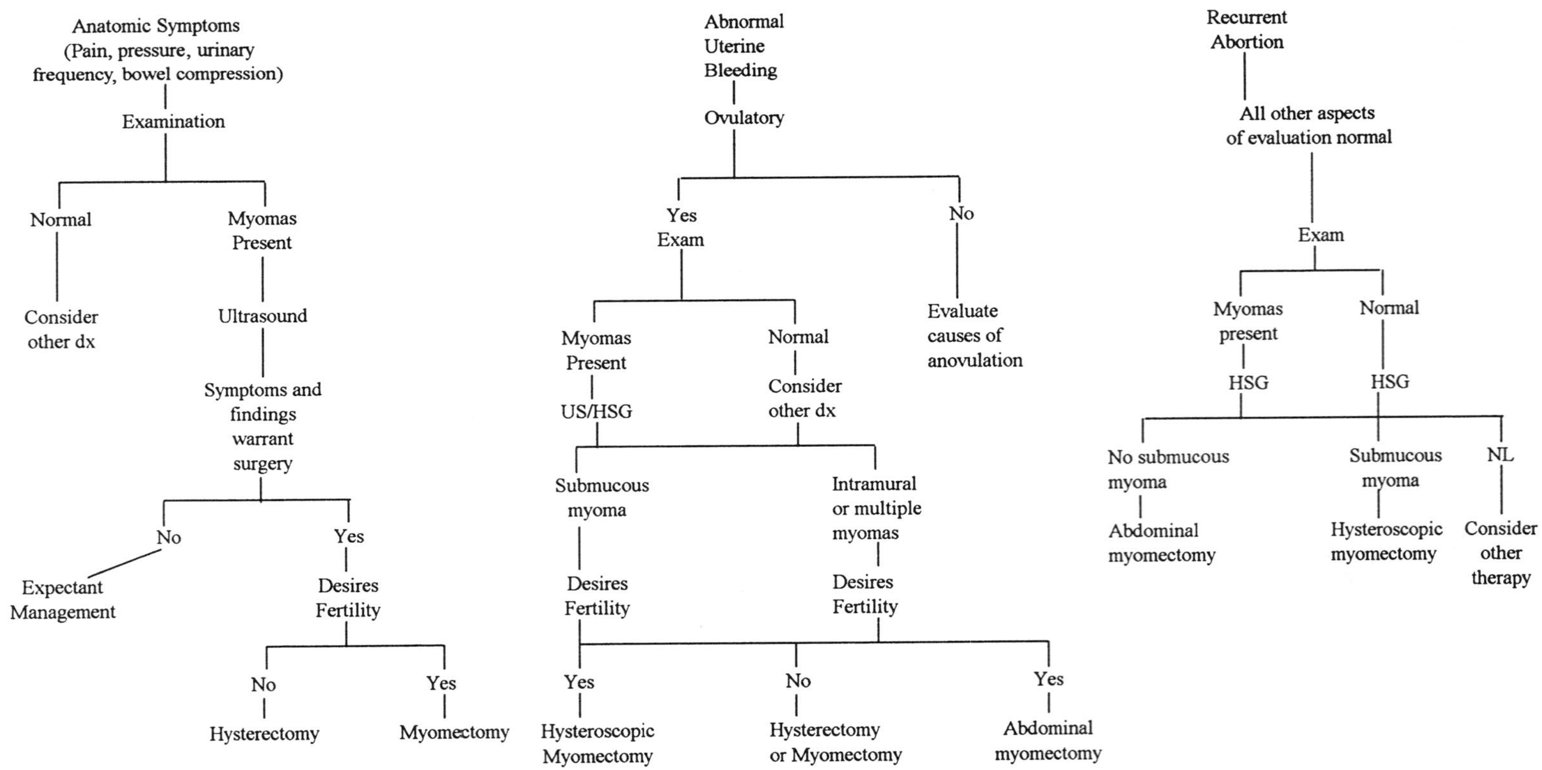

FIG. 2.1.

Preoperative evaluation of uterine fibroids. US, ultrasound; HSG, hysterosalpingography; NL, normal. (Revised and reproduced by permission from Rock JA, Schlaff WD. Decision making in reproductive endocrinology. Boston: Blackwell Science, 1993.)

orrhagia. However, actual examination of hysterectomy specimens failed to disclose ulceration of the endometrium overlying a submucous tumor (9). In addition, only about 5% of all leiomyomas are submucosal. While the incidence of menorrhagia may not be affected by the presence of submucous leiomyomas, the severity of bleeding may be increased when submucous fibroids are present (10). It has also been suggested that anovulation associated with uterine fibroids is responsible for menorrhagia (11). However, no studies have conclusively demonstrated that the incidence of anovulation in women with leiomyomas is higher than that in a control group. Correlation between severity of bleeding and increased endometrial surface area has been documented (12). The endometrial surface area of myomatous uteri may attain a size of more than 200 sq cm, as compared with 15 sq cm for normal uteri. This hypothesis does not suggest the actual mechanism of bleeding and does not explain bleeding associated with subserous and intramural leiomyomas, which may not distort the uterine cavity. Another plausible explanation for menorrhagia associated with fibroids is that the tumors interfere with normal uterine contractility (13,14). While feasible, this hypothesis also remains unsubstantiated. It is likely that patients who present with menorrhagia associated with leiomyomas have one or more combinations of the above processes that result in increased bleeding.

Infertility

A history of infertility may be commonly associated with fibroids. However, it is unusual for it to be the only factor present in infertile couples. In fewer than 3% of patients undergoing myomectomy, no other cause of infertility could be identified (5). In African Americans, however, fibroids were the sole cause of infertility in 9% of patients. Several mechanisms have been proposed by which myomas may contribute to infertility. One is that anatomic enlargement and alterations of the uterine cavity that increase the surface area may affect sperm transport (15). Alternatively, cervical displacement as a result of distorted anatomy may compromise exposure of the cervical mucus to the ejaculate (16). Additionally, leiomyomas may alter normal uterine contractility, which may potentially alter sperm transport (17). Furthermore, endometrial thinning and atrophy, inflammation, or vascular alterations that occur in the presence of leiomyomas can interfere with implantation (18–20). Leiomyomas situated in the cornual or cervical region of the uterus may impinge sufficiently on the endocervical canal or tubal lumen to cause infertility (10).

Pelvic Pain and Pressure: Urinary and Rectal Symptoms

While most patients with uterine leiomyomas are symptom free, when symptoms are present they are often related to the location of fibroids. Pain is frequently experienced in patients with pedunculated leiomyoma when a pedicle undergoes torsion. Pain may also be attributed to carneous degeneration or cervical dilatation by submucous leiomyoma protruding through the lower uterine segment. Pain in these situations is often acute and requires immediate attention. Differential diagnosis should include ectopic pregnancy, ovarian cyst, or acute pelvic inflammatory disease.

Pelvic pressure and an increase in abdominal girth are more commonly encountered than is pain. These symptoms are often more insidious, less apparent, and vaguely described by patients. Urinary frequency may result when leiomyomas are located in the subvesical region, or if they are large enough to fill the entire pelvis, and exert pressure on the bladder. Ureteral obstruction is one of the most serious consequences of chronic pressure on the urinary collecting system. This complication is usually silent and results from pressure at the pelvic brim or bladder neck leading to hydroureter or hydronephrosis. Generally renal parenchymal damage does not result and anatomic change is reversible once the pressure is alleviated. Rectal pressure is rare unless the myomatous uterus is incarcerated in the cul-de-sac or contains a solitary large posterior wall leiomyoma. Constipation and tenesmus may also be associated with a posterior leiomyoma, representing pressure of the tumor on the rectosigmoid area (21).

Pregnancy Loss

Uterine leiomyomas have been associated with an increase in spontaneous abortions. Reports in the literature of pregnancy loss rates of greater than 40% have been noted in patients with uterine fibroids (10,22,23). Spontaneous abortions can result from increased uterine irritability and contractility secondary to rapid growth/degeneration or alterations in oxytocinase activity (4). Alterations in endometrial vasculature or uterine blood flow may in some way render the blood supply of the developing placenta and fetus inadequate, and may ultimately contribute to spontaneous abortion.

MALIGNANT TRANSFORMATION AND GROWTH PATTERN

Leiomyosarcoma

Malignant transformation of benign leiomyomas is extremely rare. In a review of 13,000 leiomyomas by Montague et al (24), 38 (0.29%) cases demonstrated malignant change (24). Similarly, Corscaden and Singh (25) reported that malignant change developed in fewer than 0.13% of uterine leiomyomas. Thus, the often cited statistic that 0.5% of leiomyomas undergo malignant transformation is likely an overestimation; the true incidence is probably on the order of 0.04% (25). This overestimation has likely been made because only a small percentage of uteri that contain leiomyomas are ever surgically removed, therefore yielding a much higher denominator than that based solely on surgical procedures performed in which leiomyomas are found.

The microscopic diagnosis of malignant transformation relies on the level of mitotic activity and degree of cellular atypism. Malignant transformation is defined as evidence of greater than 10 mitotic figures per 10 high-power fields (HPF) examined (9). Tumors with fewer than 5 mitotic figures per 10 HPF examined are classified as cellular leiomyomas (9). Those with 5 to 10 mitotic figures per 10 HPF examined with no cellular atypia are referred to as "smooth-muscle tumors of uncertain malignant potential" (9). Those with cellular atypia and a high level of mitotic activity are classified as leiomyosarcomas (9).

Documented rapid growth of leiomyomas, especially postmenopausal growth, is highly suggestive of malignant transformation or development of a leiomyosarcoma. Therefore, a history of rapid growth, even in the absence of symptoms, should prompt removal. In younger patients, pregnancy should be excluded as a diagnosis in the presence of a rapidly enlarging uterus. In larger asymptomatic tumors, expectant management may also be justified, provided that ovarian neoplasm has been excluded and well documented by ultrasound, computed tomography (CT), or magnetic resonance imaging (MRI). The major indications for aggressive management of uterine leiomyomas are abnormal uterine bleeding; rapid growth; growth after menopause; infertility; recurrent pregnancy loss; pain or pressure symptoms; urinary tract symptoms or obstruction, or both; iron deficiency anemia secondary to chronic blood loss; and the possibility of ovarian neoplasia.

MEDICAL HISTORY

Anemia

The most common medical problem associated with uterine fibroids is iron deficiency anemia secondary to chronic blood loss. Clinical manifestations of anemia vary depending on the etiology, degree, and rapidity of onset. Symptoms associated with anemia include fatigue, headache, dyspnea, light-headedness, and angina. Patients may be completely asymptomatic if anemia develops gradually.

Assessment of anemia is a crucial part of the preoperative evaluation. Menstrual and gastrointestinal bleeding are the most common sources of blood loss in women, and both should be considered. A laboratory evaluation should include, at a minimum, a determination of the patient's hemoglobin and hematocrit. If anemia is confirmed, additional testing should include a reticulocyte count, mean corpuscular volume (MCV), and a manual examination of a peripheral blood smear. These additional tests will help differentiate the microcytic anemia associated with iron deficiency from the normocytic and macrocytic anemia of other disease processes (such as chronic disease, renal disease, endocrine disorders, and vitamin B_{12} and folic acid deficiency).

Therapy for iron deficiency anemia requires identifying the cause and replacing iron stores. Oral therapy with ferrous sulfate, 325 mg PO three times a day for 6 months, will usually correct the anemia and replace iron stores (26). Anemia associated with uterine fibroids may be severe enough to require transfusion preoperatively or gonadotropin-releasing hormone (GnRH) agonist therapy. Suppression of menses using a GnRH agonist can be utilized to allow time to replenish red blood cell mass and iron stores. As with all operative patients, a general assessment of health and addressing of any associated disease, such as hypertension, diabetes mellitus, and cardiovascular disease, should be routine.

If patients are not anemic, consideration should be given to autologous donation or directed donation preoperatively. While any transfusion is not without risk, this option decreases the risk of infection (such as hepatitis, human immunodeficiency virus) associated with utilizing pooled units. Although screening for human immunodeficiency virus (HIV) and hepatitis B and C is performed on all blood products, infection risks are increased with anonymously donated units. The risk of transfusion-associated infection varies with geographic location; the incidence should be obtained from the local hospital blood bank.

Papanicolaou Smear

As with any gynecologic surgical procedure, evaluation of the cervix by Papanicolaou smear is mandatory. Evaluation of any abnormal results via colposcopy or loop electrocautery excision procedure (LEEP) should be performed preoperatively.

Previous Surgery

Previous history of any surgeries, especially abdominal surgery, should be well documented. Patients with a history of bowel surgery or endometriosis may have dense adhesions and bowel preparation preoperatively may be advisable. In addition previous tubal surgery or tubal patency is a significant issue in patients who desire to maintain fertility.

Physical Examination

Pelvic examination is usually the initial step when uterine fibroids are confirmed or suspected. Characteristically, pelvic examination reveals an enlarged, often irregular, firm uterus. Individual fibroids may be palpable on bimanual examination. Subserosal, intramural, and pedunculated fibroids may be appreciated on pelvic examinations. Submucosal fibroids, however, require other modalities for detection, such as hysterosalpingography or hysteroscopy. Speculum examination may reveal a deviated cervix, displaced by fibroids in the lower uterine segment or posteriorly. While the diagnosis of fibroids is usually made on pelvic examination, the examination may be misleading. A solid ovarian tumor, uterine malformation, or pelvic kidney may be misdiagnosed as a uterine fibroid. Additional studies may be required for exclusion of ovarian neoplasm or congenital anomaly.

PREOPERATIVE TESTING

The purpose of preoperative testing in most cases is to determine if the information gained will assist in managing the patient during the peri- and postoperative periods. The extent of this evaluation is dependent on the patient's age, preoperative health status, previous response during an intraoperative procedure, and history of smoking or excessive alcohol or drug use, and the extent of the operative procedure.

Chest X-ray

It is advisable to urge a patient who smokes to decrease or stop smoking several weeks before the procedure. Chest roentgenography may prove to be necessary. The value of preoperative chest x-rays in patients being evaluated for gynecologic conditions has been assessed. Major chest x-ray abnormalities were detected in only 10% (118/1175) of patients evaluated. In patients less than 40 years of age, the age range of most patients who undergo a myomectomy procedure, only 3% of those evaluated were found to have a chest x-ray abnormality (27).

Electrocardiography

If a patient is greater than 50 years of age or if there is any reason to suspect a cardiac abnormality, an electrocardiogram may be necessary.

Laboratory Evaluation

The average blood loss during any operative procedure will vary depending on the type of surgical procedure, technical difficulty of the procedure, and the surgeon's experience in performing the technique. In a study by LaMorte et al (28) evaluating the morbidity associated with myomectomy, the average blood loss was 342 ± 37 mL, with a blood loss of greater than 1000 mL reported in 4% of the cases. Intraoperative or postoperative transfusions occurred in 20% of the cases. This amount of blood loss as well as the high percentage of patients (30%) who may present with menorrhagia (29) requires that a preoperative complete blood count (CBC) be performed in order to properly prepare for additional blood replacement during the procedure. This will, of course, necessitate that a type and screen are completed as well. Since most myomectomy procedures continue to be elective, many patients will choose to provide autologous donated blood before their surgical procedure. The standard donation is two units given at least 2 weeks prior to surgery, thereby allowing the body appropriate time for resynthesis.

It would therefore seem reasonable that the minimum preoperative laboratory evaluation should include a CBC and a type and screen. Other laboratory tests should be ordered based on the patient's history and the physician's clinical judgment.

CA-125

Einhorn et al (30) first suggested that preoperative serum CA-125 levels may be important in differentiating a benign from a malignant pelvic mass. Most centers use levels above 35 U/mL as abnormal. The usefulness of preoperative determination of CA-125 levels in patients diagnosed with leiomyomas remains obscure. Measurements of CA-125 in patients with pelvic masses have shown that leiomyoma alone will be identified to be the culprit in only 8% (6/75) of the cases with elevated CA-125 levels (31). In patients who present with leiomyomas found in concert with endometriosis or salpingitis, although the CA-125 level may be higher, the increase is probably secondary to the accompanying pathology (31). In patients who are found to have benign lesions and elevated CA-125 levels preoperatively, levels postoperatively were not found to decrease following removal of the lesion (31). This may be explained by residual unrecognized endometriosis or adenomyosis. Therefore, the usefulness of CA-125 levels in preoperative assessment of leiomyoma remains variable and should not be relied on to assess the complete excision or reoccurrence of leiomyomas.

ENDOMETRIAL BIOPSY

Leiomyomas are a well-recognized cause of abnormal uterine bleeding, particularly menorrhagia, in patients who present for myomectomy (32). Previous studies have shown that 40% of patients presenting with menorrhagia or menometrorrhagia will have abnormal pathology. In the postmenopausal patient, the most common abnormality found is hyperplasia, while in the premenopausal patient the most common lesion identified is a submucous leiomyoma, followed by endometrial polyps (33). A simple endometrial biopsy in the office provides only information in the area sampled. Blind curettage is associated with such a large error in diagnosis that it should no longer be used on its own as a routine diagnostic technique. If a malignancy or submucosal myoma is suspected the recommended procedure is hysteroscopy along with an endometrial biopsy.

HYSTEROSCOPY

Hysteroscopy used in conjunction with dilation and curettage (D&C) or endometrial biopsies when attempting to diagnose abnormal pathology associated with abnormal bleeding has been shown to increase the accuracy of diagnosis. Gimpelson (34) compared hysteroscopically directed biopsies to D&C in 66 women. He found that hysteroscopy yielded more information in 16 patients, while D&C was more useful in only 2 patients. Hysteroscopic examination following a D&C has confirmed that lesions are missed at the time of D&C. Brooks and Serden (35) hysteroscopically examined 29 patients with recurrent abnormal bleeding after a D&C and found that lesions were missed in 24 of the 29 patients.

Another benefit of inoffice hysteroscopy is that it confirms the location of a submucosal myoma, allowing the physician to better inform the patient of the suspected findings and to better plan for the surgical technique. In most cases hysteroscopy is used as a confirmatory aid following an ultrasound (US), but it can, in some cases of dysfunctional uterine bleeding, be used as a primary tool. In comparison to transvaginal ultrasound (TVUS), the sensitivity and specificity of hysteroscopy in diagnosing submucosal myomas is 100% and 96%, respectively, whereas with transvaginal ultrasound it is 100% and 94%, respectively (36). The advantage that hysteroscopy may also have over TVUS is its ability to distinguish between a polyp and a submucosal myoma.

IMAGING TECHNIQUES

Ultrasonography

Ultrasonography continues to be the most ideal method for imaging leiomyomas (Table 2.2), whether it is for diagnostic purposes or to assess changes in the size of the leiomyoma. The most common sonographic appearance is of a hypoechoic or heterogeneous uterine mass (Fig. 2.2). Submucous or small mural leiomyomas can distort the uterine cavity, thereby giving an indentation to the central endometrial echo (Fig. 2.3). If multiple myomas are present, ultrasonography may show only globular uterine enlargement (Fig. 2.4). The increased use of transvaginal ultrasonography has made detection of very small lesions easier. It also provides better differentiation between a submucous and a mural lesion, as both can produce distortion of the endometrial echo (37). The disadvantage of transvaginal versus transabdominal scanning lies in the limited field of view offered using the transvaginal approach. Subserosal or pedunculated leiomyomas may be missed. It is therefore recommended that transvaginal ultrasonography be used in conjunction with transabdominal scans when the patient is assessed before myomectomy.

When using ultrasound to follow a patient conservatively or to assess a decrease in the myoma size following hormonal treatment, many

Table 2.2

Comparison of imaging techniques for leiomyomas

Diagnostic Study	Radiation Exposure	Optimal Utilization	Cost (estimate)	Disadvantage
Abdominal US	None	Pedunculated myoma and markedly enlarged uteri	$282.00	Decreased resolution for identifying small myomas
Transvaginal US	None	Submucosal	$282.00	Limited field of view
CT	3.0 rads	Calcified	$349.00 (without contrast) $680.00 (with contrast)	Difficult to distinguish myoma from adnexa
MRI	None	Localization	$1054.00	Decreased resolution with small myomas; cost
HSG	2.2 rads	Submucosal	$379.00	Limited to submucosal myomas
UhSG	None	Submucosal vs. polyp	$250.00	Limited to submucosal myomas

US, ultrasound; CT, computed tomography; MRI, magnetic resonance imaging; HSG, hysterosalpingography; UhSG, ultrasonohysterography.

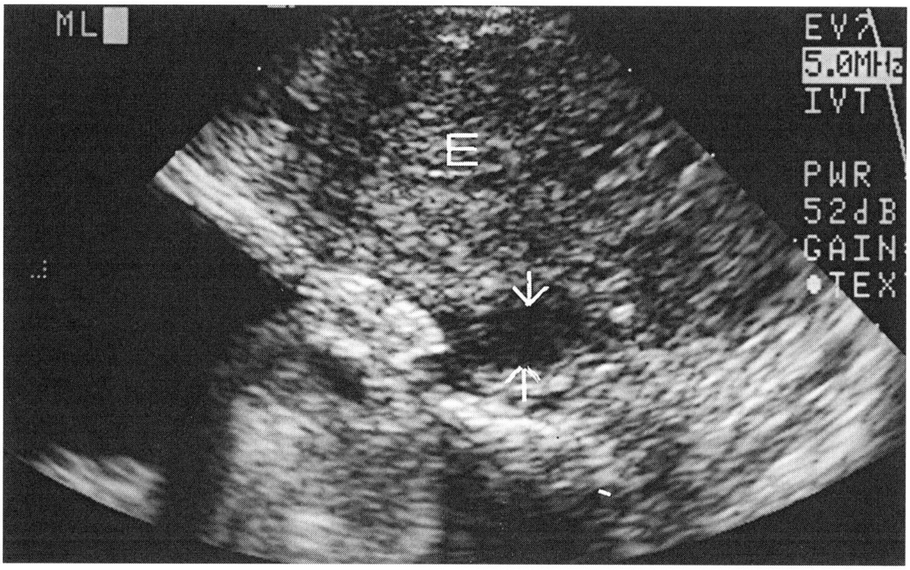

FIG. 2.2.

Transvaginal longitudinal view of a retroflexed uterus with an area of abnormal echotexture, a fibroid (*arrows*), within myometrium. E, endometrium.

authors recommend assessing leiomyoma volume to determine progress (38,39). To assess leiomyoma volume, measurements are performed on both the longitudinal and transverse dimensions. The tumor volume is then calculated by multiplying the three perpendicular diameters of each myoma by 3.14/6, the volume of a sphere (40). In a study to assess the reliability of transabdominal ultrasound in predicting uterine leiomyoma volume, Sauer et al (40) confirmed the ultrasound's ability to correctly diagnose leiomyoma, with 15 of 16 visualized tumors being confirmed at the time of surgery. However, in this evaluation of the 10 subjects presented in this study, ultrasound failed to visualize 28 of the total 43 leiomyomas removed at the time of operation. Of those 28 myomas not visualized, all were less than 2.5 cm in diameter. If these patients had undergone transvaginal ultrasound in conjunction with their transabdominal scan, many of these myomas might have been identified. This study also concluded that ultrasound was more accurate in assessing uterine volume when the leiomyoma was greater than 6 cm (40).

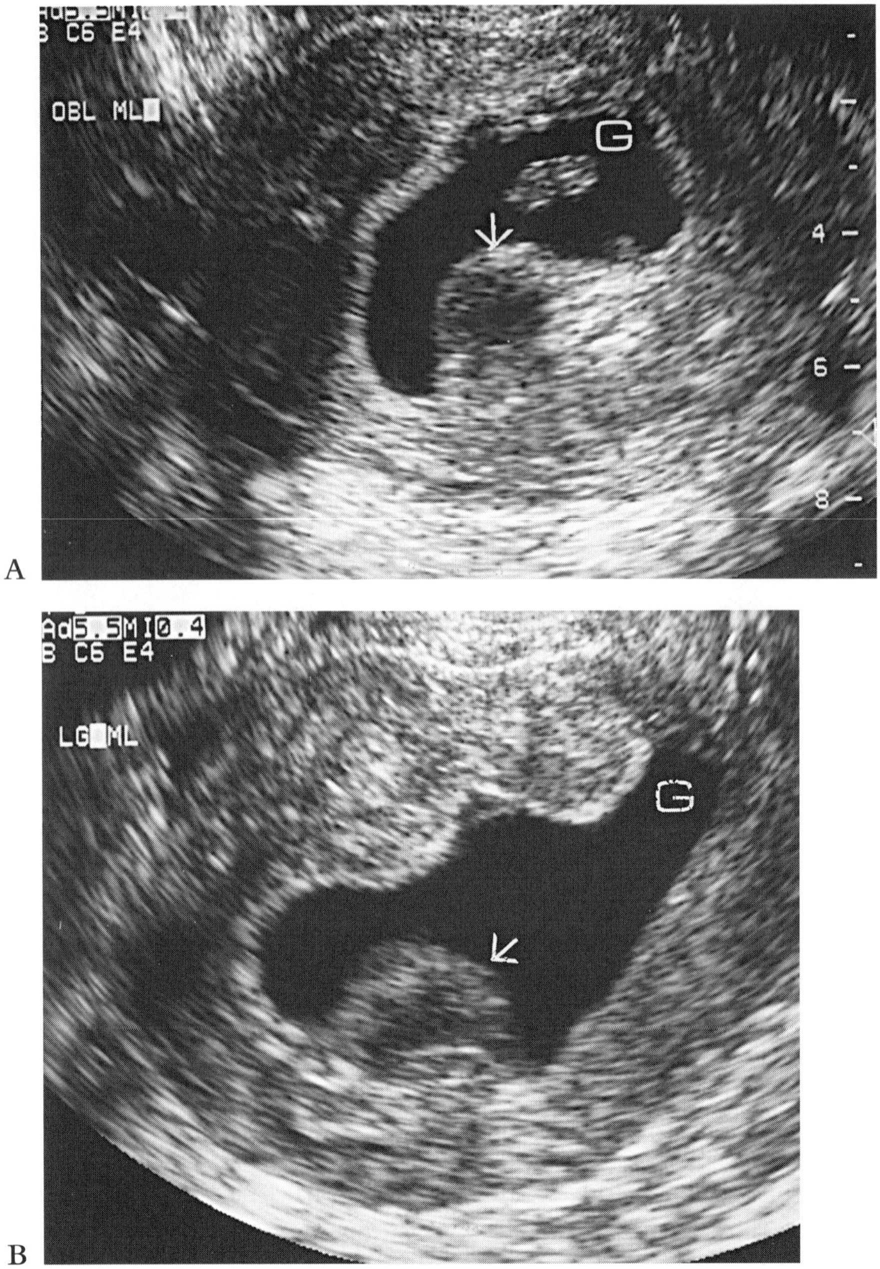

FIG. 2.3.

A. Oblique transvaginal image of the uterus with a submucous myoma (*arrow*) indenting a gestational sac (G). B. Longitudinal transvaginal view of submucous myoma (*arrow*) indenting a gestational sac (G).

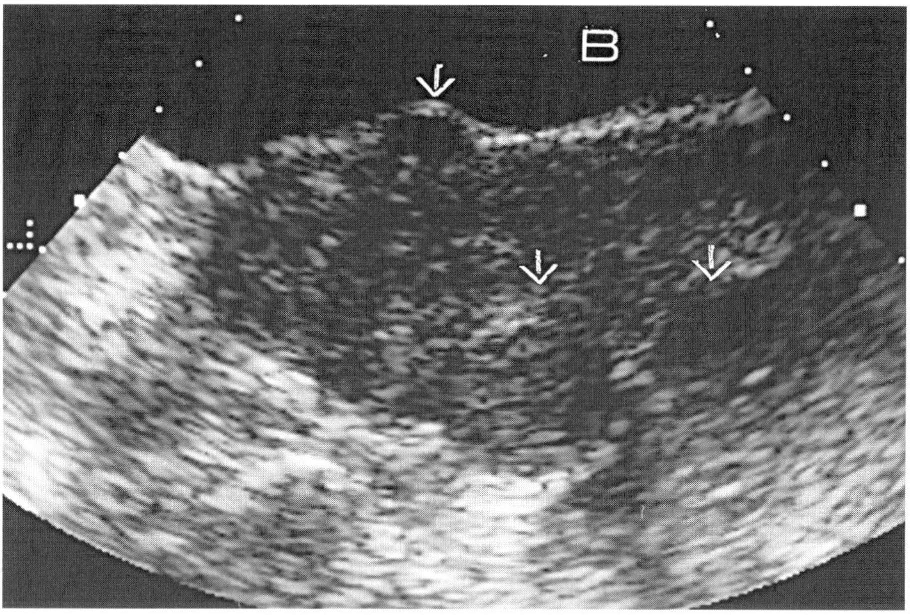

FIG. 2.4.

Transabdominal longitudinal view of the uterus with multiple leiomyomas (*arrows*). B, bladder.

Computed Tomography

Although ultrasound is the primary modality for evaluating leiomyomas, myomas are often found incidentally at the time of CT scan. Casillas et al (41) report that in their evaluation of 6000 CT scans of the abdomen and pelvis, 97 histologically proven leiomyomas were identified. Uterine enlargement and contour deformity are the most common CT findings; however, calcification is the most specific CT sign of a leiomyoma (37). When findings from US are indeterminate, magnetic resonance imaging is the next choice, because it offers greater sensitivity than CT (37).

Magnetic Resonance Imaging

Magnetic resonance imaging has recently been evaluated as a modality in which to assess leiomyomas. Its value has been particularly beneficial in cases in which ultrasound has proved to be indeterminate (37). In contrast to US or CT, the exact location of the leiomyoma can be documented (42). In infertile patients before myomectomy, Dudiak et al (43) found MRI to be more accurate than US or hysterosalpingography for the localization of leiomyoma. MRI has also been shown to permit accurate quantitative monitoring of therapeutic response to conservative medical therapy utilizing GnRH analogs (44). With the use of MRI, individual as well as total leiomyoma volume can be assessed. In a study by Zawin et al (44) that assessed the individual leiomyoma volume before and after the use of a GnRH analog, a statistically significant decrease in total and individual volume was observed in women who used the analog as compared to control subjects.

Magnetic resonance imaging has also been found to be advantageous as compared to US in attempting to assess the adnexal structures in the presence of a leiomyoma. As confirmed by Zawin et al (45), MRI correctly identifies adnexal structures separate from the uterus 96% (44/46) the time, compared to 46% (21/46) when using US.

The only disadvantage to MRI continues to be its cost and patient anxiety in performing the procedure. Estimated cost for an MRI of the pelvis at our institution is $1140.00 as compared to $233.00 for a US of the pelvis.

Hysterosalpingography

Hysterosalpingography (HSG) has mostly been utilized as a preoperative tool in the management of patients who present with menstrual abnormalities or infertility in the presence of a leiomyoma. Most recently, several studies have demonstrated the benefits of preoperative HSG in identifying submucosal myomas, and therefore in allowing increased planning of the surgical approach to myomectomy (46). Postoperative hysterosalpingography has also been found to be useful in identifying persistent filling defects, consistent with residual myomas or synechiae following resection, which could further decrease conception. In a study by Lev-Toaff et al (46) that evaluated 32 patients who were referred for HSG following a myomectomy, 4 of the 14 patients thought to have submucosal myomas preoperatively showed residual filling defects consistent with retained myomas of major synechia (46), while diverticula developed in 6 of the patients at the site of resection of the myoma. It appeared that fewer postoperative abnormalities were found when the endometrial cavity was not entered at the time of surgery (46). Although the significance of these postoperative findings as they relate to conception or pregnancy has not been studied in depth, focal weakening of the myometrial wall or failure of implantation is a possibility.

Ultrasonohysterography

Ultrasonohysterography (UhSG) is a new procedure that utilizes the visual benefit of transvaginal ultrasound along with the technical aspect of HSG, and it offers another means by which to assess the endometrial cavity. This procedure is most helpful in distinguishing a polyp from a submucosal myoma and the presence and location of such in the endometrial cavity (47). UhSG allows for the assessment of the fluid-

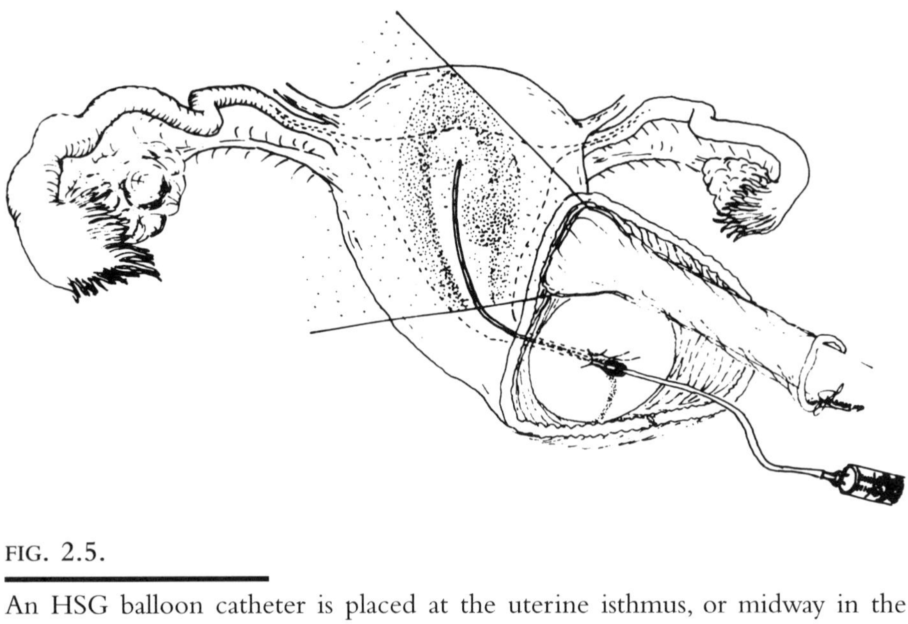

FIG. 2.5.

An HSG balloon catheter is placed at the uterine isthmus, or midway in the cervical canal to allow retention of 3 to 8 mL saline while a uterus with a patulous cervix and a polyp on the posterior uterine wall is scanned. (Reproduced by permission from Parsons AK, Lense JJ. Sonohysterography for endometrial abnormalities: preliminary results. J Clin Ultrasound 1993; 21:89.)

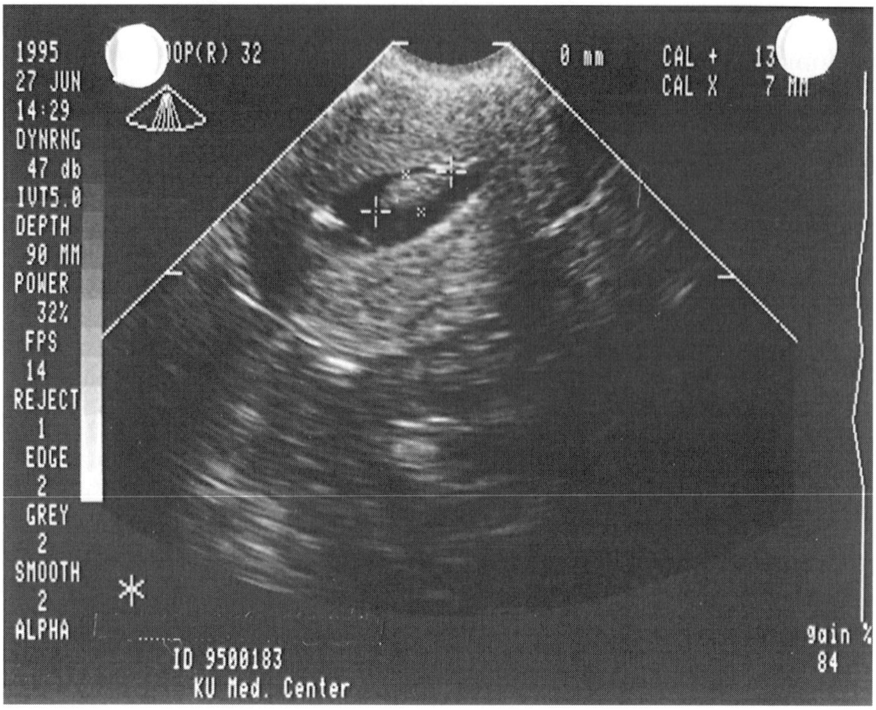

FIG. 2.6.

Oblique view of a uterus following one month of GnRH agonist therapy. During saline infusion a 13-mm × 7-mm polyp is clearly seen. This patient had undergone two previous hysteroscopic excisions of polyps before this examination.

enhanced endometrium without the need for fluoroscopy. In the office setting, during the follicular phase of the cycle, an intrauterine insemination catheter or HSG catheter is inserted, and under direct transvaginal or transabdominal examination sterile saline is slowly infused (Fig. 2.5). If present, any polyp or submucous myoma and the endometrial thickness surrounding the fluid can be measured (Fig. 2.6).

Further utilization of UhSG can assist in identifying the etiology of filling defects noted on HSG or distinguishing between polyps versus submucosal myomas indeterminately diagnosed by other radiologic procedures. It is hoped that this will assist in appropriate triage and the avoidance of some diagnostic hysteroscopy.

PREOPERATIVE COUNSELING

Medical Therapy

Medical therapy for leiomyoma before myomectomy is mostly utilized for patients who present with menorrhagia and anemia or for those with significantly enlarged myomas, greater than a 16-week–sized gestation. The goal of medical therapy for leiomyomas should be to reduce the symptoms of pain and abnormal bleeding and to decrease the size of the myoma. Patients should be counseled that these agents are only a temporary measure to prepare them for surgery. Although several agents [danazol (Danocrine) and progestational agents] have been utilized in the past to control the bleeding associated with leiomyomas and to decrease the volume of the leiomyoma, none have been as successful as the GnRH agonists (48). It is widely believed that GnRH agonists may facilitate myomectomy by reducing the volume of the myomas and vascularization of the uterus (49). Prior to prescribing a GnRH agonist for treatment, the patient's complete history, physical findings, and future fertility desires should be considered. Patients should also be counseled about the side effects experienced with GnRH agonists. The most common complaints are hot flashes, which are experienced by more than 75% of patients, beginning 3 to 4 weeks after the start of treatment. Bone loss has been observed in many patients receiving GnRH therapy, but is believed to be reversible with discontinuation of the drug (50). In patients with a submucosal myoma, significant vaginal hemorrhage has been observed when agonists are utilized preoperatively. In approximately 2% of the patients bleeding secondary to the degeneration and necrosis of the myoma occurred (51). Further information concerning the use of GnRH agonists can be found in Chapter 3.

Preoperative Antibiotics

It is well documented that the use of preoperative antibiotics in gynecologic surgery decreases morbidity (52). It has also been shown that the use of a single dose rather than multiple doses of an antibacterial agent provides the benefit of lower toxicity risk and lower selective pressure on the bacterial flora that would predispose the patient to superinfections (53). A second dose may be necessary for procedures that last longer than 2 hours.

Surgical Approach

The surgical approach utilized for a myomectomy will depend upon the preoperative location of the myoma. With the increasing use of operative hysteroscopy, submucosal myomas can be successfully removed with minimal patient morbidity. The utilization of all procedures for myomectomy is discussed in Chapters 4 to 6.

Reproductive Capabilities

The reproductive capability of a patient following a myomectomy has become even more important in this era of assisted reproductive technology. However, even with the use of sophisticated assisted reproductive technology procedures that allow pregnancies to occur without fallopian tubes or even ovaries, a successful pregnancy is not possible without a uterus. Most patients who desire a myomectomy do so because of their desire for continued reproductive capacity. Fifty women desirous of pregnancy, having undergone a myomectomy at Yale University, were observed for a median of 58.7 months to determine their capacity for conception following the procedure (54). Of these 50 patients attempting conception, 25 conceived a total of 36 pregnancies. These conceptions resulted in 24 full-term deliveries, three premature but viable pregnancies, one ectopic pregnancy, four therapeutic abortions, and four spontaneous first-trimester abortions. This study also found the indication for the procedure to be a confounding factor in the success of future fertility. Of the women who underwent exploration for a pelvic mass, 68% conceived, whereas only 16% of women with a normal infertility evaluation conceived. Women who became pregnant had fewer and smaller fibroids than those who did not. These findings are similar to those of Smith and Uhlir (55), who reported successful pregnancies in 40% of the patients who had undergone a myomectomy. The major complication associated with myomectomy that interferes with conception is postoperative adhesion formation. Gelbach et al (56) reported a 68% (13/19) documentation of pelvic adhesions in patients who had undergone previous myomectomies. Only four of these women had adhesions present and lysed at the time of their myomectomy. Postoperative adhesion formation following myomectomy has also been shown to cause intestinal obstruction. In a series by Stricker et al (57) evaluating the incidence of intestinal obstruction following gynecologic procedures, myomectomy accounted for 11% of the cases in which obstruction occurred postoperatively.

Therefore, when counseling patients who desire myomectomy, the couple's desire for future fertility should first be determined. Secondly, a minimal infertility evaluation should be employed that should include a semen analysis, preoperative HSG to determine tubal patency, and defined testing of ovulation. The impact of the leiomyoma on the patient's fertility should then be discussed. The patient should also be advised of the potential development of postoperative adhesion formation and the limitations in preventing their development.

In assessing the risk of pregnancy complications following myomectomy, the subject of uterine rupture should be stressed as a serious but extremely rare complication (58,59). The election to proceed with a cesarean delivery following a myomectomy, although limited in its foundation, is generally accepted as standard care if the uterine cavity was entered at the time of the myomectomy (60).

Risks Associated with Myomectomy

The two most significant risks associated with myomectomies are blood loss and postoperative adhesion formation. Despite preparation, excessive blood loss can occur when myomectomies are performed. Therefore, every patient undergoing a myomectomy should be counseled preoperatively of the possibility of blood transfusion and hysterectomy.

Techniques for preventing blood loss and postoperative adhesion formation are discussed in detail elsewhere. Patients should also be advised that despite using any of the techniques suggested in the text, complications still occur.

REFERENCES

1. Merrill J, Creasman W. Lesions of the corpus uteri. In: Danforth D, Scott J, eds. Obstetrics and gynecology. Philadelphia: Lippincott, 1980: 1068–1096.
2. Novak E, Woodruff J. Myoma and other benign tumors of the uterus. In: Novak E, Woodruff J, eds. Novak's gynecologic and obstetric pathology. Philadelphia: Saunders, 1967:211–226.
3. Wallach E. Myomectomy. In: Thompson J, Rock J, eds. Telind's operative gynecology. Philadelphia: Lippincott, 1992:647–662.
4. Cramer SF, Patel A. The frequency of uterine leiomyomas. Am J Clin Pathol 1990;94:435–438.
5. Buttram VC, Reiter RC. Uterine leiomyomata: etiology, symptomatology, and management. Fertil Steril 1981;36:433–447.
6. Friedman AJ, Hass S. Should uterine size be an indication for surgical intervention in women with leiomyomas? Am J Obstet Gynecol 1993; 68:751–755.
7. Baggish M. Mesenchymal tumors of the uterus. Clin Obstet Gynecol 1974;17:51–88.
8. Buttram VC, Reiter RC, eds. Surgical treatment of the infertile female. Baltimore: Williams & Wilkins, 1985.
9. Robbins S, Cotran R. Leiomyoma (fibromyoma). In: Robbins S, ed. The pathogenic basis of disease. Philadelphia: Saunders, 1979:1271.
10. Malone L, Ingersoll F. Myomectomy in infertility. In: Behrman SJ, Kistner RW, eds. Progress in infertility. Boston: Little, Brown, 1975:85.
11. Miller N, Ludovici P. Origin and development of uterine fibroids. Am J Obstet Gynecol 1955;70:720–746.
12. Sehgal N, Haskins A. The mechanism of uterine bleeding in the presence of fibromyomas. Am J Surg 1960;26:21.
13. Faulkner R. The blood vessels of the myomatous uterus. Am J Obstet Gynecol 1944;47:185–197.
14. Farrer-Brown G, Beilby J, Tarbit M. The vascular patterns in myomatous uteri. J Obstet Gynaecol Br Commonw 1970;77:967.
15. Hunt J, Wallach E. Uterine factors in infertility: an overview. Clin Obstet Gynecol 1974;17:44–64.
16. Iosif C, Akerlund M. Fibromyomas and uterine activity. Acta Obstet Gynecol Scan 1983;62:165–167.

17. Coutinho V, Maia H. The contractile response of the human uterus, fallopian tube, and ovary to prostaglandins in vivo. Fertil Steril 1971;22:539–543.
18. Deligdish L, Lowenthal M. Endometrial changes associated with myomata of the uterus. J Clin Pathol 1970;23:676–680.
19. Forssman L. Distribution of blood flow in myomatous uteri as measured by locally injected ^{133}xenon. Acta Obstet Gynecol Scand 1976;55:101–104.
20. Jacobson F, Enzer N. Uterine myomas and the endometrium. Obstet Gynecol 1956;7:206–210.
21. Wallach E. Leiomyomas. In: Wallach E, Zacur H, eds. Reproductive medicine and surgery. St. Louis: Mosby, 1995:731–746.
22. Stevenson C. Myomectomy for improvement of fertility. Fertil Steril 1964;15:367–384.
23. Ingersoll F. Fertility following myomectomy. Fertil Steril 1963;14:596–603.
24. Montague A, Swartz A, Woodruff J. Sarcoma arising in a leiomyoma of the uterus. Am J Obstet Gynecol 1965;92:421–427.
25. Corscaden J, Singh B. Leiomyoma of the uterus. Am J Obstet Gynecol 1958;75:149–155.
26. Gailani D. Anemia and transfusion therapy. In: Woodley M, Whelan A, eds. Manual of medical therapeutics. Boston: Little, Brown, 1993:341–355.
27. Umbach GE, Zubek S, Deck H-J, et al. The value of preoperative chest X-rays in gynecological patients. Arch Gynecol Obstet 1988; 243:179–185.
28. LaMorte AI, Lalwani S, Diamond MP. Morbidity associated with abdominal myomectomy. Obstet Gynecol 1993;82:897–900.
29. Lacey CG. Benign disorders of the uterine corpus. In: Pernoll ML, ed. Current obstetric and gynecologic diagnosis and treatment. Norwalk, CT: Appleton & Lange, 1991:732–738.
30. Einhorn N, Bast RC, Knapp RC, et al. Preoperative evaluation of serum CA 125 levels in patients with primary epithelial ovarian cancer. Obstet Gynecol 1986;67:414–416.
31. Vasilev SA, Schlaerth JB, Campeau J, Morrow CP. Serum CA 125 levels in preoperative evaluation of pelvic masses. Obstet Gynecol 1988; 71:751–756.
32. West CP, Lumsden MA. Fibroids and menorrhagia. Bailliere's Clin Obstet Gynecol 1989;3:357–374.

33. Loffer FD. Hysteroscopy with selective endometrial sampling compared with D&C for abnormal uterine bleeding: the value of a negative hysteroscopic view. Obstet Gynecol 1989;73:16–20.
34. Gimpelson RJ. Panoramic hysteroscopy with directed biopsies vs. dilatation and curettage for accurate diagnosis. J Reprod Med 1984;33: 872–876.
35. Brooks PG, Serden SP. Hysteroscopic findings after unsuccessful dilatation and curettage for abnormal uterine bleeding. Am J Obstet Gynecol 1988;158:1354–1357.
36. Goldstein SR. Use of ultrasonohysterography for triage of perimenopausal patients with unexplained uterine bleeding. Am J Obstet Gynecol 1994; 170:565–570.
37. Karasick S, Lev-Toaff AS, Toaff ME. Imaging of uterine leiomyomas. AJR 1992;158:799–805.
38. Fedele L, Bianchi S, Dorta M, et al. Transvaginal ultrasonography versus hysteroscopy in the diagnosis of uterine submucous myomas. Obstet Gynecol 1991;77:745–748.
39. Carr BR, Marshburn PB, Weatherall PT, et al. An evaluation of the effect of gonadotropin-releasing hormone analogs and medroxyprogesterone acetate on uterine leiomyomata volume by magnetic resonance imaging: a prospective, randomized, double blind, placebo-controlled, crossover trial. J Clin Endocrinol Metab 1993;76:1217–1223.
40. Sauer MV, Agnew C, Worthen N, et al. Reliability of ultrasound in predicting uterine leiomyoma volume. J Reprod Med 1988;33:612–614.
41. Casillas J, Joseph RC, Guerra JJ. CT appearance of uterine leiomyomas. Radiographics 1990;10:999–1007.
42. McCarthy S. Gynecologic applications of MRI. Crit Rev Diagnostic Imaging 1990;31:263–281.
43. Dudiak CM, Turner DA, Patel SK, et al. Uterine leiomyomas in the infertile patient: preoperative localization with MR imaging versus US and hysterosalpinography. Radiology 1988;167:627–630.
44. Zawin M, McCarthy S, Scoutt L, et al. Monitoring therapy with gonadotropin-releasing hormone analog: utility of MR imaging. Radiology 1990;175:503–506.
45. Zawin M, McCarthy S, Scoutt LM, Comite F. High-field MRI and US evaluation of the pelvis in women with leiomyomas. Magnetic Resonance Imaging 1990;8:371–376.

46. Lev-Toaff AS, Karasick S, Toaff ME. Hysterosalpingography before and after myomectomy: clinical value and imaging findings. AJR 1993;160:803–807.
47. Parsons AK, Lense JJ. Sonohysterography for endometrial abnormalities: preliminary results. J Clin Ultrasound 1993;21:87–95.
48. Christiansen JK. The facts about fibroids: presentation and latest management options. Postgrad Med 1993;94:129–137.
49. Fedele L, Vercellini P, Bianchi S, et al. Treatment with GnRH agonists before myomectomy and the risk of short-term myoma recurrence. Br J Obstet Gynecol 1990;97:393–396.
50. Friedman AJ, Hoffman DI, Comite F, et al. Treatment of leiomyomata uteri with leuprolide acetate depot: a double-blind, placebo-controlled, multicenter study. Obstet Gynecol 1991;77:720–725.
51. Friedman AJ, Rein MS, Harrison-Atlas D, et al. A randomized, placebo-controlled, double-blind study evaluating leuprolide acetate depot treatment before myomectomy. Fertil Steril 1989;52:728–733.
52. Shapiro M, Schuenbaum SC, Jager IB, et al. Benefit–cost analysis of antimicrobial prophylaxis in abdominal and vaginal hysterectomy. JAMA 1983;249:1290.
53. Periti P, Mazzei T, Orlandini F, Mini E. Comparision of the antimicrobial prophylactic efficacy of cefotaxime and cephazolin in obstetric and gynaecological surgery. A randomised multicentre study. Drugs 1988;35(suppl 2):133–138.
54. Berkeley AS, DeCherney AH, Polan ML. Abdominal myomectomy and subsequent fertility. Surg Gynecol Obstet 1993;156:319–322.
55. Smith DC, Uhlir JK. Myomectomy as a reproductive procedure. Am J Obstet Gynecol 1990;162:1476–1482.
56. Gehlbach DL, Sousa RC, Carpenter SE, Rock JA. Abdominal myomectomy in the treatment of infertility. Int J Gynecol Obstet 1993;40:45–50.
57. Stricker B, Blanco J, Fox HE. The gynecologic contribution to intestinal obstruction in females. J Am Coll Surg 1994;178:617–620.
58. Garnet JD. Uterine rupture during pregnancy. Obstet Gynecol 1964; 23:898.
59. Golan D, Aharoni A, Gonen R, et al. Early spontaneous rupture of the post myomectomy gravid uterus. Int J Gynecol Obstet 1990;31:167–170.
60. Egwuatu VE. Fertility and fetal salvage among women with uterine leiomyomas in a Nigerian teaching hospital. Int J Fertil 1989;34:341–346.

CHAPTER

3

Molecular Biology of Leiomyomas and Leiomyosarcomas

Lawrence C. Layman

Leiomyomas (LM) are common smooth-muscle tumors that affect at least 20% to 30% of women, and they account for significant morbidity requiring both medical and surgical management. These benign tumors respond to hormonal milieu, particularly to estrogen stimulation, and have been treated with antiestrogenic compounds, including progestins, antiprogestins, and gonadotropin-releasing hormone agonists. Leiomyosarcomas (LMS) are rare smooth-muscle sarcomas that are occasionally associated with LM, and have been suggested to arise from benign LM, although this is rare. Molecular and cytogenetic abnormalities have been increasingly elucidated in these tumors, which usually appear to be clonal in nature. An overview of some general genetics concepts, the technique of in situ hybridization, the approach to gene mapping, and clonality are provided in this chapter. The cytogenetic and molecular data for LM and LMS are then reviewed, and regions for putative genes are discussed.

PATHOLOGIC APPEARANCE OF LEIOMYOMAS AND LEIOMYOSARCOMAS

Leiomyomas are firm, white, spherical nodules in the myometrium that consist of smooth-muscle fibers with a whirled appearance, flattened nuclei, and rare mitoses (1). Leiomyosarcomas usually display hypercellularity and cellular atypia, and demonstrate greater than 5 mitoses per 10 high-power fields (HPF) (1). However, there are a variety of other recognizable pathologic classifications (Table 3.1), which are generally considered to be benign. Hypercellular leiomyomas have normal-appearing cells and 0 to 4 mitoses per 10 HPF, while atypical leiomyomas have variable cellularity with 0 to 4 mitoses. Another variant, termed *mitotically active leiomyomas*, displays normal cellularity and 5 to 15 mitoses per 10 HPF. Sometimes LM are difficult to distinguish from LMS when they are hypercellular, demonstrate minimal atypia, and have 5 or greater mitoses per 10 HPF. They

TABLE 3.1

Classification of leiomyoma-type smooth-muscle tumors

LEIOMYOMA TYPE	CHARACTERISTICS
Mitotically active	5–15 mitoses, normal cells
Cellular	<5 mitoses, normal cells
Atypical	<5 mitoses, atypical cells
Epithelioid	
Leiomyoblastoma	Round cells, eosinophilic cytoplasm
Clear-cell leiomyoma	Polygonal, clear cytoplasm
Plexiform leiomyoma	Nests of cells, scant cytoplasm
Myxoid	Amorphous myxoid material
Vascular	Numerous large vessels
Lipoleiomyoma	Significant fat
Diffuse leiomyomatosis	Many small nodules of smooth muscle
Myometrial hypertrophy	Symmetric uterine enlargement
Intravenous leiomyomatosis	Muscle nodules within vessels
Benign metastasizing leiomyoma	Smooth-muscle nodules, distant sites
Disseminated peritoneal leiomyomatosis	Multiple peritoneal nodules

Source: Zaloudek C, Norris HJ. Mesenchymal tumors of the uterus. In: Kurman RJ, ed. Blaustein's pathology of the female genital tract. 4th ed. New York: Springer-Verlag, 1994:487–528.

have been designated *leiomyomas of uncertain malignant potential* (1). A variety of other rare forms of LM are shown in Table 3.1, but of particular interest is diffuse leiomyomatosis, which does appear to have a genetic basis (see below).

CONCEPTS OF CLONALITY: SOMATIC CELL AND GERMLINE MUTATIONS

Through the study of many different types of neoplasms, it has become clear that most arise from acquired somatic cell (nongermline) mutations, that is, from the smooth-muscle cells in this case. When a smooth-muscle cell acquires a mutation, its daughter cells receive the same mutation (Fig. 3.1). This process, termed *clonality*, appears to explain the coexistence of normal myometrial cells (those without mutations) and

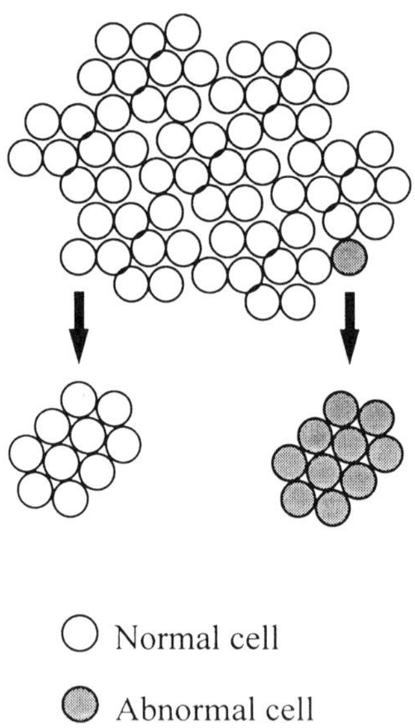

FIG. 3.1.

Clonality is demonstrated. Normal progenitor cells give rise to normal daughter cells, but if a cell acquires a mutation, it passes it on to its daughter cells.

LM (those with mutations) (2). Most benign and malignant tumors are clonal, since they arise from the same progenitor cell (2).

Cancers (and probably also benign neoplasms) are genetic, though only a small percentage, about 5%, are hereditary (2). If the mutations occur in the germline, as has been described in familial cancer syndromes, such as BRCA1 in hereditary breast-ovarian cancer, BRCA2 in hereditary breast cancer (breast cancer in females and males, prostate cancer in males), and p53 in Li Fraumeni syndrome (breast cancers, adrenocortical cancers, soft-tissue sarcomas, leukemia, osteosarcomas), transmission is usually autosomal dominant (2,3). In these situations, a germline mutation exists on one chromosome, and during the lifetime of the patient, a second mutation occurs in somatic cells, for example, in the breast with BRCA1 or in the bone marrow in Li Fraumeni syndrome (Fig. 3.2). Now both copies of these tumor suppressor genes are mutated, and therefore cellular growth becomes unchecked and tumors result. This is often termed *loss of heterozygosity* (LOH), since the germline is initially heterozygous for a mutation, but once a second somatic muta-

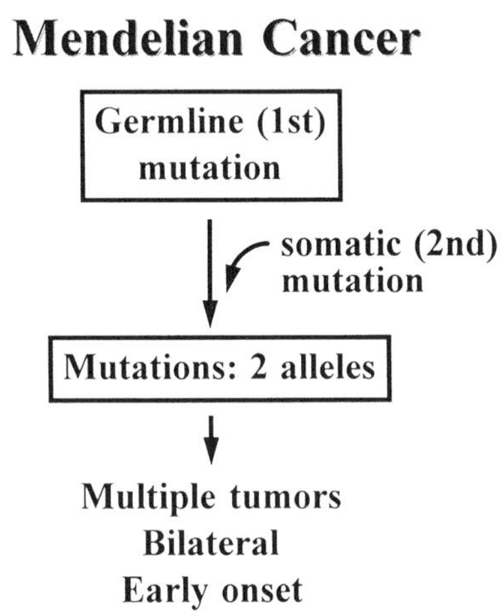

FIG. 3.2.

Mendelian inheritance of cancer occurs when one of the alleles of a tumor suppressor gene in the germline has a mutation. When a second mutation occurs, two abnormal alleles are now present, resulting in defective tumor suppression.

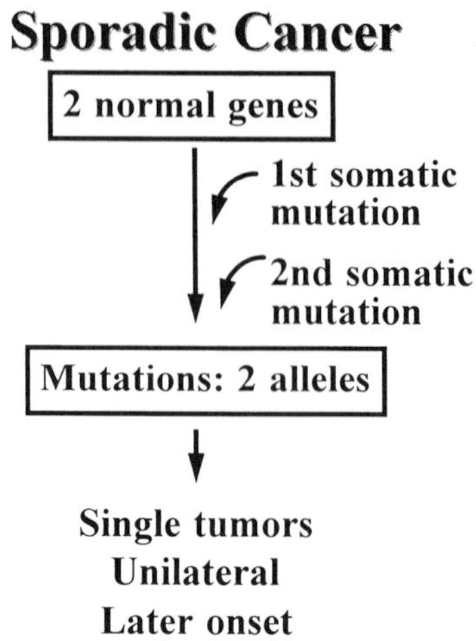

FIG. 3.3.

Sporadic cancer occurs when both germline alleles are normal. It now takes two somatic mutations to inactivate the tumor suppressor genes' protective effect.

tion occurs, the other normal allele of the tumor suppressor gene is lost (2). Familial cancer tends to produce bilateral disease, which occurs earlier in life since the probability of acquiring a single somatic cell mutation is greater than two (Fig. 3.2). If no germline mutation is present, two separate somatic cell mutations are required to produce the loss of these tumor suppressor genes. In these sporadic cases, the cancer will occur later in life and will often be unilateral (2) (Fig. 3.3).

At least three different types of genes are important in oncogenesis. Proto-oncogenes, genes that are important for normal cellular growth, may acquire activating mutations that result in unchecked cellular growth (examples are ras and myc). Mutations can also occur in tumor suppressor genes, which, when inactivated, allow for uncontrolled cellular growth (examples are p53, retinoblastoma gene, and BRCA1). The most recently recognized type of genes involved in cancer development are genes for deoxyribonucleic acid (DNA) repair enzymes. Gene mutations occur in all tissues of the body, but these enzymes function to repair the defects. When these genes acquire mutations, this protective function is lost, and cancers such as hereditary nonpolyposis coli can develop (2,3). For most sporadic cancers, a number of mutations must occur as the normal cell progresses through the transformation into adenoma to invasive cancer to metastatic tumor. The classic example is sporadic colon cancer, in which the accumulation of APC mutations and activating ras mutations, followed by the loss of tumor suppressor genes MCC (chromosome 5q), p53 (on 17p), and DCC (on chromosome 18q), produces a cancer cell (2,3). Leiomyomas and LMS are clonal tumors that arise from mutations in somatic cells, and germline mutations, if they exist, do not appear to be common. It is likely that the progression to leiomyosarcoma, if it occurs from leiomyomas, appears after multiple other chromosomal mutations are accumulated. It is also possible, through the study of the chromosomal constitution of both LM and LMS, that the potential etiologies may be elucidated.

GENETIC TECHNIQUES TO DETECT MUTATIONS IN NEOPLASMS

The explosion of molecular biologic techniques has tremendously aided investigators in studying the biology of neoplasia. *Cytogenetics* has revealed a number of different chromosomal anomalies, which accumulate in benign neoplasia and cancer. However, technical limitations include a bias for growing cells, since cells must be cultured for cytogenetic analysis, and therefore it is possible that some acquired mutations that cause necrosis might not be ascertained (4). Additionally, the resolution of chromosome banding is such that fine mapping of the putative causative gene cannot be detected with cytogenetics alone. However, the finding of a cytogenetic abnormality, such as a deletion or translocation, narrows down the region where the causative gene may reside. Instead of randomly searching the entire genome, which is often done in gene mapping, the chromosomal deletion or translocation allows for the focus of a specific region to be explored.

The technique of *fluorescent in situ hybridization* (FISH) has partly overcome the obstacles imposed by cytogenetics, and actually merges cytogenetics with molecular genetics. With FISH, either metaphase cells

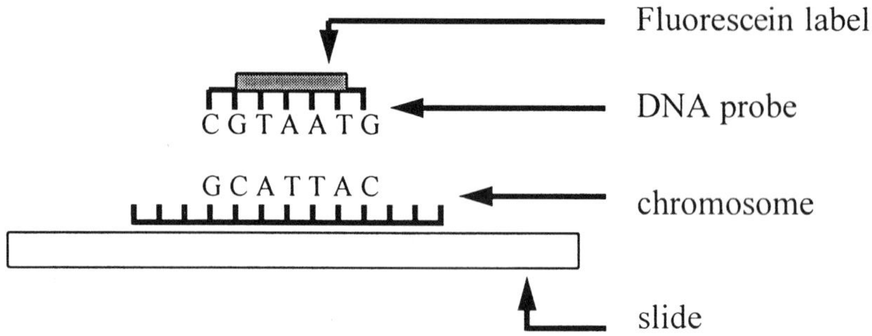

FIG. 3.4.

Fluorescent in situ hybridization. A labeled single-stranded probe joins complementary sequences in the denatured (single-stranded) template immobilized on the slide.

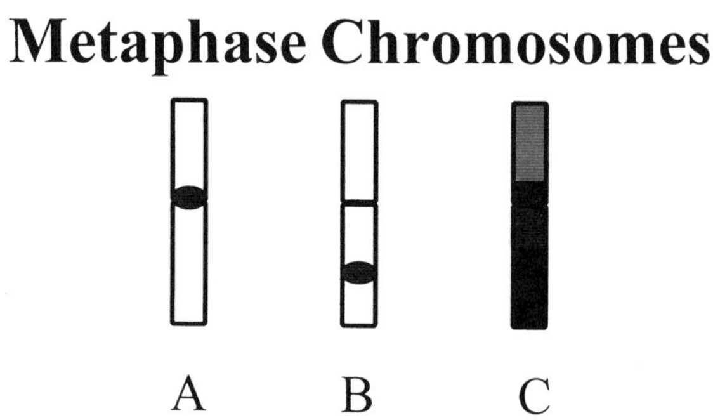

FIG. 3.5.

Examples of FISH probes. A. Alpha satellites are repetitive sequences at the centromeres of chromosomes. B. In this example, a cosmid probe is complementary to the long arm. C. Chromosome painting occurs when overlapping sequences of DNA from a specific chromosome library "paint" the whole chromosome.

or interphase cells can be studied in archival tissue to determine which sections of chromosomes are deleted, duplicated, or rearranged (4) (Fig. 3.4). In FISH, either interphase cells or metaphase chromosomal spreads are fixed onto a slide. The DNA is denatured by exposing the cells to alkali so that single-stranded DNA now exists. A single-stranded DNA [or ribonucleic acid (RNA)] probe labeled with fluorescein is then placed onto the slide, and complementary sequences of the probe join with sequences of the immobilized DNA in a process termed *hybridization*. Hybridization forms the basis of all molecular biology techniques. Different types of probes can be used for FISH, including centromeric probes, chromosome-specific cosmid probes, and sets of overlapping chromosomal probes spanning the entire chromosome that "paint" the chromosome (4) (Fig. 3.5). Centromeres must be present for a chromosome to be viable, and these centromeric probes consist of repeated sequences (called alpha satellites) that are generally chromosome specific. Often, a combination of these probes are used in FISH analysis to screen for chromosomal anomalies.

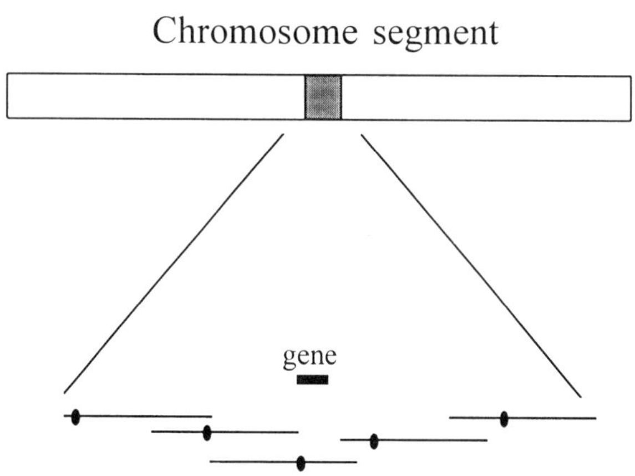

FIG. 3.6.

Gene mapping of a region of a chromosome. Large pieces of DNA (up to 1000 kb) can be cloned into yeast artificial chromosomes (YACs), indicated by the horizontal lines. Note that YACs can be mapped to cover a continuous region (contig) across the chromosomal region of interest. The putative gene (thickened line) resides somewhere within this interval. YACs can be ordered across the interval of interest using long-range restriction mapping by pulsed field gel electrophoresis; by sequence tagged sites (STS), which are unique sites on cloned fragments identified by polymerase chain reaction (STS sites shown as small ovals on the YACs); or by FISH. These methods allow a more rapid means to identify genes than older methodology.

Clonal abnormalities can be detected by using cytogenetic or molecular genetic techniques. Traditionally, the determination of X-inactivation is followed through successive generations (2,3). Normally, a given cell contains only one X chromosome (either maternally or paternally derived) since one is inactivated in somatic cells. Since inactivation is usually random, a given tissue should have populations of both cells. However, cells derived from a common cell (i.e., they are clonal) will possess the same maternal or paternal X chromosome. This type of analysis can be performed for LM or LMS in a similar fashion to determine clonality. Either Xg blood groups, which are polymorphic, or DNA polymorphisms can be used to determine clonality.

Techniques to screen large pieces of DNA have greatly facilitated the discovery and cloning of genes. DNA is cloned in large vectors, such as yeast artificial chromosomes (YACs) (5) (Fig. 3.6). By mapping these YAC clones, they can be arranged as overlapping fragments (contigs) on the physical map, determined, for example, by a chromosome deletion or translocation (5). If the breakpoint occurs within one fragment, this fragment can be studied in more detail to identify the putative gene. The combination of cytogenetic and molecular techniques complement one another in the identification of new genes.

MOLECULAR BIOLOGY OF LEIOMYOMAS

It has been nearly a decade since the first cytogenetic studies of myomas were reported. Approximately 20% to 50% of leiomyoma karyotypes reveal six major classes of cytogenetic aberrations (Table 3.2). In the series by Pandis et al (6), 90 of 96 fibroids were successfully karyotyped, and about one-third had chromosomal abnormalities. The most commonly affected chromosome is chromosome 7, with deletions of the long (q) arm, specifically in region 7q21.2q31.2, representing the most frequently encountered cytogenetic abnormality (13/31, 42%) (6). Most of these deletions were interstitial rather than terminal. The next most frequently occurring chromosomal aberration was involvement of chromosome 12q (6/31, 19%), most commonly as a translocation, t(12;14)(q14–15;q23–24) (6). In this instance breaks occur on chromo-

TABLE 3.2

Chromosomal abnormalites in LM and LMS*

LEIOMYOMA	LEIOMYOSARCOMA
7q22	1p36
12q15	1p32
14q24	1p13
13q22	1q32
10q22	7p11.1–p21
3q	7q32
6p	10q22
	13q14
	14p11
	−9
	−18
	−22

*Monosomy is indicated by the − sign.
Source: LM: (4–17); LMS: (18–29).

some 12q in the q14–15 region and on chromosome 14 in the q24–25 region. The material from chromosome 12 and 14 is then exchanged, producing the translocation. In this series, some chromosome 12q rearrangements were observed in the absence of chromosome 14 abnormalities, but no chromosome 14 rearrangements were seen when chromosome 12 abnormalities were not observed, suggesting that perhaps chromosome 12 rearrangements were more common in the genesis of LM (6). The third chromosome most commonly involved in myomas was the short (p) arm of chromosome 6, which was rearranged in 5 of 31 tumors (16%). Trisomy 12 was also seen in 2 cases, while a variety of others constituted the remainder. More than one chromosome abnormality was seen in just over half of the tumors (17/31). Half of these with two abnormalities were believed to represent clonal evolution, meaning that a new mutation evolved from the primary mutation. Occasionally biclonality was suggested in some of the tumors.

The mere identification of a chromosomal abnormality does not prove causality in the pathogenesis of leiomyomas, since it may occur by chance alone and have no role; however, when the same (or similar) karyotypic abnormalities are repeatedly demonstrated, more credence can be given to potential involvement. A variety of other studies have substantiated the chromosomal abnormalities in leiomyomas (4–17). More recently, other chromosome rearrangements, such as 13q22, 10q22, and 3q deletions have also been consistently identified in myomas (4–17). These data suggest that a variety of genes if disrupted or deleted will produce overgrowth of smooth muscle and result in the development of fibroids. Alternatively, a translocation could potentially produce a fusion gene between gene products of two genes on 12q and 14q similar to the 9;22 translocation in chronic myelogenous leukemia when the c-Abl gene on 9q34 and the BCR gene on 22q11 form a fusion gene (Philadelphia chromosome), which alters tyrosine kinase activity, resulting in uncontrolled cellular growth (3).

In a compilation of series of 191 total myomas with chromosomal anomalies, one-third demonstrated clonal changes in chromosome 7 (7). A large number of chromosome 7 deletions have centered on the 7q22 region as being the most important region of this chromosome. Either a gene deletion or a disruption of a tumor suppressor gene has been suggested as the possible etiology in this case, although no specific genes have been cloned and demonstrated causality (7). Ozisik et al (7) suggested that one of the important genes in the genesis of fibroids is located within 7q22, but it appears to be insufficient for the transformation into a sarcoma. Chromosome 7 deletions appear to be the only one of the recognized chromosomal abnormalities unique to fibroids (7).

In contrast to the unique chromosome 7 involvement with fibroids, chromosome 12q14–15 aberrations are involved in a variety of benign neoplasms, including lipomas, pleomorphic adenomas of the salivary gland, pulmonary chondroid hamartomas, cervical polyps, epithelial breast tumors, rhabdomyosarcomas, hemangiopericytomas, chondromatous tumors, diffuse astrocytomas, and giant-cell tumors of the bone

(5,14). Despite the observation that all of these tumors have involvement of the 12q13–15 region, it is currently unknown if the breakpoints are identical. The 12q14–15 region is involved in translocations in 20% of the chromosomally abnormal LMs (4,17).

Through the study of a large number of cell lines that contain different 12q14–15 breakpoints, this region, termed the *uterine leiomyoma cluster region* (ULCR), was narrowed down to a region of 260 kilobases (kb) using cytogenetic and molecular techniques (9,10). This is within a region termed the *multiple aberration region* (MAR), where breakpoints on 12q15 occur in a variety of solid tumors, including leiomyomas, endometrial polyps, fibroadenomas of the breast, lipomas, pleomorphic salivary gland adenomas, hamartomas of the breast and lung, and angiomyxomas (16,17). Recently, a putative gene termed *HMGI-C* has been cloned from this region of 12q15, and, as seen by FISH analysis of these tumors, most of the breakpoints occur within this gene (16). This gene may be the common denominator, the so-called *multitumor aberrant growth locus* (MAG), important in the genesis of many different types of tumors (16). This is only one gene, which appears to be pathogenetic for leiomyomas, but there are likely to be more genes characterized where other translocations and deletions have been identified. Now that HMGI-C has been cloned and disruption of the gene has been demonstrated, additional information concerning the biology of these tumors will be forthcoming (16,17).

MOLECULAR BIOLOGY OF LEIOMYOSARCOMAS

Leiomyosarcomas are rare tumors that comprise only about 7% of all sarcomas (1). Less information is available than for the more commonly encountered LM. From the available cytogenetic and molecular data, it appears that LM and LMS are probably distinct tumors of different origin. Evidence in favor of this hypothesis is the rarity of LM degenerating into LMS, being in the range of 0.5% to 0.7% (1), and the cytogenetic data demonstrating different chromosomal aberrations (18–29) (see Table 3.2). Whereas chromosomes 7, 12, 14, 10, 3, and 6 account for most of the abnormalities identified in LM (4–17), chromosomes 1, 7, 10, 13, and 14 per Sreekantaiah et al (18) and monosomy 9, 14, and 22 are most frequent in LMS (22). Similar to LM, LMS also display clonal chromosomal aberrations in about 40% to 50% of cases (18–29). Han et al (4), in an attempt to avoid cell selection by culture techniques, performed FISH on nuclei obtained from paraffin blocks using centromeric, cosmid, and painting probes. They identified trisomy 8, monosomies of chromosomes 6 and 1, and a 1q translocation (4). The molecular biology of LMS is likely to be more complicated than the benign LM because LMS probably evolve when a number of mutations are accumulated, similar to other sporadic cancers.

Some of the factors involved in the genesis of LMS include the activation of proto-oncogenes, deregulation of growth factors, and possibly the inactivation of tumor suppressor genes. Overexpression of p53 (21), MDM2 gene (the receptor for p53) (22), c myc (protein P62) (23), and H-ras (protein P21) (23) has been demonstrated in LMS when compared with benign LM. In the study of smooth-muscle tumors of the gastrointestinal tract by Cai et al (21), expression of p53 was found in a significantly higher proportion of LMS (90%) than smooth-muscle tumors of potentially malignant smooth-muscle tumors (75%) versus LM (14%) (21). Five-year survival rates were also better with lower p53 expression, indicating that the presence of p53 expression might be a predictor of outcome. This study suggests that tumors of indeterminate malignant potential might progress to LMS through the overexpression of p53 (21). Although the overexpression was markedly less in LM, this still raises some concern that LM could progress to the more malignant forms of smooth-muscle tumors. Whether these findings can be generalized to uterine LM and LMS remains to be determined. An activating 9 base pair insertion in the TC21 gene, a member of the ras family, was identified in a human uterine LMS cell line (24).

Altered growth factor expression has also been demonstrated in LMS in comparison with LM (25). Normally, insulin-like growth factor II (IGF-II) exhibits genomic imprinting—only the paternal allele is expressed, not the maternal allele (25). This is unlike most genes, which are expressed equally from maternal and paternal genomes. However, in LMS, this imprinting effect is lost, so that both maternal and paternal alleles of IGF-II are expressed and increased cellular growth occurs (25). The IGF-II gene is localized to a different chromosome (11p13) than those that are found to be involved in LMS (25).

DIFFUSE LEIOMYOMATOSIS

Alport's syndrome is an X-linked recessive genetic disorder characterized by progressive renal failure, ocular lesions, and sensorineural deafness (26). It is a disorder of the basement membrane caused by mutations of the gene for type α5(IV) collagen (COL4A5). Interestingly, this COL4A5 gene has been mapped adjacent to the gene for type α6(IV) collagen, COL4A6. In some families, Alport syndrome coexists with diffuse leiomyomatosis, and deletions that affect both genes appear to cause these disorders (26). These findings suggest that some disorders of smooth muscle may be caused by collagen gene mutations, and that type IV collagen may regulate smooth-muscle differentiation and morphogenesis (26).

CONCLUSION

Leiomyomas and leiomyosarcomas commonly arise as clonal chromosomal aberrations within the myometrium. For each fibroid that arises within the smooth muscle, there is a 20% to 40% chance that a chromosomal aberration will be detected, most commonly 7q22 or 12q15 abnormalities. Therefore, if a patient has multiple fibroids, it is likely that some will have no detectable chromosomal anomaly, but some will have chromosome 7q mutations, some will have 12q15 mutations, and so forth. Similarly, about 40% of LMS contain detectable chromosomal anomalies. It is apparent that genes on multiple chromosomes are important for development of LM. One gene, localized to 12q15 through a combination of cytogenetic and molecular analyses, has been recently cloned, and should provide important new information about the biology of these tumors. The biology of LMS is more complicated, and probably involves the accumulation of multiple chromosomal deletions/gene mutations. Despite our increased understanding of these benign and malignant smooth-muscle tumors, many important questions remain unanswered. Does a benign LM progress through the potentially malignant tumor with a few mitoses per 10 HPF to LMS? Though comparison of the chromosomal aberrations in LM and LMS yields different results, increased expression of p53 from the LM to borderline tumor to LMS raises some concern. If only 20% to 40% of these benign and malignant tumors possess chromosomal aberrations, what causes the other 60% to 80%? They probably arise from as yet unidentified gene mutations, which are not detected by cytogenetic techniques. Through the study of the recently cloned HMGI-C gene and the isolation of new genes, we will acquire a better understanding of the biology of these tumors within the next decade.

REFERENCES

1. Zaloudek C, Norris HJ. Mesenchymal tumors of the uterus. In: Kurman RJ, ed. Blaustein's pathology of the female genital tract. 4th ed. New York: Springer-Verlag, 1994:487–528.
2. Vogelstein B, Kinzler KW. The multistep nature of cancer. TIG 1993; 9:138–141.
3. Sandberg AA. Chromosomes and hereditary predisposition to cancer. Heme Onc Ann 1994;2:141–156.
4. Han K, Lee W, Harris CP, et al. Comparison of chromosome aberrations in leiomyoma and leiomyosarcoma using FISH on archival tissues. Cancer Genet Cytogenet 1994;74:19–24.
5. Fejzo MS, Yoon S-J, Montgomery KT, et al. Identification of a YAC spanning the translocation breakpoints in uterine leiomyomata, pulmonary chondroid hamartoma, and lipoma: physical mapping of the 12q14–15 breakpoint region in uterine leiomyomata. Genomics 1995;26:265–271.
6. Pandis N, Heim S, Bardi G, et al. Chromosome analysis of 96 uterine leiomyomatas. Cancer Genet Cytogenet 1991;55:11–18.

7. Ozisik YY, Meloni AM, Surti U, Sandberg AA. Deletion 7q22 in uterine leiomyoma: a cytogenetic review. Cancer Genet Cytogenet 1993;71: 1–6.
8. Sargent MS, Weremowicz S, Rein RS, Morton CC. Translocations in 7q22 define a critical region in uterine leiomyomata. Cancer Genet Cytogenet 1994;77:65–68.
9. Wanschura S, Hennig Y, Deichert U, et al. Molecular-cytogenetic refinement of the 12q14 → q15 breakpoint region affected in uterine leiomyomas. Cytogenet Cell Genet 1995;71:131–135.
10. Schoenmakers EFPM, Mois R, Wanschura S, et al. Identification, molecular cloning, and characterization of the chromosome 12 breakpoint cluster region of uterine leiomyomas. Genes, Chromosomes, Cancer 1994;11: 106–118.
11. Dal Cin P, Moerman P, Deprest J, et al. A new cytogenetic subgroup in uterine leiomyomata is characterized by a deletion of the long arm of chromosome 3. Genes, Chromosomes, Cancer 1995;13:219–220.
12. Ozisik YY, Meloni AM, Altungoz O, et al. Translocation (6;10)(p21;q22) in uterine leiomyomas. Cancer Genet Cytogenet 1995;79:136–138.
13. Hug K, Doney MK, Tyler MJ, et al. Physical mapping of the uterine leiomyoma t(12;14)(q13–15;q24.1) breakpoint on chromosome 14 between SPTB and D14S77. Genes, Chromosomes, Cancer 1994;11: 263–266.
14. Schoenmakers EF, Kools PF, Mols R, et al. Physical mapping of chromosome 12q breakpoints in lipoma, pleomorphic salivary gland adenoma, uterine leiomyoma, and myxoid liposarcoma. Genomics 1994;20:210–222.
15. Osisik YY, Meloni AM, Surti U, Sandberg AA. Involvement of 10q22 in leiomyoma. Cancer Genet Cytogenet 1993;69:132–135.
16. Ashar HR, Fejzo MS, Tkachenko A, et al. Disruption of the architectural factor HMGI-C: DNA-binding AT hook motifs fused in lipomas to distinct transcriptional regulatory domains. Cell 1995;82:57–65.
17. Schoenmakers EFPM, Wanschura S, Mols R, et al. Recurrent rearrangements in the high mobility group protein gene, HMGI-C, in benign mesenchymal tumours. Nature Genet 1995;10:436–444.
18. Sreekantaiah C, Davis JR, Sandberg AA. Chromosomal abnormalities in leiomyosarcomas. Am J Pathol 1993;142:293–305.
19. Bardi G, Johansson B, Pandis N, et al. Recurrent chromosome aberrations in abdominal smooth muscle tumors. Cancer Genet Cytogenet 1992; 62:43–46.

20. Laxman R, Curries JL, Kurman RJ, et al. Cytogenetic profile of uterine sarcomas. Cancer 1993;71:1283–1288.
21. Cai J, Jiang Y, Zhang Y, et al. Quantitation of P53 protein expression in gastrointestinal smooth muscle tumors. Clinicopathological correlation and prognostic significance. Chinese Med J 1995;108:669–673.
22. Patterson H, Gill S, Fisher C, et al. Abnormalities of the p53 MDM2 and DCC genes in human leiomyosarcomas. Br J Cancer 1994;69: 1052–1058.
23. Fotiou SK, Tserkezoglou AJ, Mahera H, et al. Chromosome aberrations and expression of ras and myc oncogenes in leiomyomas and a leiomyosarcoma of the uterus. Eur J Gynaecol Oncol 1992;13:340–345.
24. Huang H, Saez R, Chao L, et al. A novel insertional mutation in the TC21 gene activates its transforming activity in a human leiomyosarcoma cell line. Oncogene 1995;11:1255–1260.
25. Vu TH, Yballe C, Boonyanit S, Hoffman AR. Insulin-like growth factor II in uterine smooth-muscle tumors: maintenance of genomic imprinting in leiomyomata and loss of imprinting in leiomyosarcomata. J Clin Endocrinol Metab 1995;80:1670–1676.
26. Zhou J, Mochizuki T, Smeets H, et al. Deletion of the paired alpha 5 (IV) and alpha 6 (IV) collagen genes in inherited smooth muscle tumors. Science 1993;261:1167–1169.
27. Sait SNJ, Dal Cin P, Sandberg AA. Consistent chromosome changes in leiomyosarcoma. Cancer Genet Cytogenet 1988;35:47–50.
28. Boghosian L, Dal Cin P, Turc-Carel C, et al. Three possible cytogenetic subgroups of leiomyosarcoma. Cancer Genet Cytogenet 1989;43:39–49.
29. Nilbert M, Mandahl N, Heim S, et al. Chromosome abnormalities in leiomyosarcomas. Cancer Genet Cytogenet 1988;34:209–218.

CHAPTER

4

Gonadotropin-Releasing Hormone (GnRH) Agonist Treatment Before Myomectomy

Elizabeth Puscheck

Leiomyomas are the most commonly occurring pelvic tumor of reproductive-aged women. The incidence overall ranges from 20% to 50% in this patient population (1). Fewer than half of these women become symptomatic. Symptoms may range from menorrhagia with or without anemia, urinary frequency, pelvic pressure or pain, increased abdominal girth, and less commonly, miscarriages and infertility. A brief review of the biology of leiomyomas will help in understanding the medical therapy available for presurgical preparation.

BIOLOGY OF LEIOMYOMAS

Uterine leiomyomas are benign smooth-muscle neoplasms with interspersed fibrous tissue. These tumors rarely undergo sarcomatous degeneration (<0.7%). Leiomyomas are hormonally sensitive neoplasms that occur in women of reproductive age. The cells that make up leiomyomas express receptors for both estrogen and progesterone. The estradiol receptors in leiomyomas are greater in number than in the normal myometrium. Estrogen, whether endogenous or exogenous, promotes the growth of endometrium and leiomyomas. Similarly, hypoestrogenic states that occur naturally (menopause) or are induced (i.e., with GnRH agonists) result in reduction of leiomyoma sizes in most cases.

Greater variation in progesterone receptor numbers exists in leiomyomas than in the surrounding tissues and no statistically significant differences have been notable (2). Within the normal uterus, progesterone receptors are produced in response to estrogen stimulation. Progesterone exposure reduces the number of progesterone receptors and estrogen receptors. The latter is thought to occur by interfering with estrogen receptor recycling. Progesterone is believed to counteract estrogenic growth effects. Progesterone and androgens supposedly exert antimitotic effects on myocytes (3,4). Tiltman (5) argues that these studies mainly involve histologic assessments of endometrium. Tiltman demonstrated higher mitotic activity in leiomyomas of women treated with medroxyprogesterone. More recent clinical studies involving GnRH agonists and medroxyprogesterone show much less reduction in leiomyoma volume (6,7) and suggest a role for progesterone in leiomyoma growth. The antiprogesterone (RU 486) used in clinical trials demonstrates a reduction in leiomyoma growth similar to the effects of hypoestrogenism (8). Consequently, the mechanism for the progestin-induced myoma growth is unknown. Androgens or local growth factors may be involved.

A number of other receptors have been identified within leiomyomas that include but are not limited to a number of growth factor receptors, prostaglandin E and F receptors, human chorionic gonadotropin/luteinizing hormone (HCG/LH) receptors, and oxytocin receptors. These cellular receptors may be directly affected by medical therapy or affected via paracrine or hormonal effects. Recently, GnRH receptors were also found to be expressed in leiomyoma. This finding suggests an alternative mechanism(s) of action for GnRH agonists. GnRH agonists may directly affect the leiomyomas as well as work through the hypothalamic-pituitary-ovarian axis to cause hypoestrogenism and secondarily affect leiomyomas.

WHY PRETREAT?

Pretreatment of the leiomyomatous uterus before myomectomy surgery is optional but often beneficial. The development of GnRH agonists allowed for the first truly effective medical therapy for leiomyomas. However, previous medical therapies revolved around treating the symptoms of menorrhagia and thinning the endometrial lining without having much effect on the leiomyomas. There are several benefits and few disadvantages to pretreating leiomyomatous women prior to endoscopic leiomyoma resection or abdominal myomectomy. The goals of pretreatment are to decrease symptomatic bleeding, to restore iron reserves and normalize the hemoglobin preoperatively, to decrease vascularity and intraoperative bleeding, to decrease operative time, to improve ease of surgery, to improve visualization in hysteroscopic cases, and to increase flexibility in scheduling surgery for busy operating rooms. Pretreatment with GnRH agonists can actually shrink leiomyomas in most cases and possibly convert the abdominal myomectomy into a hysteroscopic or laparoscopic approach. Such pretreatment increases the feasibility and success.

A variety of agents have been used for pretreatment, including progestational agents, oral contraceptives, androgens, and GnRH agonists. All of these medications often achieve the goal of symptomatic relief from menorrhagia and an atrophic endometrium through a variety of different mechanisms. The symptom and side effect profiles differ based on the agent used. This chapter briefly reviews the pretreatment regimens for all of these agents, but concentrates on GnRH agonists in depth, and concludes with future therapeutic directions.

MEDICAL PRETREATMENTS

Progestins

Progestins are common to gynecologic practice. These agents are cheap and accessible. Therapy with progestins allows for timed withdrawal bleeding, which will facilitate operating room scheduling and control of bleeding. These progesterone-like agents initially cause pseudodecidualization of the endometrium and, later, endometrial atrophy. Progestins succeed by inhibiting mitoses, which stabilizes the endometrium and counteracts the estrogenic growth of endometrium.

Typical progestins in use are oral medroxyprogesterone acetate, depomedroxyprogesterone (DMPA), and norethindrone. Doses vary depending on the study. Oral medroxyprogesterone can be given as 10mg daily to three times a day for 10 to 60 days. Depomedroxyprogesterone is given intramuscularly in a 150-mg dose every 3 months. Its advantage is that it is also an effective contraceptive. Approximately 50% of patients become amenorrheic within one year; the amenorrheic patient demonstrates the extreme of endometrial atrophy. The disadvantage is that as many as 10% of patients may have persistent menorrhagia despite therapy. An alternative progestin is norethindrone acetate, which is given orally in doses of 5 to 10mg daily. The side effects for the oral progestins include breakthrough bleeding, weight changes, edema, depression, and insomnia/somnolence. Additional side effects of the DMPA include the above side effects and the following in 5% or more of patients: headache, nervousness, abdominal discomfort, dizziness, weakness, and fatigue.

Oral Contraceptives

Oral contraceptives work in a similar manner to the progestins as a pretreatment. The combined oral contraceptives contain progestin in every pill as well as an estrogen component. As with the progestin therapy, the endometrium is stabilized and atrophies. Clinically, the menstrual flow decreases by greater than 40% (9). The additional advantage is that ovulation is inhibited.

However, the estrogenic component is not completely antagonized by the progestin. Amenorrhea rarely occurs on the usual cyclic regimen. On the continuous regimen or the cyclic regimen, breakthrough bleeding is one of the more common side effects. This unpredictable bleeding can interfere with surgical scheduling and visualization if one starts the procedure. Although the endometrium thins on oral contraceptives, a variable portion remains proliferative. Visualization may be impaired. Leiomyomas have been reported to grow in size while the patient is taking oral contraceptives. This medication is only a temporizing measure to control bleeding. High-dose pills may be successful at controlling menorrhagia for a limited time.

Androgens

Danazol is a synthetic derivative of 17-alpha ethinyl testosterone. Clinically, it suppresses the endometrium so that it becomes inactive or atrophic. It controls the symptomatic menorrhagia associated with leiomyomas. Estradiol levels are decreased to the low follicular level through direct inhibitory effects on the gonad and interference with sex steroid receptors. Gonadotropin levels also are reduced either subsequently or directly. Dosages used are 200 to 800 mg daily for 3 to 6 months. The androgenic symptoms limit the patient's tolerance of this therapy.

GnRH Analogs

The topic of GnRH analogs is discussed exclusively during the rest of this chapter under the title GnRH Agonists.

GnRH AGONISTS

GnRH and GnRH Agonists

GnRH analogs were created by modifying the GnRH peptide by one or two amino acids. But first let us review the natural hormone. Gonadotropin-releasing hormone is a naturally occurring hormone, produced by the hypothalamus in a pulsatile fashion. The pulsatile release of GnRH stimulates the pituitary gonadotrophs to synthesize and secrete follicle-stimulating hormone (FSH) and luteinizing hormone (LH), which then stimulates the ovaries to secrete sex steroids and folliculogenesis. The porcine form of this hormone was first isolated in 1971 by Schally et al (10). It is the decapeptide: pyro-Glu^{1}-His^{2}-Trp^{3}-Ser^{4}-Tyr^{5}-Gly^{6}-Leu^{7}-Arg^{8}-Pro^{9}-Gly^{10}-NH_2.

In the 1980s, Knobil (11,12) demonstrated that GnRH must be secreted in a pulsatile form to initiate and maintain normal ovulatory function in rhesus monkeys. The half-life of GnRH is very short (2–4 min), which makes it difficult to obtain human samples to study. The chief characteristics of the GnRH peptide include a receptor activation region around amino acids 1–3, a metabolic stability region with affinity to receptors at amino acids 5–6, and biologic activity at amino acids 9–10. Although the biologic activity of the GnRH molecule is conferred by both ends of the peptide, the proteolytic effect of enzymes on amino acids 5–6 eliminates the action of the GnRH molecule and keeps the half-life short.

GnRH agonists have been developed to be resistant to enzymatic cleavage and to have longer half-lives. All of the GnRH agonists have a substitution of the sixth amino acid (glycine) from the native GnRH peptide by a d-isomer. This substitution increases the half-life and stability dramatically. The second amino acid change in some GnRH agonists is the removal of the tenth amino acid. Without substitution this

TABLE 4.1

GnRH analogs

GENERIC NAME	TRADE NAME	AMINO ACID SUBSTITUTIONS	ROUTE
Buserelin	Suprefact	a.a. #6 = d-Ser(tBu) a.a. #10 = N-EtNH$_2$	Intranasal or SQ
Goserelin*	Zoladex	a.a. #6 = dSer(tBu) a.a. #10 = Aza-Gly-NH$_2$	Implant
Histrelin	Supprelin	a.a. #6 = imbzl-d-His a.a. # 10 = N-EtNH$_2$	SQ
Leuprolide*	Lupron	a.a. #6 = d-Leu a.a. #10 = N-EtNH$_2$	SQ or IM
Nafarelin*	Synarel	a.a. #6 = d-Nal$_2$ a.a. #10 = N-EtNH$_2$	Intranasal
Tryptorelin	Decapeptyl	a.a. #6 = d-Trp	SQ or IM

*Available in the United States.
SQ, subcutaneous; IM, intramuscular; a.a. #, amino acid number in GnRH peptide sequence.

deletion would result in the loss of 90% of the GnRH biologic activity. However, the substitution of an NH-ethylamide restores the GnRH biologic activity to the GnRH agonist (13). The biologic potency for most GnRH agonists is 100 times or more greater than that of the native GnRH molecule. Table 4.1 enumerates the currently available GnRH agonists, their molecular structures, and their route of administration. Two agonists are available in intranasal forms (buserelin and nafarelin) and two are available in a monthly depot form (leuprolide and goserelin). Typical GnRH agonist protocols are listed in Table 4.2.

As mentioned above, the native GnRH is secreted in a pulsatile fashion for normal ovulatory function. However, the GnRH agonists have a longer half-life and can be administered in intervals as far apart as a month. These drugs expose the body to a continuous form of a GnRH-like molecule. When this drug is given in the early follicular phase, there is a "flare" in the secretion of gonadotropins (i.e., FSH and LH) that can last for 3 to 10 days. GnRH agonists work by occupying the GnRH receptors for a prolonged time. While the GnRH receptor is occupied with the GnRH agonist, it is not available for endogenous GnRH. This GnRH agonist-receptor complex may undergo pinocyto-

TABLE 4.2

Typical GnRH agonist protocols

GENERIC	ROUTE	DOSE AND INTERVAL
Buserelin	SQ	0.2–0.5 mg/day
	Intranasal	0.2–0.5 mg SQ t.i.d. × 14 days, then 0.4 mg intranasal t.i.d.
	IM	0.9–1.2 mg/day
Goserelin	Implant	3.6 mg/mo
Leuprolide	SQ	0.5–1.0 mg/day
	IM	3.75–7.50 mg/mo
Naferelin	Intranasal	400 mg b.i.d.
Tryptorelin	SQ	0.25–0.50 mg/day
	IM	3.75 mg/mo

sis and enzymatic degradation, resulting in fewer GnRH receptors. Desensitization of GnRH caused by GnRH agonists occurs by down-regulation of GnRH receptors and probably postreceptor mechanisms. The final result is a reversible, medical castration. The gonadotropins (FSH and LH) and the sex steroids (estrogen and progesterone) remain low. This hypoestrogenic environment leads to shrinkage of leiomyomas and many other advantages before myomectomy; these are discussed later in this chapter.

GnRH Agonist Side Effects

GnRH agonists essentially cause a reversible, medical "menopause." The side effects or adverse symptoms experienced by a high percentage of patients on GnRH agonists are similar to menopausal symptoms: hot flushes, vaginal dryness, and mood lability. (See Table 4.3 for the commonly reported side effects.) Most of these symptoms are tolerable and the patient will remain on the GnRH agonist. Uncommon side effects

TABLE 4.3

Common side effects of GnRH agonists

SIDE EFFECTS	ESTIMATED OCCURRENCE
Hot flushes	80–90%
Headaches	30–55%
Vaginal dryness	14–37%
Irregular bleeding	20–40%
Emotional lability	20–45%
Weight change (Gain or loss)	15–30%
General pain	10–16%
Nausea/vomiting	15%
Dizziness	10–12%
Decreased libido	10–14%
Skin reactions	10%

Table 4.4

Uncommon side effects of GnRH agonists (<10% incidence)

Neuromuscular complaints
Breast tenderness/changes
Gastrointestinal disturbances
Paresthesias
Fatigue
Insomnia
Asthenia
Edema
Acne
Memory disorder
Ophthalmologic disorder

are listed in Table 4.4. A few rare side effects reported are anaphylaxis (14) and severe menorrhagia (15). Essentially, all of the side effects are self-limited and resolve within a few months after cessation of the GnRH agonist.

The intranasal GnRH agonists have a few other annoyances (16). The patient controls the administration of the medication. Compliance may be an issue for prolonged therapy. A wet or runny nose may irritate the patient. Patients will call if their allergies are bothering them. They need clarification from the beginning of treatment that allergic rhinitis does not interfere with intranasal absorption of the GnRH agonist.

Long-term use of GnRH agonists is limited by the long-term side effects of menopause; that is, the risk for cardiovascular disease increases with the lipid changes that are common to gonadal suppression without hormone replacement. Bone loss has been reported during as little as 24 weeks of therapy and may not be entirely recoverable. For pretreatment therapy for myomectomy, the GnRH agonist therapy can be limited to

3 months to get the maximum benefits and the fewest disadvantages. However, the perimenopausal woman may wish to have prolonged medical therapy to avoid a hysterectomy (see Chap. 13).

GnRH Agonist Benefits

GnRH agonists used as pretreatment for myomectomies take advantage of the reversible, medical menopause. As in menopause, a woman who is taking GnRH agonists enters a hypoestrogenic state, and she becomes amenorrheic. If anemia is present, it may resolve during the amenorrheic time period. Autologous blood can be donated, if desired. The endometrium becomes atrophic. Scheduling of surgery can be more flexible. Visualization will be improved during the operation since the endometrium is thin. Vascularization is decreased, and less bleeding will occur during surgery. Leiomyomas shrink in size during GnRH agonist pretreatment. This latter attribute may make some cases more feasible hysteroscopically or laparoscopically. Smaller leiomyomas typically result in higher success rates during the first surgical procedure.

Decrease in Leiomyoma Size: Multiple reports have demonstrated that GnRH agonists significantly decrease the size of all leiomyomas (Table 4.5). The leiomyoma volumes were calculated from three ultrasound measurements in most cases. A couple of studies have used magnetic resonance imaging (MRI). The range of leiomyoma size reduction varies from 32% to 84% over the duration of GnRH agonist therapy. The mean average reduction in size of leiomyomas is 50.7%. The duration of therapy ranged from 2 to 6 months. The maximum reduction of leiomyoma size occurred by the third month of GnRH agonist therapy.

In a couple of papers, no change was noted in leiomyoma size. Serra et al (17) reported that approximately 18% of leiomyomas did not regress in size. The intranasal preparation of leuprolide was ineffective in the regression of leiomyomas and allowed leiomyomas to continue to grow in size (18). This preparation of leuprolide did not reduce estradiol to menopausal levels. The size reduction of leiomyomas correlates well with the patient's estradiol levels. Postmenopausal estradiol levels are required to reduce leiomyoma sizes maximally.

TABLE 4.5

GnRH agonist therapy reduces leiomyoma size

YR	REFERENCE	AGONIST	PTS	DURATION	REDUCTION
1983	Filicori et al (37)	Tryptorelin	1	3 mo	77%
1984	Maheux et al (38)	Buserelin	3	6 mo	84%
1985	Maheux et al (39)	Buserelin	10	6 mo	80%
1987	Maheux et al (40)	Buserelin	9	6 mo	71%
1987	Perl et al (41)	Tryptorelin	10	3 mo	62%
1989	Donnez et al (42)	Buserelin	20	2 mo	32%
1992	Serra et al (17)	Leuprolide	110	4 mo	>50%
1996	Benagiano et al (43)	Goserelin	168	3 mo	44%
Average					62.5%

Reduction in Uterine Volume: Several papers measure the uterine volume pre- and posttherapy. The uterine volume decreased in most cases described. The range of decreased uterine volumes is 35% to 85% (Table 4.6), and the average is 50.7%. In a couple of cases, no change in uterine size or an increase in uterine volume was shown. These latter cases again demonstrate the significance of the estradiol level. In each instance, the estradiol levels were not suppressed to those seen at menopause. The uterine size directly correlates to the estradiol level. Similarly, the uterine cavity shrinks with sufficiently low estradiol levels.

Friedman et al (6) reported that using medroxyprogesterone in addition to GnRH agonist leuprolide was associated with less of a reduction in uterine volume. This study was a randomized, prospective, double-blind trial with the GnRH agonist leuprolide and medroxyprogesterone study arm (14% reduction in uterine volume) versus GnRH agonist and placebo study arm (40–50% reduction in uterine volume). Similar results were reported by Carr et al (7), who treated all patients with the GnRH agonist leuprolide (subcutaneous) and were prospectively randomized with a double-blind crossover approach using

TABLE 4.6

GnRH agonist therapy reduces uterine volume

Yr	Reference	Agonist	Pts	Duration	Reduction
1984	Healy et al (44)	Buserelin	1	4 mo	85%
1986	Healy et al (45)	Buserelin	5	2–3 mo	55%
1986	Coddington et al (46)	Histrelin	6	6 mo	57%
1986	Van Leusden (47)	Tryptorelin	6	4 mo	55%
1987	Friedman et al (18)	Leuprolide	7	6 mo	53%
1987	West et al (48)	Goserelin	12	6 mo	55%
1987	Lumsden et al (21)	Goserelin	14	3 mo	40%
1988	Andreyko et al (24)	Naferelin	10	6 mo	57%
1988	Friedman et al (6)	Leuprolide	8	6 mo	51%
1989	Friedman et al (29)	Leuprolide	18	6 mo	40%
1989	Matta et al (49)	Buserelin	10	6 mo	44%
1991	Friedman et al (30)	Leuprolide	63	6 mo	45%
1991	Nakamura et al (33)	Buserelin	25	4 mo	35%
1993	Vercellini et al (22)	Goserelin	41	6 mo	52%
1996	Benagiano et al (43)	Goserelin	168	3 mo	37%
	Average				50.7%

placebo or medroxyprogesterone. However, Carr et al used MRI to make the measurements and were able to dissect the effects of medroxyprogesterone on the leiomyomas versus the "nonmyoma" uterine tissue. Carr et al postulate that the "nonmyoma" uterine volume increases in response to medroxyprogesterone as measured by MRI. The mechanism for inhibiting the reduction in uterine volume is not clear. Additional evidence is provided by the limited data on the effects of an antiprogesterone, RU 486. Leiomyoma volume decreases by 49% after 3 months of RU 486 therapy (8). This study does not assess the nonmyoma uterine volume. Whatever the mechanism, RU 486 may be an alternative therapy for pretreatment in the future.

Increase in Hemoglobin Levels: GnRH agonist therapy causes amenorrhea in a majority of cases and hypomenorrhea (or spotting) in the rest (19). The bleeding-free time period allows for natural recovery of blood counts. Several reports document significant increases in hemoglobin levels by the end of GnRH agonist therapy (Table 4.7). Occasionally, the hemoglobin level has risen high enough for the patient to donate autologous blood for potential transfusion during the myomectomy.

Operative Benefits: Theoretically, a smaller uterus presenting for myomectomy will result in less intraoperative blood loss, fewer blood transfusions, ease of surgery, and shorter operative times. From the literature, the first premise appears to be true. Three prospective studies with placebo controls demonstrate less blood loss intraoperatively in the GnRH agonist treatment group compared to the control group (19–21). The former study was statistically significant (235 mL in the GnRH agonist goserelin group with 13 subjects vs. 350 mL in the placebo group with 14 subjects; $p < .01$). The study by Friedman et al (19) was only statistically significant when the patients were additionally stratified by

TABLE 4.7

GnRH agonist therapy increases hemoglobin levels

YR	REFERENCE	AGONIST	PTS	DURATION	HGB (PRE/POST)
1983	Filicori et al (37)	Tryptorelin	1	3 mo	7.4/12.8 g/dL*
1988	Friedman et al (6)	Leuprolide	7	6 mo	12.7/14.1 g/dL*
1989	Friedman et al (19)	Leuprolide	9	3 mo	12.7/12.2 g/dL
1989	Donnez et al (42)	Buserelin	9	2 mo	10.4/13.6 g/dL*
1991	Nakamura et al (33)	Buserelin	25	4 mo	9.5/13.0 g/dL*
1993	Golan et al (20)	Tryptorelin	29	2 mo	11.3/12.2 g/dL
1993	Vercellini et al (22)	Goserelin	41	6 mo	8.5/13.3 g/dL*
1996	Benagiano et al (43)	Goserelin	168	3 mo	10.1/12.7 g/dL

*Statistically significant.

uterine size: Then, the operative blood loss was less in women receiving GnRH agonists who had a uterine volume of greater than 600 mL (189 mL blood loss in the GnRH agonist leuprolide group consisting of 5 women vs. 390 mL in the placebo group consisting of 6 women; $p < .01$). The numbers in each of these studies are small.

The most recent study includes myomectomy and hysterectomy patients (53 total patients), and it confirms that the intraoperative blood loss was significantly lower in all the patients of the GnRH agonist tryptorelin group (320 mL in the 12 subjects of the GnRH myomectomy group vs. 476 mL in the 9 subjects in the control myomectomy group). Vercellini et al (22) also report significant reduction in blood loss in their patients who underwent hysterectomy (41 subjects), both abdominally and vaginally, who were pretreated with the GnRH agonist goserelin versus similar controls (92 subjects). Doppler studies by Matta et al (23) also support these findings. They found that uterine leiomyomas have significantly increased arterial impedance to blood flow after 4 months of GnRH agonist therapy. These myomectomy studies are limited by their small numbers.

The incidence of blood transfusions was significantly reduced in the GnRH agonist groups versus control subjects in two of the above studies (20,22); these studies are abdominal cases. Hysteroscopic cases should have markedly reduced incidence of blood loss and blood transfusion rates. Further studies are needed to demonstrate the benefit in hysteroscopic and laparoscopic cases.

GnRH agonist pretreatment increases the ease of surgical myomectomies according to Andreyko et al (24), Moghissi (25), and Coddington et al (26). Operative planes were easily identified and the vascularity was visibly decreased. However, operative times were not significantly different for any of the above studies. The overall postoperative complication rate is decreased in patients who receive GnRH agonist pretreatment (22,25).

Postoperatively, the hospital stays are comparable in duration when abdominal approaches are compared (20,22). Obviously, if a case can be converted to a laparoscopic or hysteroscopic procedure by the mere addition of the GnRH agonist, the hospital stay, home recuperation, and overall morbidity will be decreased.

GnRH Agonist Potential Disadvantages

As mentioned previously, GnRH agonists work in patients with leiomyomas by their ability to cause hypoestrogenism and possibly by direct action on the GnRH receptor in the leiomyomas (27). During such therapy, one needs to consider the risks of hypoestrogenism. The estrogen levels during GnRH agonist therapy are similar to postmenopausal estrogen levels without hormonal replacement. The concerns of changes in lipids and bone density must be addressed; the literature is reviewed in detail below. Additional disadvantages of GnRH agonist therapy are the extra cost and the delay of 3 months to surgery. These latter disadvantages are outweighed by the benefits noted previously.

Several studies of short-term GnRH agonist therapy have addressed lipid levels. Most report no statistically significant changes in the lipids overall and specifically in the total cholesterol, high-density lipoprotein, or low-density lipoproteins during the 2- to 6-month duration of treatment (6,7,26,28). Two studies by Friedman et al in 1989 (29) and 1991 (30) do show statistically significant changes in the GnRH agonist leuprolide group when compared with the pretreatment levels. Total cholesterol increased (1989—203 ± 9 vs. 219 ± 11 mg/dL; 1991—192 ± 5 vs. 205 ± 3 mg/dL). Low-density lipoprotein increased (1989—127 ± 8 vs. 139 ± 11 mg/dL; 1991—118 ± 5 vs. 126 ± 4 mg/dL). The mean high-density lipoprotein decreased in 1989 (59 ± 3 vs. 54 ± 3 mg/dL) but was not significantly different in the 1991 study. The numbers overall do not appear clinically significant over the short course. This result may change over long-term therapy without add-back hormones (see Chap. 13).

Bone densitometry is another critical aspect to assess before any consideration is given to long-term therapy with GnRH agonists. Several studies have evaluated bone densitometry by a variety of methods during GnRH agonist studies that ranged from 4 to 6 months. Single-photon absorptiometry (6,29) and dual-photon absorptiometry (DPA) (20,28,31,32) demonstrated no significant difference in bone densitometry over this short time period. Nakamura et al (33,34) used a quantitative x-ray assessment of bone density and also noted no decrease in bone mineral density. However, quantitative computed tomography

(CT) revealed a significant loss of 5.9% trabecular bone density from the lumbar vertebrae at the end of GnRH therapy with buserelin that was completely restored within 6 months to the pretreatment value (35).

Friedman et al (30) noted a mean decrease in trabecular lumbar bone density in the patients receiving GnRH agonist leuprolide who were assessed by DPA (3.8% decrease vs. controls with a 0.2% decrease) and assessed by CT of the lumbar spine (13.5% vs. 2.8% in controls). It is concerning to see some report considerable decreases in bone densitometry over such a short time. One must keep in mind that most of these studies involve small numbers of patients and the testing is performed over a relatively short time interval in regard to bone densitometry testing. It is somewhat reassuring to see that Matta's study (35) demonstrated bone density restoration. The other studies did not assess bone densitometry at any time interval after the GnRH agonist therapy was completed. These data still need to be collected, however. Another caveat is that reliability of bone densitometry testing varies considerably with the type of testing performed. Most recommend dual-energy x-ray absorptiometry (DEXA), with a 1% to 5% accuracy, over a 1- to 2-year time interval between tests. Perhaps, urinary tests of bone resorption would be more sensitive and predictive to changes over the shorter time interval.

SUMMARY AND FUTURE DIRECTIONS

Overall, GnRH agonists have made a dramatic improvement in preoperative preparation for myomectomy, abdominally and particularly endoscopically. There appears to be no significant difference in benefits between various types of GnRH agonists. Dosing interval may be a more clinically relevant factor for compliance issues. The depot formulations may be preferred. With 3 months of GnRH agonist pretreatment, the maximal benefits of leiomyoma and uterine volume reduction occur. The endometrium is atrophic and vascularization is reduced. These attributes provide the best opportunity for visualization hysteroscopically. Pretreatment also allows for normalization of the hemoglobin levels in those individuals affected with anemia and may offer the ability for autologous blood donation. Intraoperative blood loss is decreased. The incidence of blood transfusions decreases with pretreatment. The surgery is easier to perform due to easily identifiable planes and reduced vascularization. Postoperatively, the complication rate is also reduced with GnRH pretreatment.

Given all of these benefits, the disadvantages of increased cost and a 3-month delay in surgical scheduling seem minor. However, some patients do not respond with a decrease in leiomyoma volume or an amenorrheic time period. There have been rare reports of anaphylactic response to GnRH agonists as well as severe hemorrhage associated with necrosis of submucous leiomyomas and GnRH agonist therapy. In these cases, the pretreatment would obviously need to be abandoned.

The future directions for pretreatment therapy will probably involve maintaining the benefits while decreasing the delay to surgery. GnRH antagonists are currently in clinical trials. Since they produce no "flare" effect, as there is with GnRH agonists, the pretreatment duration can be reduced. One report of seven subjects noted a 50% reduction in leiomyoma volume within 4 weeks of therapy (36). Another alternative for individuals who cannot take GnRH analogs may be RU 486. Over a 3-month trial, a 49% reduction was found in leiomyoma volume and 100% amenorrhea (8). Further studies will be needed before the current recommendations can be changed.

Finally, the near future may offer a completely medical approach to the treatment of some individuals with symptomatic leiomyomas in the perimenopausal years. The GnRH analog with physiologic hormonal replacement may serve this use in the near future. As our understanding of the etiology and mechanisms of leiomyoma development and growth improves and our medical approaches follow suit, the future may make the myomectomy an archaic procedure.

REFERENCES

1. Buttram VC, Reiter RC. Uterine leiomyomata: etiology, symptomatology, and management. Fertil Steril 1981;36:433–445.

2. Wilson EA, Yang F, Rees ED. Estradiol and progesterone binding in the uterine leiomyomata and in normal uterine tissues. Obstet Gynecol 1980;55:20–24.
3. Goldzieher JW, Maqueo M, Ricaud L, et al. Induction of degenerative changes in uterine myomas by high dose progestin therapy. Am J Obstet Gynecol 1966;96:1078.
4. Goodman AL. Progesterone therapy in uterine fibromyoma. J Clin Endocrinol Metab 1946;6:402–408.
5. Tiltman AJ. The effect of progestins on the mitotic activity of uterine fibromyomas. Int J Gynecol Pathol 1985;4:89–96.
6. Friedman AJ, Barbieri RL, Doubilet PM, et al. A randomized, double-blind trial of a gonadotropin-releasing hormone (leuprolide) with or without medroxyprogesterone acetate in the treatment of leiomyomata uteri. Fertil Steril 1988;49:404–409.
7. Carr BR, Marshburn PB, Weatherall PT, et al. Evaluation of the effect of gonadotropin-releasing hormone analogs and medroxyprogesterone acetate on uterine leiomyomata volume by magnetic resonance imaging: a prospective, randomized, double blind, placebo controlled, crossover trial. J Clin Endocrinol Metab 1993;76:1217–1223.
8. Murphy AA, Kettel LM, Morales AJ, et al. Regression of uterine leiomyomata in response to the antiprogesterone RU 486. J Clin Endocrinol Metab 1993;76:513–517.
9. Nisson L, Rybo G. Treatment of menorrhagia. Am J Obstet Gynecol 1971;110:713–720.
10. Schally AV, Nair RM, Redding TW, Arimura A. Isolation of the luteinizing hormone and follicle-stimulating hormone-releasing hormone from porcine hypothalami. J Biol Chem 1971;246:7230–7236.
11. Knobil E, Plant TM, Wildt L, et al. Control of the rhesus monkey menstrual cycle: permissive role of hypothalamic gonadotropin-releasing hormone. Science 1980;207:1371–1373.
12. Knobil E. The neuroendocrine control of ovulation. Hum Reprod 1988;3:469–472.
13. Henzyl MR. Gonadotropin-releasing hormone and its analogs: from bedside to laboratory. Clin Obstet Gynecol 1993;36:617–635.
14. Letterie GS, Stevenson D, Shah L. Recurrent anaphylaxis to a depot form of GNRH analog. Obstet Gynecol 1991;78:943–946.

15. Friedman AJ. Vaginal hemorrhage associated with degenerating submucous leiomyomata during leuprolide acetate treatment. Fertil Steril 1989; 52:152–154.
16. Henzyl MR. Gonadotropin-releasing hormone analogs: update on new findings. Am J Obstet Gynecol 1992;166:757–761.
17. Serra GB, Panetta Z, Colosimo M, et al. Efficacy of leuprolide acetate depot in symptomatic fibromatous uteri: the Italian Multicenter Trial. Clin Ther 1992;14(suppl A):57–69.
18. Friedman AJ, Barbieri RL, Benacerraf BR, Schiff R. Treatment of leiomyomata with intranasal or subcutaneous leuprolide, a gonadotropin-releasing hormone agonist. Fertil Steril 1987;48:560–564.
19. Friedman AJ, Rein MS, Harrison-Atlas D, et al. A randomized, placebo-controlled, double-blind study evaluating leuprolide acetate depot treatment before myomectomy. Fertil Steril 1989;52:728–733.
20. Golan A, Bukovsky I, Pansky M, et al. Perioperative gonadotropin releasing hormone agonist treatment in surgery for uterine leiomyomata. Hum Reprod 1993;8:450–452.
21. Lumsden MA, West CP, Baird DT. Goserelin therapy before surgery for uterine fibroids. Lancet 1987;1:36–37.
22. Vercellini P, Bocciolone L, Colombo A, et al. Gonadotropin-releasing hormone agonist treatment before hysterectomy for menorrhagia and uterine leiomyomas. Acta Obstet Gynecol Scand 1993;72:369–373.
23. Matta WH, Stabile I, Shaw RW, Campbell S. Doppler assessment of uterine blood flow changes in patients with fibroids receiving the gonadotropin-releasing agonist buserelin. Fertil Steril 1988;49:1083–1085.
24. Andreyko JL, Blumenfeld Z, Marshall LA, et al. Use of agonistic analog of gonadotropin-releasing hormone (nafarelin) to treat leiomyomas: assessment by magnetic resonance imaging. Am J Obstet Gynecol 1988;158: 903–910.
25. Moghissi KS. Hormonal therapy before surgical treatment for uterine leiomyomas. J Surg Gynecol Obstet 1991;172:497–502.
26. Coddington CC, Brizyski R, Hansen KA, et al. Short term treatment with leuprolide acetate for colitis as a successful adjuvant to surgical therapy for leiomyomas of the uterus. J Surg Gynecol Obstet 1992;175:57–63.
27. Chegini N, Rong H, Dou Q, et al. Gonadotropin-releasing hormone (GnRH) and GnRH receptor gene expression in human myometrium and leiomyomata and the direct action of GnRH analogs on myometrial

smooth muscle cells and interaction with ovarian steroids in vitro. J Clin Endocrinol Metab 1996;81:3215–3221.
28. Schlaff WD, Zerhouni EA, Huth JA, et al. A placebo-controlled trial of a depot gonadotropin-releasing hormone analog (leuprolide) treatment of uterine leiomyomata. Obstet Gynecol 1989;74:856–862.
29. Friedman AJ, Harrison-Atlas D, Barbieri RL, et al. A randomized, placebo-controlled, double-blind study evaluating the efficacy of leuprolide acetate depot in the treatment of uterine leiomyomata. Fertil Steril 1989; 51:251–256.
30. Friedman AJ, Hoffman DI, Comite F, et al. Treatment of leiomyomata uteri with leuprolide depot: a double-blind, placebo-controlled, multicenter study. Obstet Gynecol 1991;77:720–725.
31. Damewood MD, Schlaff WD, Hesla JS, Rock JA. Internal bone mineral density with long term gonadotropin releasing hormone agonist suppression. Fertil Steril 1989;52:596–599.
32. Tummon IS, Ali A, Pepping ME, et al. Bone mineral density in women with endometriosis before and during ovarian suppression with gonadotropin-releasing hormone agonists or danazol. Fertil Steril 1988;49:792–796.
33. Nakamura Y, Yoshimura Y, Yamaba H, et al. Treatment of uterine leiomyomata with luteinizing hormone-releasing hormone agonist: the possibility of nonsurgical management in selected perimenopausal women. Fertil Steril 1991;55:900–905.
34. Nakamura Y, Yoshimura Y. Treatment of uterine leiomyomas in perimenopausal women with gonadotropin-releasing hormone agonists. Clin Obstet Gynecol 1993;36:660–667.
35. Matta WH, Shaw RW, Hesp R, Evans R. Reversible trabecular bone density loss after induced hyperestrogenism with the GnRH analogue buserelin in perimenopausal women. Clin Endocrinol 1988;29:45–51.
36. Kettel LM, Murphy LA, Morales AJ, et al. Rapid regression of uterine leiomyomas in response to daily administration of gonadotropin releasing hormone antagonist. Fertil Steril 1993;60:642–646.
37. Filicori M, Hall DA, Loughlin JS, et al. A conservative approach to the management of uterine leiomyoma: pituitary desensitization by a luteinizing hormone-releasing hormone analog. Am J Obstet Gynecol 1983; 147:726–727.
38. Maheux R, Guilloteau C, LeMay A, et al. Regression of leiomyomata uteri following hypoestrogenism induced by repetitive luteinizing hormone-

releasing agonist treatment: preliminary reports. Fertil Steril 1984;42: 644–646.

39. Maheux R, Guilloteau C, LeMay A, et al. Luteinizing hormone-releasing hormone agonist and uterine leiomyomata: a pilot study. Am J Obstet Gynecol 1985;152:1034–1038.
40. Maheux R, LeMay A, Marat P. Use of intranasal luteinizing hormone-releasing hormone agonist in uterine leiomyomas. Fertil Steril 1987;47:229–233.
41. Perl Z, Marquez J, Schally AV, et al. Treatment of leiomyomata uteri with D-TRP^6-luteinizing hormone-releasing hormone. Fertil Steril 1987;48: 383–389.
42. Donnez J, Schrurs B, Gillerot S, et al. Treatment of uterine fibroids with implants of gonadotropin-releasing hormone agonist: assessment by hysterography. Fertil Steril 1989;51:947–950.
43. Benagiano G, Kivinen FT, Fadini R, et al. Zoladex (goserelin acetate) and the anemic patient: results of a multifibroid study. Fertil Steril 1996; 66:223–229.
44. Healy DL, Fraser HM, Lawson SL. Shrinkage of a uterine fibroid after subcutaneous infusion of a LHRH agonist. Br Med J 1984;289: 1267–1268.
45. Healy DL, Lawson SR, Abbot M, et al. Toward removing uterine fibroids without surgery: subcutaneous infusion of a luteinizing hormone-releasing hormone agonist commencing in the luteal phase. J Clin Endocrinol Metab 1986;63:619–625.
46. Coddington CC, Collins RL, Shawker TH, et al. Long acting gonadotropin-releasing hormone analogs used to treat uteri. Fertil Steril 1986;45:624–629.
47. van Leusden HAIM. Rapid reduction of uterine myomas after short-term treatment with microencapsulated D-TRP^6-LHRH. Lancet 1986;2:1213.
48. West CP, Lumsden MA, Lawson S, et al. Shrinkage of uterine fibroids during therapy with goserelin (Zoladex): a luteinizing hormone-releasing hormone agonist administered as a monthly subcutaneous depot. Fertil Steril 1987;48:45–51.
49. Matta WH, Shaw RH, Nye M. Long-term follow-up of patients with uterine fibroids after treatment with LHRH agonist buserelin. Br J Obstet Gynaecol 1989;96:200–206.

CHAPTER

5

Myomectomy by Laparotomy

Eric J. Bieber

Long before we investigated the performance of hysteroscopic or laparoscopic myomectomy or evaluated the idea of medical treatment of myomas, laparotomy was successfully employed. Today, it remains the gold standard by which other treatment modalities, both surgical and nonsurgical, are compared. This chapter focuses on the method of myomectomy by laparotomy and addresses issues of preoperative evaluation, including patient consent, preoperative medical treatment, noninvasive or minimally invasive imaging, and blood donation. Surgical aspects, such as exposure, myoma extraction techniques, and options for myoma bed closure, are described.

HISTORIC PERSPECTIVE

Myomectomy has advanced significantly since 1890, when Martin first reported on the use of the procedure for uterine conservation, boasting a mortality of 19% (1). Although this was no higher than the mortality for hysterectomy at that time, there was little interest in the procedure. Victor Bonney (2) later stated, "Myomectomy is therefore one of the oldest of the abdominal operations, but its development has been very slow." Bonney was one of the innovators in describing methodologies for securing hemostasis and described the nuances of the procedure. His statement, "Since cure without deformity or loss of function must ever be surgery's highest ideal, the general proposition that myomectomy is a greater surgical achievement than hysterectomy is incontestable," seems no less appropriate or controversial today than it did in 1931 (2). He believed that neither fibroid number nor uterine size was a strict contraindication to myomectomy, having reported on the removal of 125 myomas from a single uterus. Other authors in subsequent years reported on large series of patients who underwent myomectomy successfully. Davids (3), in reporting on his extensive series of myomectomies, stated, "The number of successful myomectomies will be in proportion to the enthusiasm of the surgeon for the procedure." He also stated in the same article, "The psychological impact of the loss of the uterus may be so profound as to affect the entire life pattern." These views were certainly consistent with those of Dr. Bonney two decades earlier. These discussions continue today at gynecology conferences and prompted inclusion of the chapter Myomectomy in the Nonreproductive Woman, (Chap. 11).

PREOPERATIVE EVALUATION

Noninvasive Imaging

Regardless of the route, it is critical that one have a detailed understanding of myoma size and location before performing a myomectomy. With laparoscopy we lose the ability to palpate fibroids, whereas with hysteroscopy we may only be seeing the tip of the iceberg. Even during laparotomy it may be challenging to differentiate a submucous myoma from underlying myometrium. We have seen a number of such cases, in which a laparotomy was performed for menorrhagia and fibroids without evaluation of the endometrial cavity, only to have the patient return with continued menorrhagia, and, with subsequent evaluation, demonstrate an intracavitary lesion that requires a second operation.

Ultrasound

By optimizing preoperative imaging, we may be able to decrease the chance of missing myomas and facilitate intraoperative management. Ultrasound may be the most cost-effective method for evaluating the uterus and pelvis. Multiple studies have demonstrated high sensitivity and specificity, especially for transvaginal scanning (4–6). There is, however, occasional difficulty in evaluating the endometrial canal as well as defining the extent of intracavitary myoma involvement using this modality. The advent of liquid instillation into the uterine cavity contemporaneous with the performance of ultrasound, known as sonohysterography (SHG), has improved our ability to evaluate the endometrial canal (see Sonohysterography, below). Occasionally, clinical evaluation of the adnexa in patients with large myomatous uteri may be difficult. Ultrasound can be used to rule out concomitant adnexal abnormalities in these patients.

Several studies have addressed the difficulty of diagnosing leiomyosarcoma preoperatively. Some authors have suggested that a decreased resistance index may increase suspicion of malignancy. The significant intrinsic variability of myoma vascularity, however, may reduce the predictive value. Finally, as with all testing, the skill of the sonographer or sonography technician may well determine the adequacy of the evaluation.

Hysterosalpingography

Hysterosalpingography (HSG), in which a liquid medium, either water or oil based, is instilled under fluoroscopic guidance, provides excellent information about the endometrial canal and fallopian tubes. Multiple studies have documented the high sensitivity of HSG in demarcating intrauterine abnormalities (7,8). Like ultrasonography, hysterosalpingography has significant limitations, including the inability to define the extent of intramural or subserosal involvement as well as occasional difficulties in determining the extent of submucous myoma protrusion.

Sonohysterography

Sonohysterography has only recently been employed as a minimally invasive diagnostic tool for evaluation of the uterine cavity. The procedure is simple to perform in the office setting. The patient is sterilely prepped and an intrauterine catheter is placed into the uterus. We have used a number of insemination-type catheters successfully, and recently procedure-specific catheters have been introduced by several companies (Fig. 5.1). After removal of the speculum a transvaginal probe is placed. Initial reports evaluated transabdominal sonohysterograms; however, use of transvaginal imaging may improve sensitivity and specificity. Sterile saline is then used to distend the cavity during real-time sonography (Figs. 5.2 to 5.4).

Turner and colleagues (9) noted improved visualization of submucous myomas and endometrial polyps with sonohysterography in 17 of 19 patients compared with routine vaginal sonography. Gaucherand et al (10) compared sonohysterography with transvaginal sonography and hysterosalpingography. Using histology as their gold standard they found sonohysterography to have a higher sensitivity and specificity than either transvaginal sonography or hysterosalpingography.

Romano and partners (11) evaluated the use of abdominal and vaginal sonohysterograms. They noted that the combination of the abdominal and vaginal route yielded a sensitivity of 95% and a

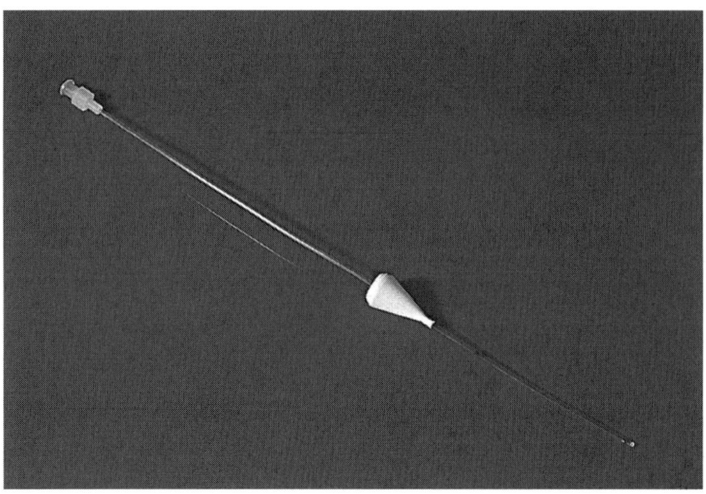

FIG. 5.1.

An example of a catheter that is useful for performance of sonohysterography.

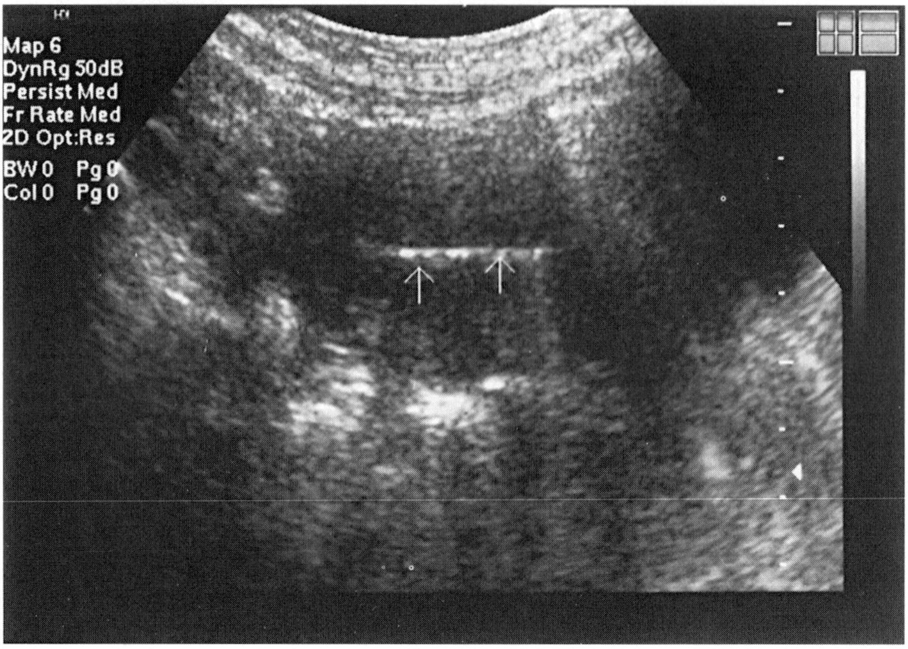

FIG. 5.2.

An insemination catheter is easily visualized in the uterine cavity with transvaginal sonography.

specificity of 100%, with the predictive value of an abnormal test being 100% (11).

The advantage of sonohysterography is the ease of performance of the procedure. Since many clinicians have ready access to ultrasound in their offices, there may be no significant financial outlay. Patients seem to tolerate sonohysterography with less cramping and discomfort than even well-performed hysterosalpingograms without the exposure to radiation.

Magnetic Resonance Imaging and Computed Tomographic Scan

Both magnetic resonance imaging (MRI) and computed tomography (CT) offer an expensive but extensive evaluation of abdominal and pelvic

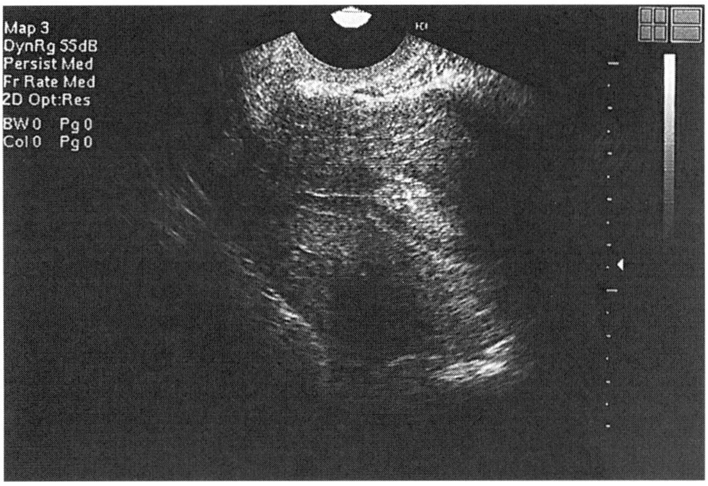

FIG. 5.3.

Transvaginal sonogram of a patient with menorrhagia and a thickened stripe.

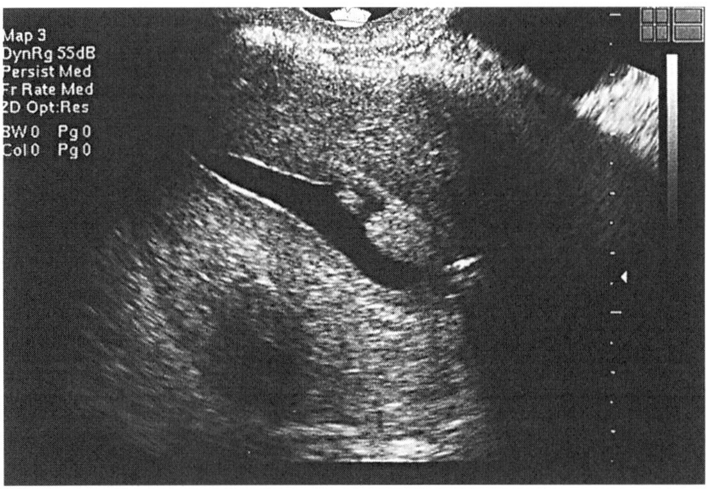

FIG. 5.4.

The same patient from Fig. 5.3 undergoes sonohysterography with intracavitary instillation of normal saline. Two separate lesions with intracavitary projection are now identified distinct from the endometrium.

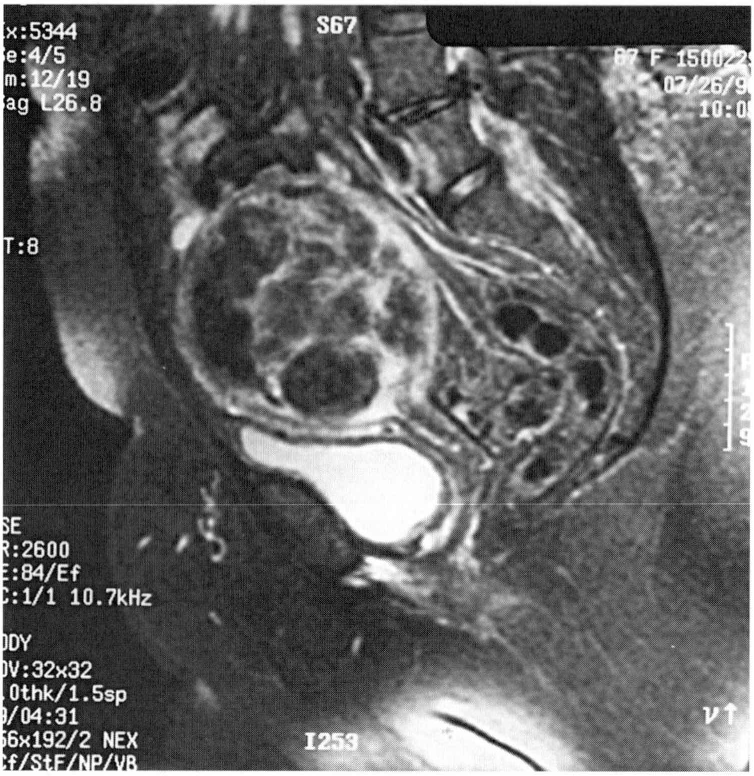

FIG. 5.5.

MRI demonstrates an enlarged uterus with multiple myomas.

structures (12). Some authors have suggested that MRI allows a more accurate determination of myoma size, location, and number (13) (Fig. 5.5). MRI does not have the ability to investigate in real time like ultrasound, but does allow an evaluation of adnexal or abdominal structures when the uterus is large. In addition, MRI may be better suited for attempting delineation of adenomyosis versus myomas (Fig. 5.6).

Hysteroscopy

Hysteroscopy is the gold standard for evaluation of the uterine cavity. Multiple studies have documented the superiority of the hysteroscope versus dilation and curettage (D&C) (14,15). In addition, hysteroscopy provides the most comprehensive evaluation of the

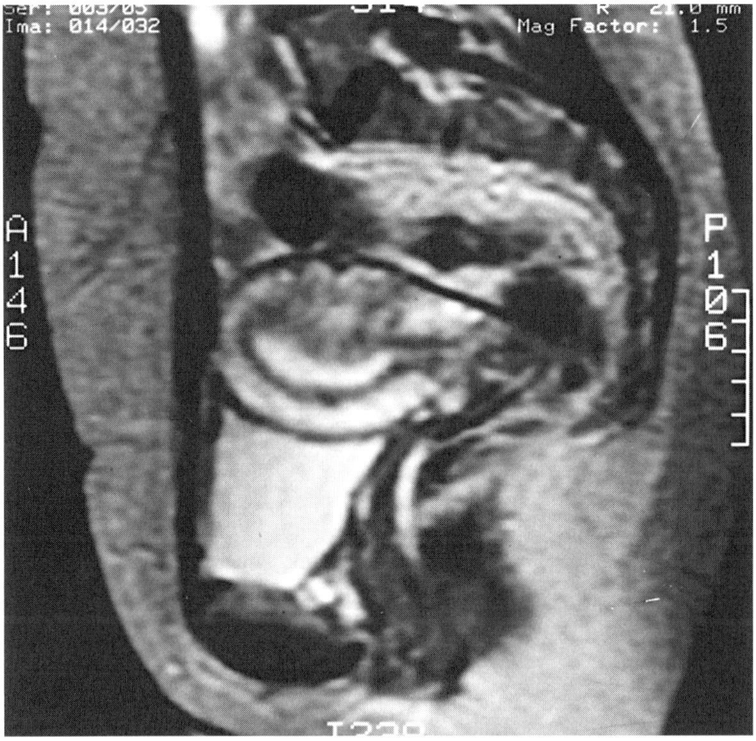

FIG. 5.6.

MRI of an enlarged uterus with no identifiable focal lesions consistent with adenomyosis.

cavity, allowing optimal planning strategies preoperatively. The majority of physicians do not have the ability to perform office hysteroscopy as they do ultrasound. In addition, hysteroscopy is occasionally misleading, as not all myomas are concentrically shaped, with some being bilobed or oblong. In these situations the surgeon may believe that more than 50% of the myoma is intracavitary when in reality it may be mostly intramural and thus better addressed abdominally instead of transvaginally.

X-Ray

Once the main imaging modality, x-ray has today been replaced by the previously discussed modalities. Calcifications of myomas present a

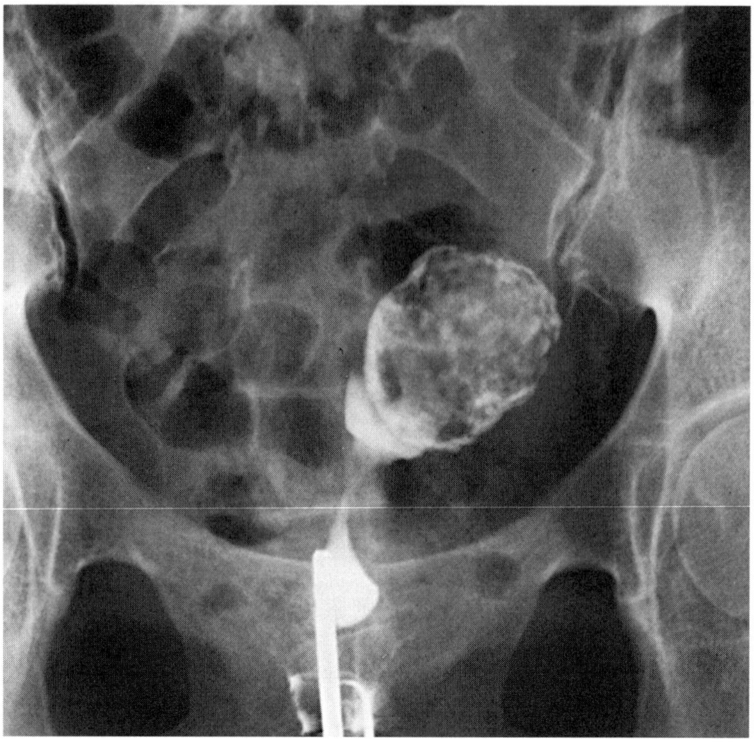

FIG. 5.7.

Pelvic radiograph demonstrating a highly calcified uterine fibroid.

striking appearance but generally do not change our clinical management (Fig. 5.7).

Intravenous Pyelography

Intravenous pyelography (IVP) may be intermittently useful when myomas are located laterally in the broad ligament or paracervically. However, even in the very large leiomyomatous uterus without adnexal pathology, lateral or retroperitoneal dissection is rarely necessary in performing a myomectomy. Excretory urograms and renal ultrasound may document hydronephrosis or renal pelvis dilatation, but again this rarely alters surgical management.

Blood Workup

Generally, we order a complete blood count on all patients who present with symptomatic myomas. It is often surprising that patients will deny significant abnormal bleeding, but present with very low hemoglobins. A dramatic example of this was a patient who presented to our office with "minimal increased bleeding" who had a hemoglobin of 5.2g/dL, all secondary to a small 1- to 2-cm completely intracavitary myoma. The hemoglobin/hematocrit allows us to gauge what time interval might be required to optimize the patient's hemodynamic status before surgery. With low hemoglobin values, patients are offered the option of gonadotropin-releasing hormone (GnRH) analog suppression in addition to iron therapy, as discussed in detail in Chapter 4. Especially for laparotomy myomectomy procedures, we also encourage patients to donate autologous blood (see below).

Medical Pretreatment

Multiple regimens have been used to suppress bleeding and improve hematocrit before surgery. They are discussed in detail in Chapter 4. Briefly, oral contraceptives can be used to control bleeding in the short term using the classic regimen of a low dose two to four times a day for 5 to 7 days, then decreasing the dose to once a day until the bleeding has stopped or is controlled. We generally concomitantly administer a GnRH analog (GnRHa) at the start of therapy. Analogs are of little value in the acute situation since downregulation and desensitization occur over a 7- to 10-day period. Once the hemoglobin has reached an acceptable level and downregulation has occurred, we stop the oral contraceptive and allow what may be a large withdrawal bleed. Depomedroxyprogesterone acetate (DMPA) has also been used to decidualize endometrial tissue and decrease bleeding. The long period of action (3mo) and the unpredictable effect on bleeding make this a less acceptable regimen in the acute situation. In the anovulatory menorrhagic patient, the situation is quite different and a timed withdrawal bleed with oral progestins is preferable prior to surgery (especially with hysteroscopy).

GnRH analogs have also been used to successfully decrease myoma and uterine size before surgery (16–18). Maximal reduction is seen after a 3- to 4-month course. However, there may be a differential response from one myoma to another. Recently, Stovall et al (19) reported on a large, multicenter, randomized double-blind study in which patients received the GnRH analog leuprolide acetate or placebo and all patients received iron. They noted a statistically significant increase in patients who were able to achieve a hemoglobin of greater than 12g/dL in the GnRHa and iron group (74%) versus the placebo group (46%)

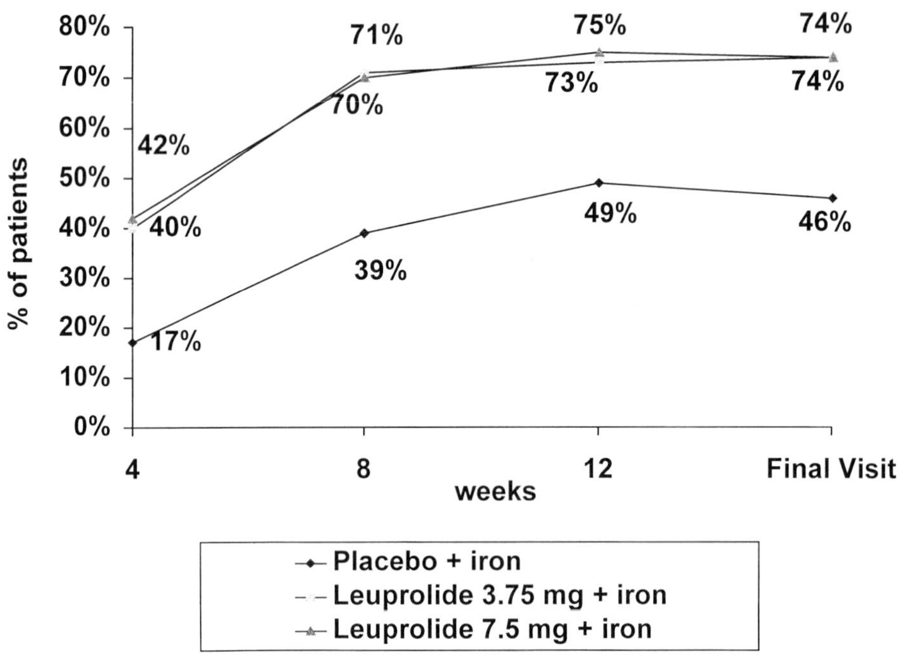

FIG. 5.8.

Patients presenting with hematocrit ≤30% and/or hemoglobin ≤10.2g/dL and uterine fibroids. Patients received either placebo and iron; leuprolide acetate, 3.75mg per month ×3, and iron; or leuprolide acetate, 7.5mg per month ×3, and iron. The graph represents the percent of patients who attained a hemoglobin level of at least 12g/dL and a hematocrit of at least 36%. (Adapted from Stovall TG, Muneyyirci-Delale O, Summitt RL, et al. GnRH agonist and iron versus placebo and iron in the anemic patient before surgery for leiomyomas: a randomized controlled trial. Obstet Gynecol 1995;86:65–71.)

TABLE 5.1

Use of GnRH analogs in patients with myomas

	Leuprolide, 7.5 mg	Leuprolide, 3.75 mg	Placebo
% change in uterine volume after 3 mo	−31	−39	+10
% change in myoma volume after 3 mo	−23	−27	+8
% of patients receiving nonautologous transfusion	8	2	13

Source: Stovall TG, Muneyyirci-Delale O, Summitt RL, et al. GnRH agonist and iron versus placebo and iron in the anemic patient before surgery for leiomyomas: a randomized controlled trial. Obset Gynecol 1995;86:65–71.

(Fig. 5.8). In this large trial they also found significant decreases in myoma and uterine volume in the GnRHa groups consistent with the reports of other investigators (Table 5.1). They noted no difference in myoma or uterine shrinkage when the higher dosage of leuprolide, 7.5 mg per month, was compared to the lower dosage of 3.75 mg per month.

In general, we consider GnRHa as presurgical adjuncts and discuss with patients that, although they may have improved symptomatology secondary to decreased bleeding and fibroid shrinkage, symptoms will return and fibroids will increase to their pretreatment size without surgical intervention. It is interesting that Stovall et al (19) noted that 47 of 265 patients (17.7%) chose not to have surgery after treatment. This underscores the need for very frank discussion with the patient before GnRH analog therapy is initiated.

Endometrial Sampling

It has been recommended that patients who present with abnormal bleeding be evaluated with D&C before undergoing definitive myomectomy. In the young patient, this is probably unnecessary and if needed an office endometrial biopsy or directed biopsy at the time of hysteroscopy can be performed. Indeed, D&C can actually be very difficult in the patient with intracavitary distortion or cervical displacement, requiring ultrasound guidance to ensure adequacy of the sample. Leiomyosarcoma may occasionally be picked up from D&C but is certainly not excluded on the basis of a negative sample.

Rate of Uterine Enlargement

Historically, we have been taught that rapid uterine enlargement is a potential sign of leiomyosarcoma. As we presently follow many patients without symptoms, we have begun to appreciate the natural history of myomas. The lack of predictability is demonstrated by periods of growth followed by periods of stability. Parker and colleagues (20) reported on the lack of correlation between rapid fibroid growth and an actual histologic diagnosis of leiomyosarcoma. In patients who met the criteria of rapid growth (an increase of 6 gestational weeks during 1 year), 0 of 198 patients actually had uterine sarcoma. In patients treated with GnRHa, a lack of appreciable response over 2 to 3 months should lead the clinician to proceed to surgery, as additional months of treatment are unlikely to yield a substantial benefit. Whether this group of patients is at a higher risk of sarcoma is as yet unknown.

Autologous Blood Banking

As part of the preoperative discussion with patients, they are offered the option of autologous blood donation before surgery. Our laboratory requires a hemoglobin of 11 g/dL or greater before autologous donation is allowed. The first unit is donated 4 to 5 weeks prior to surgery and the second unit is donated 1 week or more later. Although patients are allowed to donate up to 3 days before surgery, this may not allow optimization of the preoperative hematocrit. Patients are given ferrous sulfate, 325 mg three times a day, and a concomitant multivitamin with B_{12} and folate to improve iron absorption. If surgery is delayed, donated units can be frozen for prolonged periods. It is important to note that, once thawed, these units must be used within 24 hours.

Consent Before Surgery

As with all surgeries it is important to discuss with patients surgical options as well as the risks and benefits of the various options. It is particularly important when discussing myomectomy that patients be counseled regarding the possibilities of further surgery secondary to myoma recurrence. As recurrence may require the patient to undergo a subsequent laparotomy this may be important in the patient choosing between conservative therapy versus definitive management. In addition, the risks of blood loss and adhesion formation are important issues of which the patient should be made aware.

The risk of possible hysterectomy should also be addressed with all patients who are contemplating laparotomy myomectomy. Historically, the risk of conversion of myomectomy to hysterectomy has been reported as greater than 10%. However, LaMorte et al (21) reported only one hysterectomy in their retrospective review of 128 planned myomectomies. Classic indications for conversion have included an inability to reconstruct a functional uterus and excessive blood loss. The first should occur infrequently, as even large uteri or uteri with multiple myomas can generally be reconstructed given adequate time. Issues of blood loss exist for every surgery but additional surgical time may be gained by having several units of autologous blood available, thereby giving the surgeon a maximal "cushion" before having to resort to hysterectomy. Occasionally, a large adenomyotic uterus may be encountered when myomas have been reported on ultrasound. At this point, depending on the clinical setting and patient desires, hysterectomy may be the most reasonable choice.

In our series, no patient with a fibroid uterus, including cases of up to 34-week size and more than 40 myomas, has had to undergo hysterectomy. In spite of this, all patients are counseled that the risk exists.

ABDOMINAL MYOMECTOMY

In selected cases of abdominal myomectomy in which substantial numbers of myomas are involved or a patient may have a borderline hemoglobin, it may be worthwhile to consider use of the cell saver. The cell saver allows salvage of blood during the course of the proceduce. It is difficult to predict which patients will have excessive blood loss before these procedures are begun. LaMorte and colleagues (21) reported a 4% incidence of blood loss of greater than 1000 mL in reviewing the records of 128 women who underwent abdominal myomectomy. Twenty percent of patients received transfusions, of which 70% were autologous. This underscores the advantages of preoperative autologous donation as well as presurgical optimization of hematocrit. However, at times more than two units would be required. The cell saver is connected before the procedure is begun and is used once the skin incision has been made. If the cavity is entered the salvage is discontinued secondary to the risk of contamination and possible sepsis. Although no specific data exist in this regard, we believe that the potential for infectious morbidity outweighs the risk of blood at this point.

Prophylactic antibiotics have been advocated by some. Unfortunately, few or no data exist in regard to actual efficacy. Because of uterine manipulation and especially in cases in which the uterine cavity is entered, we have chosen to give one preoperative dose of antibiotics as well as several postoperative doses of broad-spectrum antibiotics.

During our initial evaluation, if the patient has had a hysterosalpingogram that is abnormal, we will generally perform a hysteroscopy immediately preceding the laparotomy to locate and best define the intracavitary lesions. If the patient has had no such evaluation, a hysteroscopy can be performed to rule out the possibility of submucous involvement. Unfortunately, there may be cases in which significant uterine distortion exists and hysteroscopy may be quite difficult because of canal distortion. We have rarely needed to perform significant operative hysteroscopic or resectoscopic procedures at this time, although if one notes a completely intracavitary myoma, this could be resected before the laparotomy is done to avoid entry into the uterine cavity. More often we have found that performance of hysteroscopy allows optimization of the surgical plan because it enables us to know specifically where fibroids are located within the cavity and where, if cavity entry is necessary, this would need to be performed.

Classically a vertical skin incision has been recommended in patients with total uterine size of 12 or more weeks' gestation. However, in many cases myomas that are larger than this can easily be removed through Pfannenstiel's incision. If necessary a muscle-splitting incision can also be utilized to gain additional exposure. It is surprising how a large myomatous uterus can be delivered through a relatively small incision and once some of the myomas have been resected the uterine size may become more manageable. In addition, this may decrease the rate of later adhesion formation. We presently prefer to "deliver" the uterus through the incision and perform the majority of the procedure extracorporeally if possible (Fig. 5.9). Interestingly, this is often easier with a larger uterus. By bringing the uterus extra-abdominal, we limit unnecessary trauma to the bowel that is incurred by placement of self-retaining retractors and laparotomy packs. Often patients with minimal bowel trauma have excel-

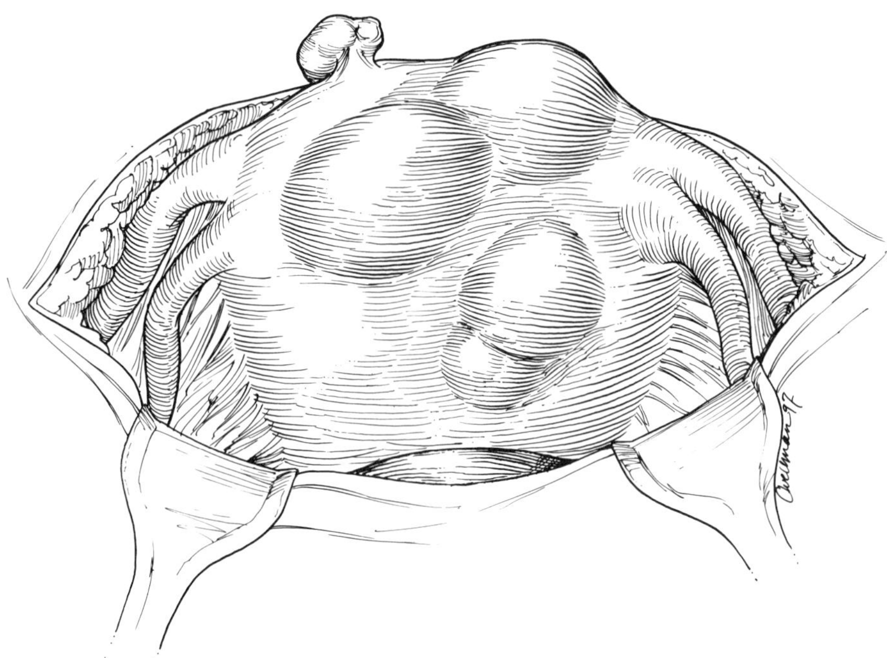

FIG. 5.9.

The uterus has been delivered through the abdominal incision.

lent bowel function even in the first 12 to 24 hours following laparotomy. It is hoped that by limiting bowel trauma and tissue dissection subsequent adhesion formation can be decreased, although no data exist in this regard. With the uterus extracorporeal it is important to continuously irrigate the tissue so as not to allow serosal injury. For this reason we use a cesarean section type of drape that contains collecting bags on each side of the table and limits fluid on the floor and on the surgeon.

Optimizing Hemostasis

It is critically important during the performance of myomectomy to optimize hemostasis. Limiting blood in the field improves visualization while decreasing patient morbidity, allowing the surgeon to take the necessary time to remove all the myomas as well as achieving excellent tissue reapproximation. Multiple methodologies have been proposed over the last century to aid in achieving hemostasis. The most common solution presently used is vasopressin (Pitressin), in a mixture of 20 units or one ampule of Pitressin mixed with 20 to 50 mL normal saline. When it is injected into the myometrium, significant vasoconstriction and tissue blanching occur. Bleeding is markedly decreased following injection but is time limited. Care should be taken when injecting vasopressin into tissues to avoid intravascular injection. Several recent publications have evaluated the use of intramyometrial vasopressin during the performance of myomectomy. Frederick and colleagues (22) noted in a randomized placebo trial a marked difference in blood loss between the placebo group and vasopressin group. Patients who received vasopressin had a median blood loss of 225 mL compared with a loss of 675 mL in the placebo group. In this small trial, 50% of the patients in the placebo group received blood transfusions whereas no patients in the vasopressin arm were transfused. In contrast to what is commonly perceived, Frederick et al also noted no change in pulse and blood pressure between the two groups.

Mechanical techniques have also been used to achieve hemostasis. Penrose drains or catheters can be used as tourniquets to compress the uterine vasculature, as well as devices to compress the infundibulopelvic ligaments. Multiple authors have suggested the use of rubber shods applied over various clamps and jaws as a means of protecting tissues yet achieving vaso-occulsion. Delancey (23) described a technique in which the broad ligament is pierced above the level of the uterine artery bilaterally and a urethral catheter is placed around the uterus. This effectively occludes the ascending branches of the uterine arteries. He then used a Bainbridge vascular clamp bilaterally to occlude the more superior uterine blood flow. The advantage of the Bainbridge clamp is a cutout that exists within the clamp where the fallopian tube can be placed, thereby causing no injury to the tube but allowing compression of uterine and ovarian vessels.

Few studies exist comparing these various techniques. In one study, Ginsburg et al (24) performed a randomized trial comparing vasopressin injection (20 units in 20 mL normal saline) and mechanical vaso-occlusion with a Penrose drain placed through the broad ligaments at the level of the internal os and vascular clamps placed on the infundibulopelvic ligaments. No significant differences in blood loss, transfusion rates, or morbidity were found between the two groups. The authors did, however, note an increased blood loss in larger uteri with volumes greater than or equal to 600 mL and found a correlation between patient weight and total blood loss. Interestingly, mean arterial pressure, which was monitored throughout the operation in all subjects, was no different between the two groups. In addition to preoperative uterine size, blood loss was additionally correlated with the total time spent performing myomectomy as well as the total weight of fibroids removed. While mechanical techniques for hemostasis are effective, they may require additional dissection in the broad ligament. This has the potential to add time and risk to the procedure. It also leaves an additional traumatized area that is at risk for postsurgical adhesion formation.

Sacks and Hoyne (25) previously described a case that underscores the need for hemostasis. They reported a patient with a large, 36-week fibroid uterus who underwent resection of 52 myomas. Total blood loss for the procedure was 2500 mL with intraoperative replacement of red blood cells and administration of Hespan. Disseminated intravascular coagulation, oliguria, hematuria, and acute renal failure developed secondary to myoglobinemia and the patient required hemodialysis and a 24-day hospitalization.

Uterine Incision Choice and Myoma Extraction

It is important to choose the appropriate incisions into the uterus. In general, vertical incisions in the midline offer the greatest opportunity for maximizing multiple myoma removal through a single incision versus multiple small incisions placed throughout the uterus. A vertical incision may also decrease the chance of inadvertent tubal injury and uterine artery transection (Fig. 5.10). If incisions are required in the lateral margins of the uterus, a transverse incision has been recommended, as such incisions parallel the majority of the vasculature and potentially would limit the number of transected vessels (Fig. 5.11). Historically, there had been a concerted effort to avoid placement of posterior inci-

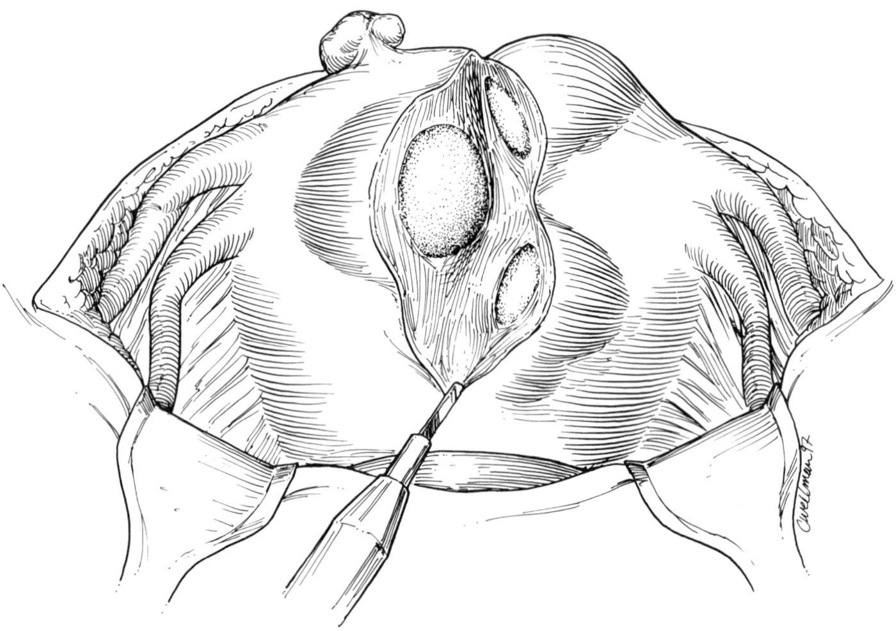

FIG. 5.10.

A uterine incision has been made in the midline in an area where multiple myomas can be extracted through the single incision and the risk of tubal injury is minimized.

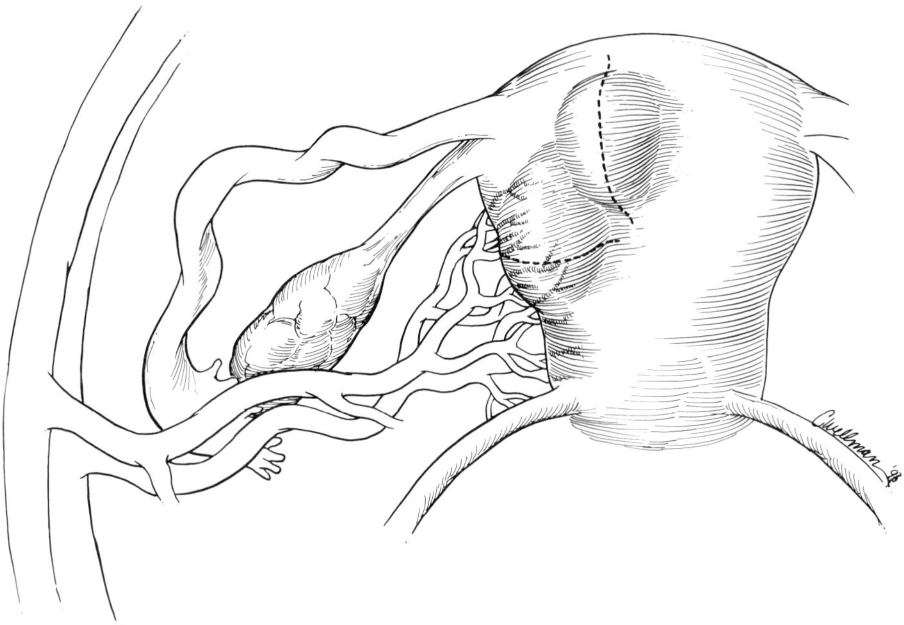

FIG. 5.11.

This illustration demonstrates the advantage of an incision parallel to the vasculature if a lateral incision is required for myoma removal.

sions on the uterus for fear of adhesions forming postoperatively and involving the adnexa. Bonney (2) advocated the "Hood operation," in which a horizontal incision was made just posterior to the tubes. Posterior myomas would then be extracted and the excess myometrium and serosa that had covered the myomas would be brought over the fundus and attached to the anterior uterus. The concept was again to minimize the amount of incision on the posterior surface of the uterus. There are no studies to assess whether this technique decreased adhesion formation and some authors have concerns regarding postoperative distortion of the myometrium. Other investigators have advocated anterior entry into the uterine cavity with subsequent extraction of posterior myomas through a posterior endometrial cavity incision, thus limiting the number of posterior serosal incisions (2). While well intentioned, this may increase the risk of intracavitary adhesions forming after the operation.

More recent data have not supported the hypothesis that the anterior cul-de-sac and anterior uterine incisions are protected from adhesion formation; indeed a similar incidence of adhesions was seen in the anterior and posterior uterus postmyomectomy in a study by Diamond et al (26). We believe that when necessary a posterior incision on the uterus should be made similar to that made in the anterior uterine surface, with an incision placed to allow the greatest number of myomas to be removed through the smallest sized incision.

After an incision through the myometrium is made, it is important to find the appropriate dissection plane. A common mistake is to believe that the correct layer has been reached and to begin the dissection only to find increased bleeding and no discernible fibroid. In these cases, the incision has usually not gone completely through the myoma pseudocapsule. A simple way to avoid this error is to incise through the capsule until a portion of the fibroid is identified and then to back away and find the appropriate cleavage plane. This avoids starting the dissection outside the margin of the pseudocapsule. Dissection in the appropriate plane decreases blood loss and facilitates extraction. At the point of myoma identification, a towel clip or tenaculum can be applied to the fibroid to improve traction and facilitate development of the appropriate plane (Fig. 5.12). Using the combination of sharp and blunt dissection, the fibroid attachments between the pseudocapsule and myoma can be incised. Monopolar or bipolar electrocautery can be utilized to achieve improved hemostasis on more vascular attachments. Some surgeons have described a "feeder vessel" at the base of the myoma. In general we have not been able to localize these types of discrete vessels and data suggest that multiple vessels may perforate through the pseudocapsule providing blood to the myoma (27). This may limit our ability to effectively place a suture at the base of the myoma and achieve hemostasis in many cases.

Once the myoma has been removed, palpation allows identification of further myomas that can be extracted through the same incision. It is surprising how difficult small myomas may be to differentiate from the underlying myometrium. However, a concerted effort should be made to detect and remove all myomas including possible seedlings, while attempting to maintain as much myometrium as possible. In fact,

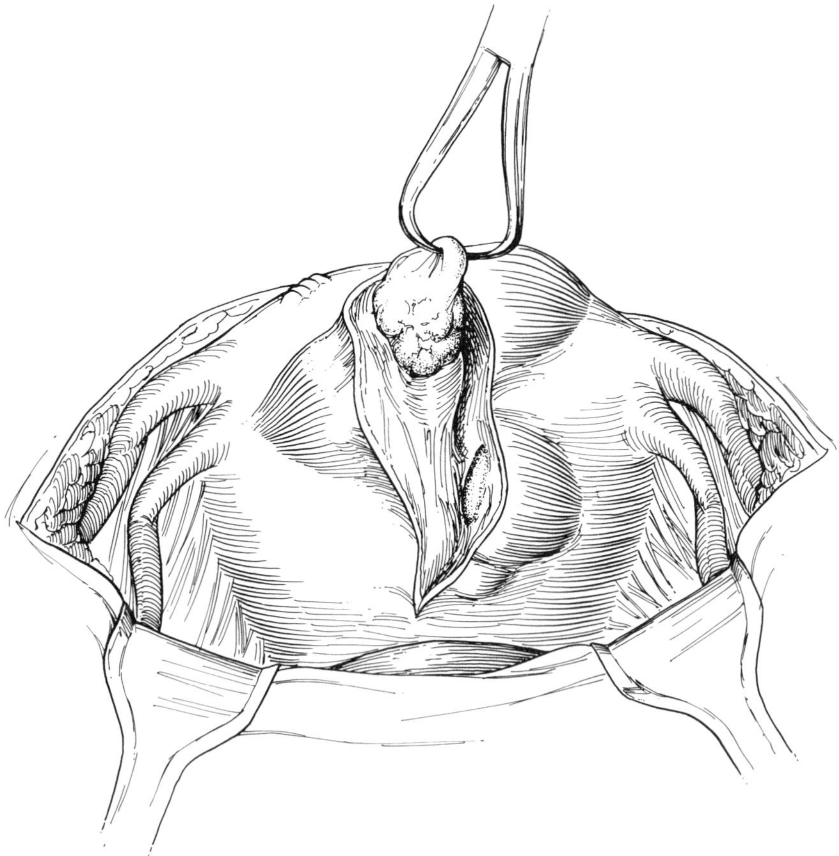

FIG. 5.12.

Towel clips or any device that provides traction facilitates identification and further development of the plane between the myoma and pseudocapsule. Multiple myomas can be extracted through a single myometrial incision, thereby diminishing the need for multiple serosal incisions. Continuous palpation for additional myomas with the thumb and index finger aids in identifying all myomas.

myometrium should not be resected if possible during the course of myomectomy. Fibroid enlargement often causes marked uterine hypertrophy such that after myomectomy with removal of all fibroids, the uterus is still markedly enlarged. This hypertrophy will regress over 3 to 6 months following surgery. Beyth and colleagues (28) followed 10 patients ultrasonographically who underwent myomectomy. They noted the greatest decrease in size during the initial 2 to 3 months following surgery with gradual decreases in some patients up until 6 months. Larger uteri did shrink to a greater extent than smaller uteri.

Occasionally, there is a desire to intraoperatively rule out the possibility of leiomyosarcoma when performing a myomectomy. Unfortunately, this may be difficult for even experienced histopathologists. Scurry and Sumithran (29) reviewed 203 gynecologic surgeries in which frozen section was performed, 11 during myomectomy. In this series they noted no false positives or negatives, but did have one case in which the reading was deferred and one inaccurate reading. For an accurate evaluation a formal mitotic count from a number of regions of the specimen is required and this is difficult in an acute setting.

It has been suggested that patients treated with GnRHa have more difficult planes to identify creating an anatomic challenge for the surgeon. A retrospective study by Gutmann et al (30) compared the histologic characteristics of patients treated with leuprolide acetate for 3 to 6 months versus no treatment. They noted no significant histologic changes, such as fibrosis, calcification, cellular atypia, or mitotic activity.

Incision Closure

Once all myomas have been extracted through the incision, closure is begun. When multiple myomas have been removed, there may be a need to close smaller defects before closure of the main incision is begun (Fig. 5.13). If the cavity has been entered, a 4-0 or 5-0 absorbable suture should be used to close the endometrium, taking care not to evert it. It has been suggested that instillation of a contrasting agent such as methylene blue into the endometrial cavity before the procedure can facilitate identification of the endometrial cavity and aid in closure (31). The remainder of the closure can be performed with a 2-0 or 3-0 absorbable suture such as polyglycolic acid (Vicryl or Dexon). Several layers may be required to close the dead space and allow the serosa to be closed with minimal tension. An alternative to a layered closure is concentric suture in a purse-string fashion around the defect (Fig. 5.13). This also effectively closes the dead space while concomitantly securing hemosta-

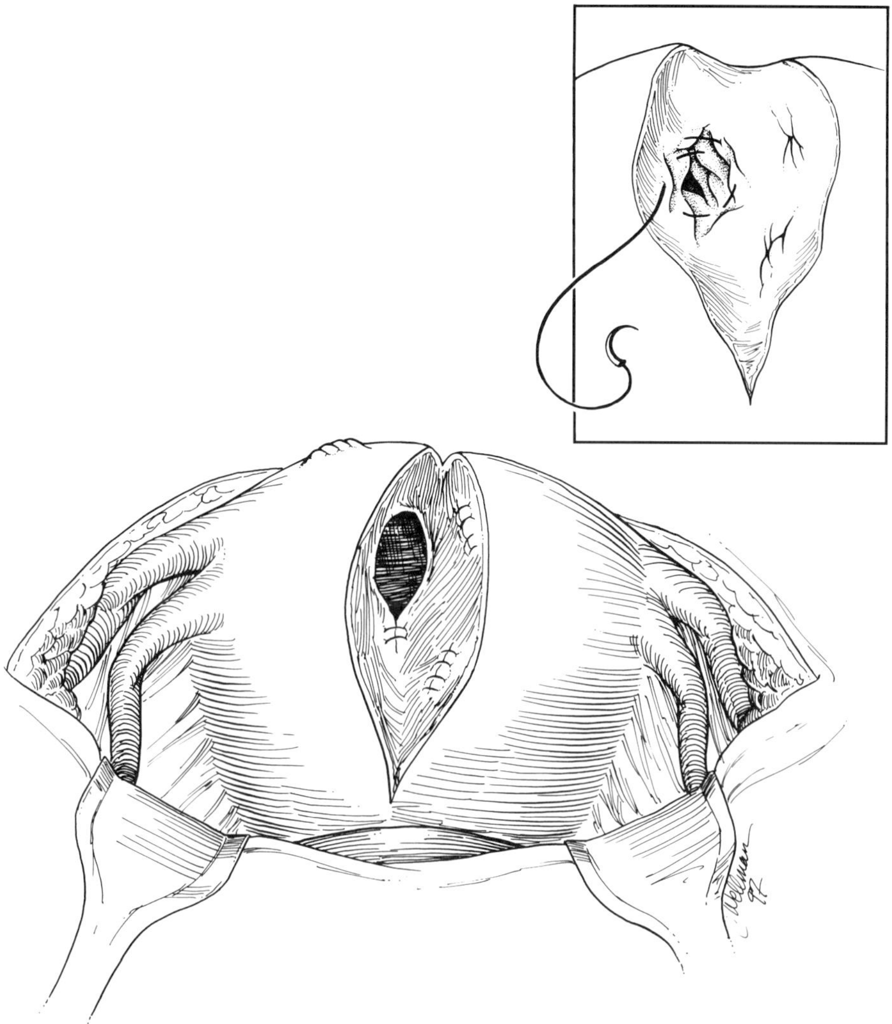

FIG. 5.13.

Areas of myoma dissection separate from the main incision must be closed to reduce the chance of hematoma formation. Incisions can be closed in a running fashion with a multilayer closure. Alternatively, a purse-string suture can be used to obliterate the dead space and close the defect (*inset*).

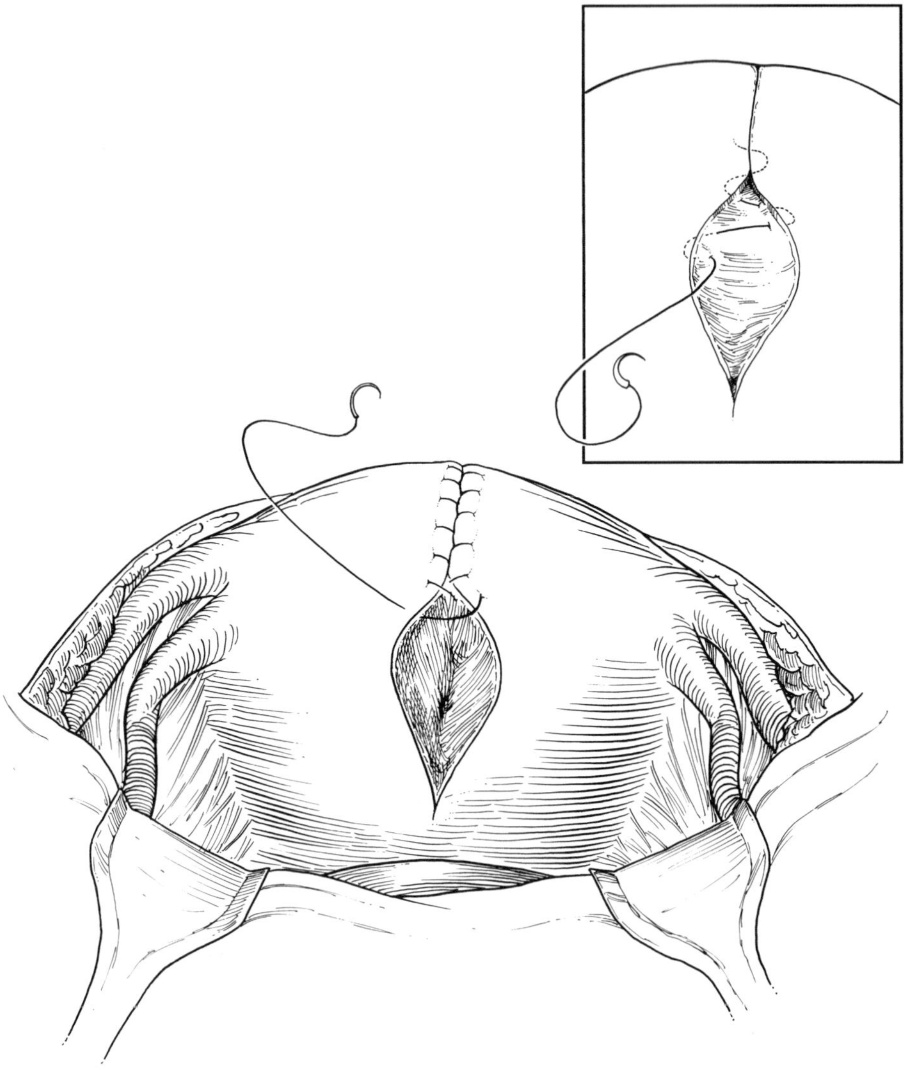

FIG. 5.14.

Serosal closure should be performed with a minimally reactive suture. Either a baseball-type stitch or a completely subserosal stitch can be used to achieve serosal approximation and limit external suture exposure.

sis. Recent reports of uteroperitoneal fistulas and uterine rupture during pregnancy after laparoscopic myomectomy point to the need for a good closure of the myometrium (32,33).

For serosal closure we have begun to use monofilament suture such as 4-0 or 5-0 poliglecaprone 25 (Monocryl) or polydioxanone (PDS) II. This final layer is likely the most important from the standpoint of adhesion formation. Closures such as the modified baseball running suture limit the amount of exposed suture material, or alternatively a completely subserosal running suture can be placed (Fig. 5.14).

Occasionally, after serosal closure bleeding may persist or there may be evidence for a hematoma. If the hematoma is small and not enlarging, no further treatment is necessary; however, continued bleeding from the bed or an enlarging hematoma mandates removal of the serosal suture line and re-exploration of the myometrial bed to attain hemostasis.

Postoperative Management

The length of postsurgical hospitalization may depend in part on incisional size as well as bowel manipulation during surgery. We have noted decreased numbers of patients with ileus since limiting bowel handling by performing the operation extracorporeally.

Often patients were noted to have small temperature elevations without evidence for underlying infection. This may be due to the many microhematomas, which likely occur throughout the myometrial dissection bed. In an effort to diminish the temperature spikes, as well as decrease the inflammatory response, we have used nonsteroidal anti-inflammatory agents such as ketorolac tromethamine (Toradol) and ibuprofen in the postoperative setting. Toradol does inhibit platelet function and probably should not be used in patients with incomplete hemostasis or very large blood loss.

Fayez and Dempsey (34) previously reported on short hospital stays in patients who had gynecologic laparotomy. They described 148 patients who underwent myomectomy and were discharged home within 24 hours. They also advocated exteriorization of the uterus and limited bowel manipulation. No postoperative complications or readmissions occurred in this series.

In contrast to the usual preoperative administration of GnRHa, Acien and Quereda (35) described the use of these medications after surgery. They suggested that GnRHa may reduce myometrial hypertrophy, myometrial scar size, and uterine size. Little other information is available about this novel application in the postsurgical setting.

One of the most common questions asked by patients and their subsequent caregivers concerns the need for elective cesarean section. We are aware of the increased rates of uterine rupture in patients with classic cesarean section incisions versus a low uterine segment transverse incision. Likewise, reports have been published of uterine rupture following laparotomy myomectomy (36,37). Historically, it has been suggested that if the cavity is entered during the course of myomectomy the patient should have a subsequent cesarean section. Unfortunately, there are limited data on which to make recommendations, and unlike cesarean section, in which a classic incision is somewhat similar from patient to patient, myomectomy incisions are markedly different, requiring deep incisions in some patients and superficial cuts in others, with wide variation throughout the uterus depending on myoma position. Given these limitations and until further data become available, we suggest cesarean section in patients who have had extensive dissections within the myometrium regardless of cavity entry.

RECURRENCE OF MYOMAS AFTER MYOMECTOMY

As discussed previously one of the most significant risks of undergoing myomectomy is the possibility of myoma recurrence. The literature is replete with publications giving a wide range of rates of myoma recurrence from under 10% to over 50%. Malone, in a 1969 publication (38), reported on 125 women who had undergone myomectomy. In his patient population he noted that approximately one-third of women had only a solitary myoma and that only 11% of this group required a subsequent hysterectomy secondary to fibroid recurrence. The remaining patients had undergone multiple myomectomy procedures; 26% of this group underwent subsequent surgery secondary to myoma recurrence.

More recent publications have addressed concerns regarding myoma recurrence and the use of GnRH analogs. Fedele and colleagues (39) reported on patients randomized to treatment with buserelin for 3 months followed by myomectomy versus an immediate myomectomy. Six months following surgery patients underwent ultrasonography. Of patients treated with GnRHa, 63% were noted to have recurrent fibroids versus only 13% of the immediate surgery group. Unfortunately the numbers in the two groups (only 8 in the group treated with analog and 16 in the patients undergoing immediate surgery) limit the ability to access clinical significance. Friedman et al, in another publication that addressed the same issue (40), noted no difference in recurrence rates between patients treated with GnRHa versus immediate surgery without agonist. Interestingly, in this study, which used high-resolution ultrasound, the recurrence rate in the GnRHa group was 67% versus 56% in the no treatment group, which was not statistically significant. It is unclear what percent of these patients will actually become clinically symptomatic or require further surgery.

Candiani et al (41) followed patients over extended periods of time and noted a 10-year recurrence rate of 27%. Consistent with previous authors they found a steady increase in recurrence over the entire period of observation. In addition, patients with only an isolated myoma tended to have lower recurrence rates, and those who gave birth following surgery had a recurrence rate one-half that of patients who never became pregnant. Fedele and colleagues (42) also reported an increasing cumulative recurrence risk in their study, which reached 51% at 5 years. They similarly noted that parity decreased recurrence following myomectomy. It is unclear how pregnancy plays a role in decreasing the risk of recurrence. It has been hypothesized that it may have a protective effect by inhibiting growth of fibroids, or that patients who have subsequent pregnancies may be more likely to use oral contraceptives and thus decrease the likelihood of a subsequent presentation (43).

It seems likely given the more recent reports suggesting higher rates of recurrence that technologic advancements in imaging may account for our increased ability to detect previously undetectable myomas. It remains to be seen what level of clinical significance such small myomas have in this patient population. It does, however, underscore the need for significant patient-physician discussions regarding the possibility of recurrence after surgery.

ADHESIONS FOLLOWING MYOMECTOMY

Adhesions may develop in a significant percentage of patients who have undergone myomectomy and may subsequently interfere with reproductive outcome. It is imperative that during myomectomy surgical technique be optimized by use of microsurgical techniques and that appropriate steps be taken at the conclusion of the operation in an attempt to minimize the potential for adhesions.

Tulandi et al (44) evaluated 26 infertile women who underwent myomectomy for large fibroid uteri followed by a second-look laparoscopy 6 weeks later. All patients in the study had uterine fibroids of at least 16 weeks in size. Myomectomy was successfully performed, in all cases, and the serosal incisions were closed with 4-0 Vicryl. At the time of second-look laparoscopy, patients with posterior uterine incisions had a 93.7% incidence of adnexal adhesions, whereas anterior uterine incisions were only associated with adnexal adhesions in 55% of patients. The cumulative pregnancy rate in this small group of patients was 66% at 12 months following the initial procedure and subsequent second-look laparoscopy with adhesiolysis. Other studies have also documented the high prevalence of adhesions following myomectomy surgery. The Myomectomy Adhesion Multicenter Study Group (45) reported on the use of expanded polytetrafluoroethylene (Gore-Tex) barrier. In this study, patients also underwent myomectomy with subsequent second-look laparoscopy 2 to 6 weeks following surgery. At the time of second-look laparoscopy, 92% of the control patients had adhesions versus only 45% in the group in which incisions were covered with the Gore-Tex barrier.

In another study, a hyaluronic acid–containing membrane, Seprafilm, was placed in 59 of 127 patients who underwent myomectomy (26). This study required a minimum of a 1-cm posterior uterine incision for study inclusion. Again, all patients underwent second-look laparoscopies. The hyaluronic acid film was used to cover the incision and the anterior and posterior uterus but was not specifically placed on tubes or ovaries. The anterior uterus was noted to have adhesions present in 94% of the patients who received no treatment versus 39% of the patients treated with the membrane. No significant difference was seen in the extent of adhesions on the posterior uterus, although the control group was noted to have a 92% incidence of adhesions to this area with the most common site of adherence being the large bowel. What may be important from a reproductive standpoint is that adhesions to the adnexa were present in 69% of the no treatment group versus 52% of the treatment arm.

Little clinical information exists regarding specific correlation between adhesion presence and causation of infertility, although clinically we recognize the importance both of the adnexa being free from adhesions and of tubo-ovarian pickup. An additional area that has been incompletely investigated is the issue of bowel adhesions and potential for bowel obstruction in these patients. Strickler and colleagues (46) noted in a retrospective chart review that myomectomy was identified as the cause of intestinal obstruction in a greater incidence than what would be expected based on the low number of procedures performed. Interestingly, in 9 of the 100 patients' charts evaluated, the site of the bowel obstruction was a region of reperitonealization.

MYOMAS AND MYOMECTOMY IN PREGNANCY

It has long been believed that fibroids will cause significant morbidity during pregnancy because of increases in myoma size. As myomas are known to shrink during menopause and with GnRH agonist treatment, and are known to contain estrogen receptors, the concept that they might respond to elevated estrogen during pregnancy has seemed reasonable. However, several studies have cast doubt on this hypothesis in the majority of patients. Lev-Toaff and colleagues (5) followed a group of 113 patients for fibroid changes during pregnancy. They found that in the second trimester smaller fibroids (less than 6 cm) increased in size whereas fibroids larger than 6 cm decreased in size. In the third trimester regardless of the initial size, myoma dimensions decreased. They also found that ultrasonic changes such as development of a heterogeneous pattern or anechoic/cystic spaces were associated with patients undergoing myoma degeneration, as a significant number of these women presented with increased abdominal pain. Davis and coworkers (47) similarly evaluated 85 patients through pregnancy who were known to have myomas. In this study patients were matched to similar patients without myomas and the groups were followed throughout pregnancy. Gestational age at delivery was significantly lower: 37.5 weeks in the group of patients with myomas versus 39.6 weeks in the control population. While the incidence of preterm premature rupture of membranes, preterm labor, and preterm delivery were all increased in the leiomyoma group, the small number of cases did not allow these values to reach statistical significance.

Exacoustos and Rosati (4), in a more recent study, also compared a group of over 12,000 pregnant patients, of whom 492 had myomas. This study demonstrated a statistically significant increase in placental abruption, pelvic pain, preterm labor, and threatened abortion. These authors additionally noted an increase in abruption in patients with myoma volume above 200 mL and, like Davis' group, observed increased pelvic pain in patients with a myoma volume greater than 200 mL and heterogeneous echo patterns with cystic areas.

There is great concern about performance of myomectomy during pregnancy secondary to issues of increased blood loss. This is due to the marked increase in vascularity during pregnancy as well as the subsequent risk of hysterectomy. Davids (3), in an early case report, described myomectomy during pregnancy in 35 patients from 6 to 18 weeks' gestation. Sixty-six percent of patients carried to term and in one case 15 fibroids were removed. Finn and Muller (31) reported a 43% abortion rate in 14 patients who underwent myomectomy during pregnancy but did not state when in pregnancy the procedure was performed.

In the modern literature, Maker et al (48) reported the performance of a myomectomy during the fourteenth week of pregnancy in a patient who presented with pain and a 12-cm mass in the posterior cul-de-sac. This myoma was noted to be degenerative and on a short pedicle. The patient's pregnancy progressed routinely following surgery. In another case report, Michalas et al (49) described a 31-year-old patient who underwent myomectomy during her fifteenth week of pregnancy. In this instance the myoma was 23 cm in diameter but was again attached on a stalk. This patient subsequently delivered by cesarean section at 39 weeks, when eight additional myomas obstructing the lower uterine segment were resected. The patient did not undergo hysterectomy. In a larger study, Burton et al (50) reviewed the experience at Los Angeles County Hospital. During the time period of their retrospective review, there were 123,492 deliveries, and they noted 14 patients who underwent surgery during pregnancy for myomas and 13 incidental myomectomies at the time of cesarean section. This yielded an antepartum operation rate of 1.1 per 10,000. Histopathologic analysis from specimens obtained during both pregnancy and cesarean section found 70% of myomas to have degenerative changes. Carneous degeneration and cystic degeneration were each seen in 6 of 23 cases. In another series review, Exacoustos and Rosati (4) described nine myomectomies performed at the time of cesarean delivery. Unfortunately, three cases were complicated by severe hemorrhage with resultant hysterectomy.

Chung et al (51) reported an interesting case of a patient who was noted to have postpartum hemorrhage following normal vaginal delivery. The patient was treated in a routine fashion in an attempt to improve uterine contractility without success. At the time of examination under anesthesia, the patient was noted to have a uterine cavity that was completely filled with an intracavitary myoma. Subsequently laparotomy was performed with entry into the cavity and removal of the myoma. As expected, following myoma removal, excellent contraction of the uterine cavity was noted and hysterectomy was avoided.

It is clear that most physicians choose not to surgically intervene with myomectomy during pregnancy, but instead manage patients conservatively. Likewise, at the time of cesarean section relatively few myomectomies are performed. Based on the limited data that currently exist, the risk of myomectomy at the time of cesarean section may be increased.

UNUSUAL MYOMA PRESENTATIONS

Leiomyomatosis peritonealis disseminata (LPD) is a rarely seen disease in which multiple, small granular nodules are identified throughout the abdomen and pelvis. Initially, the clinician may believe this to be metastatic disease but histopathology shows smooth-muscle cells usually without atypia and with a low mitotic index as well as collagen and fibroblasts. These tumors have been associated with recent pregnancy, granulosa cell tumors, and oral contraceptive use. In fact, their most common presentation may be at the time of cesarean section. A sample of the nodules should be sent for histology to rule out malignancy. The condition usually regresses after pregnancy and thus attempting to debulk the many nodules is unnecessary.

Intravenous leiomyomatosis is another rare disease in which benign smooth-muscle cells grow into and within venous channels. Interestingly, arterial vessels are not affected by this process. Worm-like masses grow by direct extension throughout the pelvic veins. The median age for presentation is 45 years, with abnormal bleeding, pelvic mass, and pelvic pain being common symptoms and findings (51).

Extensions of the lesions into the vena cava have been reported in upwards of 10% of patients. Rarely lesions will progress to the tricuspid valve or the right atrium with extension to the pulmonary veins. Like leiomyomatosis peritonealis disseminata, this disease is benign histologically but unlike LPD it may cause clinical problems because of the growth. Total abdominal hysterectomy with bilateral salpingo-oophorectomy and excision of extrauterine lesions has been the standard treatment. If the lesions have progressed to the vena cava or other major vessels, vascular surgeons should be consulted.

Benign metastasizing leiomyoma (BML) is another rare disease in which smooth-muscle tumors in lung, brain, or lymph nodes are found in association with uterine fibroids. These are also benign lesions with a low number of mitoses. Barter and colleagues (52) reported a case of BML with retroperitoneal lymph node involvement. Because so few cases exist in the literature, no specific treatment recommendation can be made, although some authors have recommended bilateral oophorectomy.

Parauterine myomas may be more common than any of the previous entities. Honoré (53) reported an incidence of 2.4% in 928 patients undergoing hysterectomy, with pericornual, parametrial, and parasalpingeal locations seen. These tumors were often found in association with intrauterine myomas and were removed at the time of surgery.

CONCLUSION

Myomectomy remains an excellent surgical option for women who desire to retain their uterus for whatever reason. In spite of surgical advances, the number of hysterectomies performed in the United States each year is far greater than the number of myomectomies.

It is important to optimize the hematocrit in patients who are anemic and to facilitate the opportunity for autologous blood donation. A thorough understanding of the location, size, and number of myomas that will be removed during surgery, as well as meticulous surgical techniques, may improve the likelihood of surgical success and postoperative outcome.

The basic tenets of myomectomy have changed little over the years. Issues such as limiting the number of incisions while maximizing exposure, decreasing blood loss, and obtaining adequate myometrial closure are just as important today as they were 50 years ago. As Bonney suggested, myomectomy is a high ideal, but is worth the extra effort in the appropriate patient.

REFERENCES

1. Verkauf BS. Myomectomy for fertility enhancement and preservation. Fertil Steril 1992;58:1–15.
2. Bonney V. The technique and result of myomectomy. Lancet 1931;1: 171–177.

3. Davids AM. Myomectomy: surgical technique and results in a series of 1150 cases. Am J Obstet Gynecol 1952;63:592–604.
4. Exacoustos C, Rosati P. Ultrasound diagnosis of uterine myomas and complications in pregnancy. Obstet Gynecol 1993;82:97–101.
5. Lev-Toaff AS, Coleman BG, Arger PH, et al. Leiomyomas in pregnancy: sonographic study. Radiology 1987;164:375–380.
6. Gross BH, Siver TM, Joeffe MH. Sonographic features of uterine leiomyomas: analysis of 41 proven cases. J Ultrasound Med 1983;2: 401–406.
7. Lev-Toaff AS, Karasick S, Toaff ME. Hysterosalpingography before and after myomectomy: clinical value of imaging findings. AJR 1993;160:803–807.
8. Weinstein D, Aviad Y, Polishuk WZ. Hysterography before and after myomectomy. AJR 1977;129:899.
9. Turner RT, Berman AM, Topel HC. Improved demonstration of endometrial polyps and cavity: preliminary investigations. J Clin Ultrasound 1995;23:339–348.
10. Gaucherand P, Piacenza JM, Salle B, Rudigoz RC. Sonohysterography of the uterine submucous myomas using saline-enhanced vaginal sonohysterography. J Am Assoc Gyne Lap 1995;2:421–425.
11. Romano F, Cicinelli E, Anastasio PS, et al. Sonohysterography versus hysteroscopy for diagnosing endouterine abnormalities in fertile women. Int J Gynecol Obstet 1994;45:253–260.
12. Tada S, Tsukioka M, Ishii C, et al. Computed tomographic features of uterine myoma. J Comput Assis Tomogr 1981;5:866–869.
13. Mitchell DG, Outwater EK. Benign gynecologic disease: applications of magnetic resonance imaging. Top MRI 1995;7:26–43.
14. Loffer FD. Hysteroscopy with selective endometrial sampling compared with D + C for abnormal uterine bleeding: the value of a negative hysteroscopic view. Obstet Gynecol 1989;73:16–20.
15. Gimpelson RJ, Rappold HO. A comparative study between panoramic hysteroscopy with directed biopsies and dilatation and curettage. Am J Obstet Gynecol 1988;158:489–492.
16. Golan A, Bukovsky I, Pansky M, et al. Preoperative gonadotrophin-releasing hormone agonist treatment in surgery for uterine leiomyomata. Hum Reprod 1993;8:450–452.
17. Friedman AJ, Rein MS, Harrison-Atlas D, et al. A randomized, placebo-controlled, double-blind study evaluating leuprolide acetate depot treatment before myomectomy. Fertil Steril 1989;52:728–733.

18. Friedman AJ, Hoffman DI, Comite F, et al. Treatment of leiomyomata uteri with leuprolide acetate depot: a double-blind placebo-controlled multicenter study. Obstet Gynceol 1991;77:720–735.
19. Stovall TG, Muneyyirci-Delale O, Summitt RL, et al. GnRH agonist and iron versus placebo and iron in the anemic patient before surgery for leiomyomas: a randomized controlled trial. Obstet Gynecol 1995;86:65–71.
20. Parker WH, Fu YS, Berek JS. Uterine sarcoma in patients operated on for presumed leiomyomata and rapidly growing leiomyoma. Obstet Gynecol 1994;83:441–418.
21. LaMorte A, Lalwani S, Diamond MP. Morbidity associated with abdominal myomectomy. Obstet Gynecol 1993;82:897–900.
22. Frederick J, Fletcher H, Simeon D, et al. Intramyometrial vasopressin as a haemostatic agent during myomectomy. Br J Obstet Gynaecol 1994; 101:435–437.
23. Delancey JOL. A modified technique for hemostasis during myomectomy. Surg Gynecol Obstet 1992;174:153–154.
24. Ginsburg ES, Benson CB, Garfield JM, et al. The effect of operative technique and uterine sizes on blood loss during myomectomy: a prospective randomized study. Fertil Steril 1993;60:956–962.
25. Sacks PC, Hoyne PM. Disseminated intravascular coagulation, hemolytic anemia, and acute renal failure associated with extensive multiple myomectomy. Obstet Gynecol 1992;79:835–838.
26. Diamond MP, et al. Reduction of adhesions after uterine myomectomy by Seprafilm membrane (HAL-F): a blinded, prospective, randomized, multicenter clinical study. 1996;66:904–910.
27. Vollenhoven BJ, Lawrence AS, Healy DL. Uterine fibroids: a clinical review. Br J Obstet Gynaecol 1990;97:285–298.
28. Beyth Y, Jaffe R, Goldberger S. Uterine remodeling following conservative myomectomy: ultrasonographic evaluation. Acta Obstet Gynecol Scand 1992;71:632–635.
29. Scurry JP, Sumithran E. An assessment of the value of frozen sections in gynecological surgery. Pathology 1989;21:159–163.
30. Gutmann JN, Thornton KL, Diamond MP, Carcangiu ML. Evaluation of leuprolide acetate treatment on histopathology of uterine myomata. Fertil Steril 1994;61:622–626.
31. Finn WF, Muller PF. Abdominal myomectomy: special reference to subsequent pregnancy and to reappearance of fibromyomas of the uterus. Am J Obstet Gynecol 1950;60:109–116.

32. Dubuisson JB, Chavet X, Chapron C, et al. Uterine rupture during pregnancy after laparoscopic myomectomy. Hum Reprod 1995;10:1475–1477.
33. Harris WJ. Uterine dehiscence following laparoscopic myomectomy. Obstet Gynecol 1992;80:545–546.
34. Fayez JA, Dempsey RA. Short hospital stay for gynecologic reconstructive surgery via laparotomy. Obstet Gynecol 1993;81:598–600.
35. Acien P, Quereda F. Abdominal myomectomy: results of a simple operative technique. Fertil Steril 1996;65:41–51.
36. Golan D, Aharoni A, Gonen R, et al. Early spontaneous rupture of the post myomectomy gravid uterus. Int J Gynaecol Obstet 1990;31:167–170.
37. Georgakopoulos PA, Bersis G. Sigmoido-uterine rupture in pregnancy after multiple myomectomy. Int Surg 1981;66:367–368.
38. Malone LJ. Myomectomy: recurrence after removal of solitary and multiple myomas. Obstet Gynecol 1969;34:200–203.
39. Fedele L, Vercellini P, Bianchi S, et al. Treatment with GnRH agonists before myomectomy and the risk of short term myoma recurrence. Br J Obstet Gynaecol 1990;97:393–396.
40. Friedman AJ, Daly M, Juneau-Norcross M, et al. Recurrence of myomas after myomectomy in women pretreated with leuprolide acetate depot or placebo. Fertil Steril 1992;58:205–208.
41. Candiani GB, Fedele L, Parazzini F, Villa L. Risk of recurrence after myomectomy. Br J Obstet Gynaecol 1991;98:385–389.
42. Fedele L, Parazzini F, Luchini L, et al. Recurrence of fibroids after myomectomy: a transvaginal ultrasonographic study. Hum Reprod 1995;10:1795–1796.
43. Anonymous. Recurrence of fibroids after myomectomy. Lancet 1991;338:548.
44. Tulandi T, Murray C, Guralnick M. Adhesion formation and reproductive outcome after myomectomy and second-look laparoscopy. Obstet Gynecol 1993;82:213–215.
45. Myomectomy Adhesion Multicenter Study Group. An expanded polyfluoroethylene barrier (Gore-Tex surgical membrane) reduces post-myomectomy adhesion formation. Fertil Steril 1995;63:491–493.
46. Strickler B, Blanco J, Fox HE. The gynecologic contribution to intestinal obstruction in females. J Am Coll Surg 1994;178:617–620.
47. Davis J, Ray-mazumder S, Hobel C, et al. Uterine leiomyomas in pregnancy: a prospective study. Obstet Gynecol 1990;75:41–44.

48. Maker AP, Schatteman EA, Vergote IB, Desmedt E. Myomectomy during pregnancy: uncommon case report. Acta Chir Belg 1989;89:212–214.
49. Michalas SP, Oreopoulou IV, Papageorgiou IS. Myomectomy during pregnancy and cesarean section. Hum Reprod 1995;10:1869–1870.
50. Burton CA, Grimes DA, March CM. Surgical management of leiomyomata during pregnancy. Obset Gynecol 1989;74:707–709.
51. Chung TKH, Chan MYM, Stock AI. Myomectomy in the treatment of post partum haemorrhage. Br J Obstet Gynaecol 1994;101:73–74.
52. Barter JF, Szpak C, Creasman WT. Uterine leiomyomas with retroperitoneal lymph node involvement. South Med J 1987;80:1320–1322.
53. Honoré LH. Parauterine leiomyomas in women: a clinicopathologic study of 22 cases. Eur J Obstet Gynecol Reprod Biol 1981;11:273–279.

CHAPTER

6

Hysteroscopic Myomectomy

Rafael F. Valle

Uterine leiomyomas are benign solid tumors that occur in about 20% to 25% of women in their reproductive years. Of these, submucous leiomyomas cause excessive uterine bleeding usually during menses; they can cause dysmenorrhea and may interfere with normal reproduction (1–3). Because these tumors frequently cannot be palpated during examinations, or felt during blind intrauterine manipulations, they may go undetected until the abnormal bleeding is severe enough to cause anemia. Methods used to evaluate these tumors are hysterosalpingography; magnetic resonance imaging (MRI); sonography, particularly with vaginal probes; and direct visualization of the uterine cavity by hysteroscopy (4–7).

With improvements in instruments designed for visualizing the uterine cavity and performing transcervical surgery, symptomatic tumors have been approached transcervically, avoiding hysterotomies and concomitant laparotomy.

BASIC ANATOMIC AND PHYSIOLOGIC CONSIDERATIONS

Uterine leiomyomas arise in the muscle cells of the uterus; as they grow, they usually migrate to a place of less resistance, toward the abdominal cavity, becoming subserous, or following the path of the intrauterine cavity and becoming submucous. Most intracavitary tumors usually have a portion of the tumor penetrating the uterine wall and are termed *sessile submucous leiomyomas*. In contrast, those that have a pedicle are termed *pedunculated*. These tumors vary in size from less than 1 cm to more than 8 to 9 cm. Because these tumors usually lack a normal endometrium, the superficial vascularization can easily be observed under hysteroscopic view. Thin-walled vessels that cross the surface of the tumor can easily be occluded on contact with a probe. The lumen fills immediately with blood. If the vessel wall is disrupted, a burst of blood can be seen erupting from these vessels, which lack self-hemostastic mechanisms (8).

Some tumors show a small portion protruding into the uterine cavity like a tip of an iceberg. Removal of mainly intramural tumors requires a transabdominal approach by hysterotomy. Other myomas protrude completely into the uterine cavity (pedunculated) and still others have a portion of their body penetrating the uterine wall.

These tumors, by distorting the symmetry of the uterine cavity and the uniform contractility of the uterine wall, do not allow a muscular contractile hemostasis when disruption of the vessels occurs. Because the vascular network has been disrupted, vascular ectasis and stagnation of surrounding vessels contribute to prolonged, abnormal bleeding (1,9).

Most submucous tumors occur at the corporeal sites of the uterine cavity. Some are fundal, and others are anterior, posterior, or laterally situated. Small tumors may also arise at the cornual regions, interfering with the uterotubal junction lumen. A few are located at the cervical canal.

INDICATIONS FOR TREATMENT AND PATIENT SELECTION

While many uterine leiomyomas are totally asymptomatic, submucous tumors usually produce heavy abnormal uterine bleeding, particularly during menstruation. This abnormal symptomatology requires removal of the tumor.

Pelvic pain, particularly severe dysmenorrhea, may accompany the symptomatology, requiring treatment. Because these tumors distort the uterine cavity and may impede implantation and the normal growth and development of the conceptus, acting as a foreign body inside the uterine cavity, infertility and pregnancy wastage may occur (1,2).

For patients in their reproductive years who desire fertility, myomectomy is the treatment of choice to preserve the uterus. Should other uterine myomas contribute to symptomatology, additional concomitant surgery may be required. In women who do not desire further childbearing and have only submucous leiomyomas, the transcervical approach is most appropriate, as hysterectomy can be avoided. Should other associated pathologic conditions require treatment, a hysterectomy can be seriously considered.

The decision to approach a leiomyoma by myomectomy in a patient who has completed her childbearing requires clinical judgment, patient counseling, and understanding of benefits and limitations.

INSTRUMENTATION AND OPERATIVE HYSTEROSCOPIC METHODS

Hysteroscopic Scissors

An operative hysteroscope, with a 7- to 8-mm outer diameter and No. 7 French operative channel, can be useful for submucous leiomyomas that are pedunculated and smaller than 3 cm. Their supporting pedicle should be well visualized and the manipulation simple. These leiomyomas can easily be transected, with or without previous coagulation of the pedicle, utilizing an electrode to deliver the electrical current at the tip. The transection is performed with semirigid scissors. The cervix is dilated and the tumor removed transcervically utilizing grasping or toothed forceps (9). The uterine cavity is distended with fluids that contain electrolytes, specifically sodium (NaCl). Normal saline, dextrose 5% in 1/2 normal saline (NaCl 0.45%), or Ringer's lactate is most appropriate. Use of these fluids prevents hyponatremia, if excessive fluids

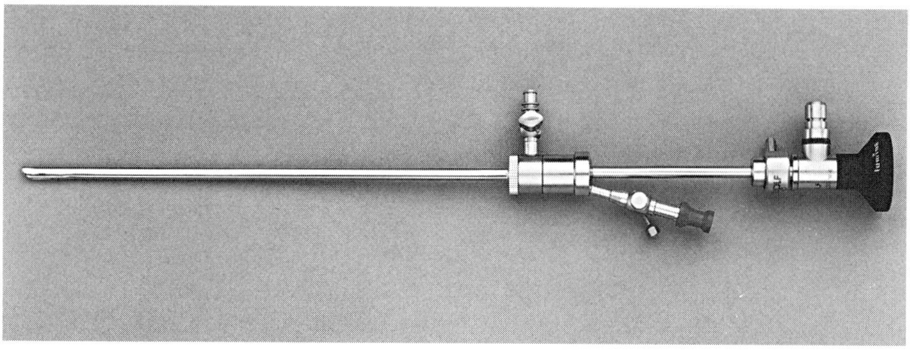

FIG. 6.1.

Assembled operative hysteroscope (Richard Wolf Medical Instruments, Corp., Vernon Hills, IL).

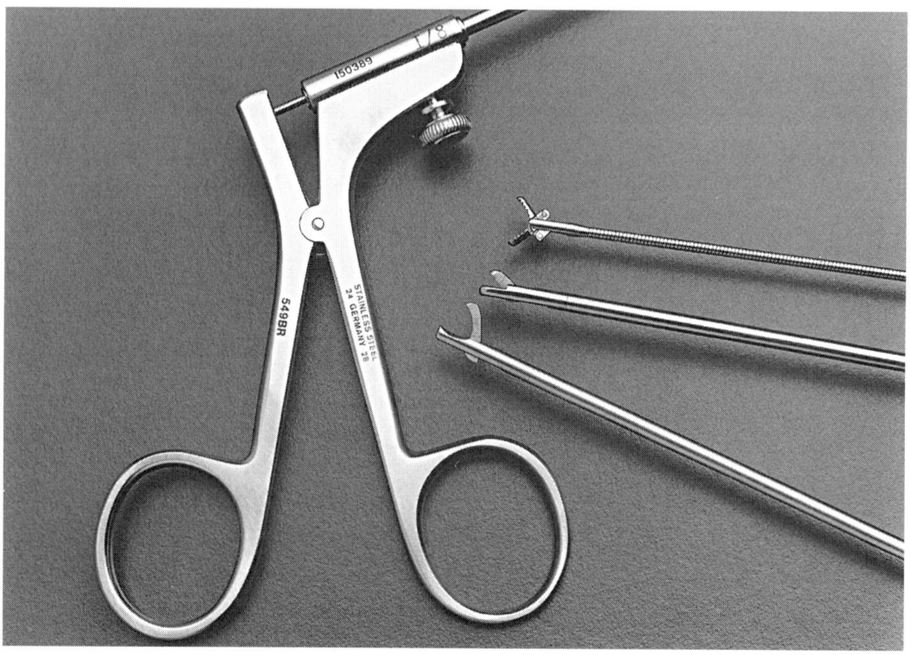

FIG. 6.2.

Hysteroscopic operative instruments: on right, from top to bottom: grasping forceps, biopsy forceps, hook scissors.

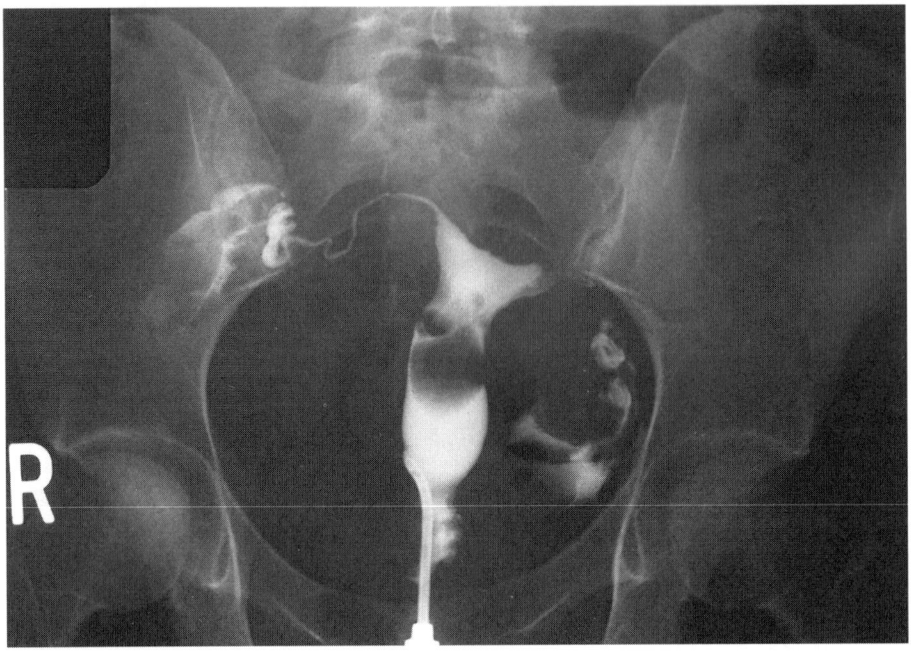

FIG. 6.3.

Hysterosalpingogram shows occupying lesion in lower portion of uterus compatible with submucous myoma.

(1.5–2.0 liters) are not recovered and are suspected of being absorbed by the patient (Figs. 6.1 to 6.6).

Resectoscopic Myomectomy

The use of a gynecologic resectoscope has markedly improved and facilitated a submucous myomectomy, particularly when the leiomyoma has a thick pedicle or is of the sessile type. In these situations, the leiomyoma is systematically shaved, utilizing a cutting loop to reduce its size, and then to remove the tumor fragments.

The resectoscope includes a straightforward telescope (0 degrees) or a slightly foreoblique 12- to 20-degree telescope with an outer diameter of 3.5 to 4.0mm. This telescope can be encased in a sheath of 8- to 9-mm outer diameter. The instrument has a built-in system that provides motion by means of a spring and moves the distal cutting loop

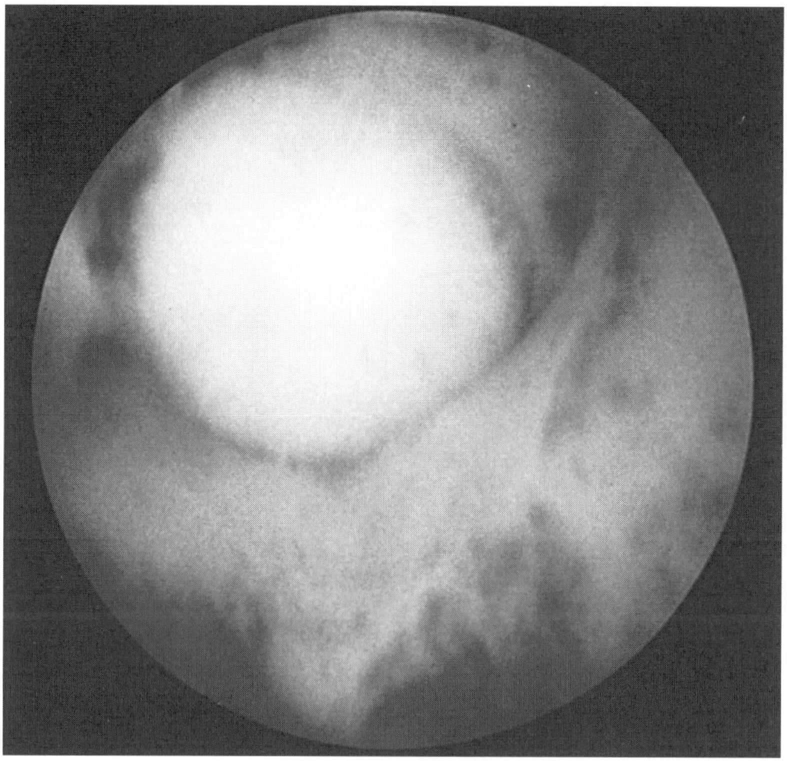

FIG. 6.4.

Hysteroscopic localization of submucous myoma.

forward and backward to shave and resect lesions by electrical cutting. The outer sheath provides an outflow by small distal perforations that permit the fluid to exit once the uterine cavity is distended, while the inner sheath provides the inflow, which enters the uterine cavity directly for continuous irrigation. The outer sheath has a short, distal insulated beak to protect against contact of the activated electrode with the outer metallic sheath. These two concentric sheaths are fitted to permit the introduction of an optical system and bridge for manipulation of various electrodes. To facilitate introduction, an obturator is available that fits the assembled two concentric sheaths. After introduction and bypassing of the cervical canal, the obturator is removed and the telescope is introduced with its bridge and the chosen electrode. Although the cutting

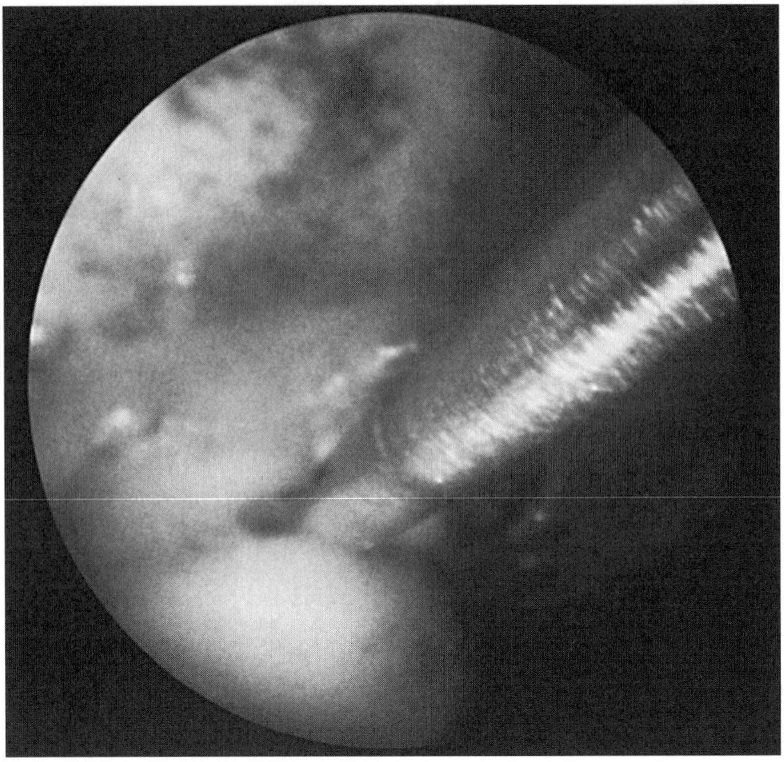

FIG. 6.5.

Hysteroscopic removal of pedunculated submucous myoma with scissors.

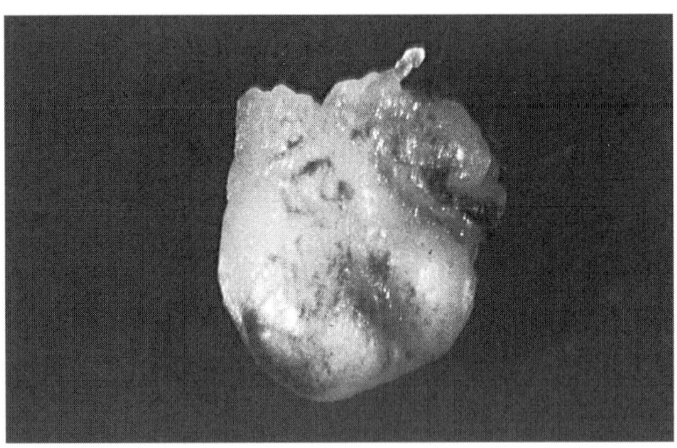

FIG. 6.6.

Myoma specimen following hysteroscopic removal.

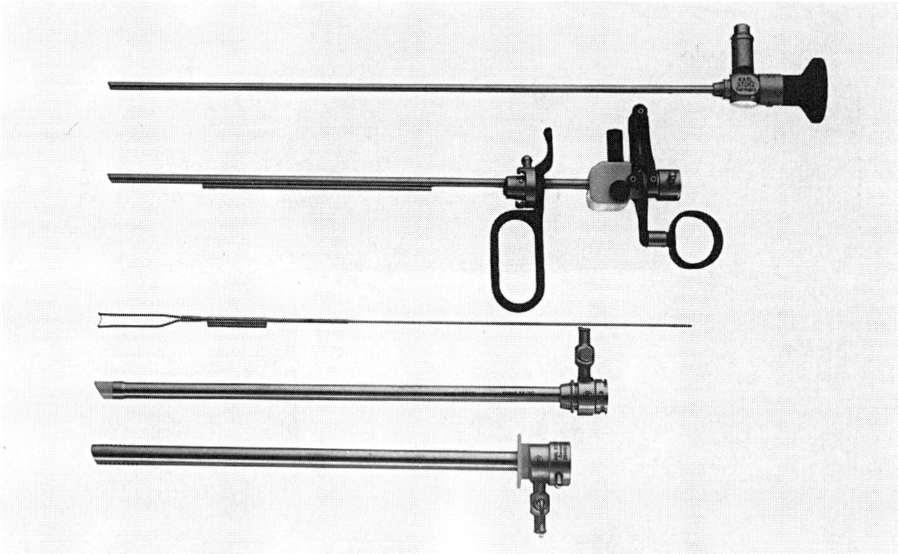

FIG. 6.7.

Unassembled resectoscope. Top to bottom: telescope, bridge, loop electrode, inner sheath, outer sheath (Storz).

loop can be manipulated directly and moves about 4 cm within the visual field of the objective lens, a clear and unobstructed panoramic view of the lesion and its surrounding normal endometrium is essential to avoid accidental perforation. The resectoscopes are manufactured by several companies (e.g., Karl Storz Endoscopy America, Inc., Culver City, CA; Wolf, Vernon Hills, IL; Olympus, Lake Success, NY; Circon-ACMI, Santa Barbara, CA) (Figs. 6.7 to 6.9).

All resectoscopes have similar features with minor modifications. The cutting loop is activated by connecting it with a high-frequency electrosurgical unit; therefore, proper grounding of the patient is required. An electrolyte-free solution should be used for distention of the uterine cavity to avoid conduction. Of the various nonconductive media available, the most commonly used are sorbitol 3%, glycine 1.5%, dextrose 5% in water, and mannitol 5%. A combination of sorbitol 2.6% and mannitol 0.5% has also been used.

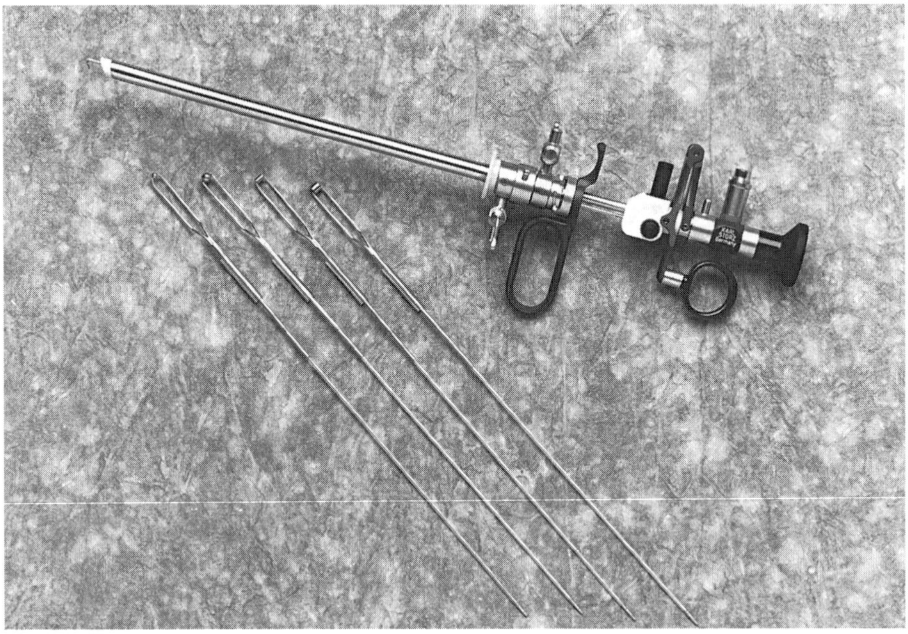

FIG. 6.8.

Assembled resectoscope with loop electrode in place (*top*). Various coagulating electrodes (*bottom*) (Storz).

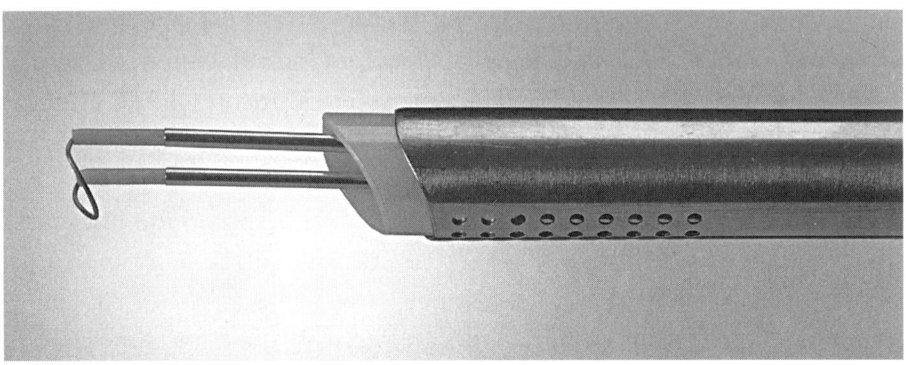

FIG. 6.9.

Close-up view of distal end of resectoscope with cutting loop in place (Storz).

Whether these fluids are delivered into the uterine cavity by pumps or by gravity pressure, it is important to monitor the fluid injected and the fluid recovered. The deficit will indicate whether fluid has been retained by the patient. It is most important to observe these patients throughout the operation, as excessive fluid absorption can occur. Careful monitoring of vital signs and pulse oximetry is conducted by the anesthesiologist and if the fluid deficit exceeds 700 to 800 mL, appropriate measures should be taken. Serum sodium determinations and monitoring of urine output to detect early fluid overload are also important.

Once the system has been assembled, the resectoscope is fitted with a cutting loop and the proper electrical cord is attached, along with the large-bore urologic tubing to permit the injection of the fluid and tubing in the outflow port to recover the circulated fluid. The cervix is dilated to the size or slightly above the size of the resectoscope and the resectoscope is introduced with or without an obturator, depending on the difficulty encountered in dilating the cervix. The stopcocks are opened and the fluid is left to circulate and cleanse the cavity of debris and blood clots. This is important, as the uterine cavity usually has several clots from bleeding during cervical dilatation. Because blood clots may obstruct the outflow perforations of the resectoscope, this sheath must be carefully cleaned until a good circulating fluid system is obtained. The resectoscope is then used to evaluate the uterine cavity, determining size and situation of leiomyomas, their relationship to the tubal openings, and their vascularization. The electrical power to be used is usually set at about 90 W to 100 W of unmodulated current (cutting current) blended with 30 W to 40 W of modulated current (coagulating current). This permits use of the cutting current for resection and the coagulating current for selective coagulating of vessels that bleed during resection by pressing the appropriate foot pedal (cutting or coagulating).

Tissue fragments from the resection can be left in the uterine cavity as long as they do not obstruct the view; otherwise, they can be easily removed with polyp forceps or suction cannulas. Should specific myoma fragments obstruct the view by attaching to the telescope, the inner sheath or the spring-loaded mechanism can be removed for cleaning without removing the whole instrument. The stopcocks are occluded, avoiding loss of fluid and making the operative field wet. This maneuver is also performed when debris adheres to the resecting loop. The myoma resection is performed as far as the level of the uterine wall, avoiding deep penetration to prevent uterine perforation. Once the resection is complete, the inflow pressure can be decreased by partially occluding the stopcock and then selectively coagulating those bleeding points that may be observed during this maneuver (Figs. 6.10 to 6.12; see also Plates 2 and 3).

Loffer (10) and others (11) have observed that while resecting submucous myomas, those with a shaved intracavitary component protrude as the uterine wall contracts and pushes the intramural portion of the

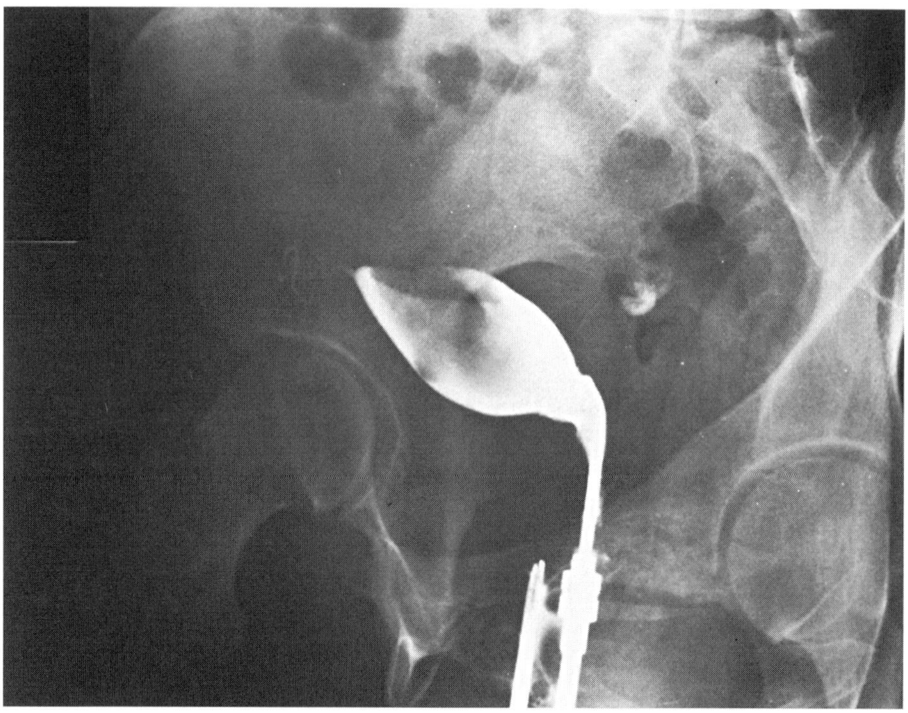

FIG. 6.10.

Hysterosalpingogram (lateral view) shows occupying lesion in uterine cavity compatible with submucous myoma.

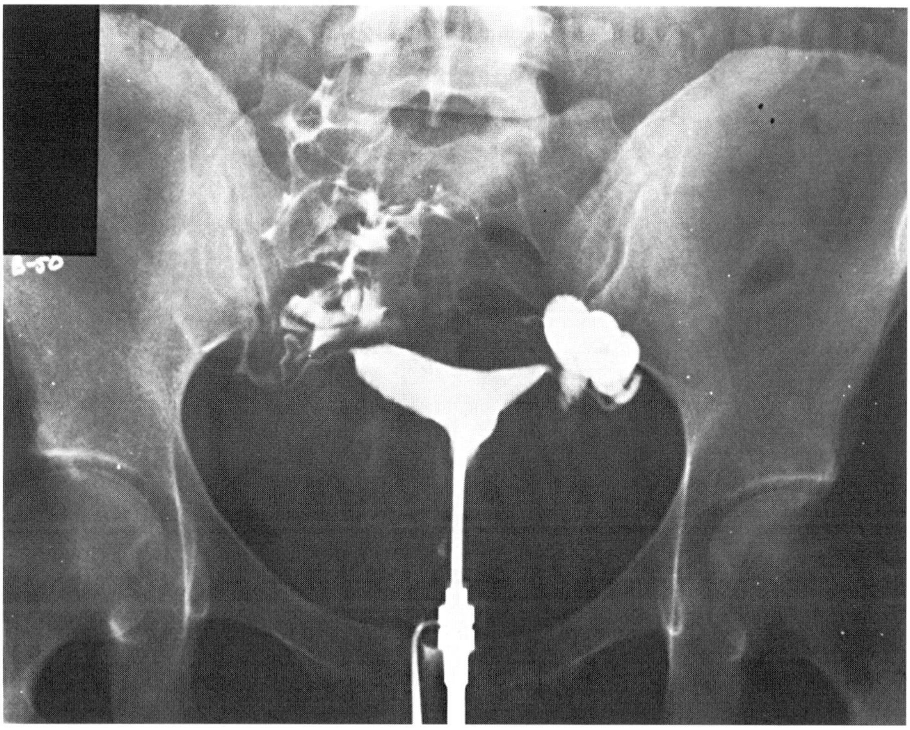

FIG. 6.11.

Hysterosalpingogram following resection of myoma.

myoma to the uterine cavity, permitting the complete resection of the myoma if the intramural portion does not involve the entire uterine wall (12).

The hysteroscopist can use two important anatomic landmarks in the removal of submucous leiomyomas: 1) the consistency and texture of the fibrous tissue of the myoma determined by gently touching the tissue with the inactivated loop (the pseudocapsule can be easily felt) and 2) while the resection comes in contact with the juxtaposed myometrium, the fascicularis myometrial tissue can easily be seen making contrast with the fibrous myomatous tissue. Also, the softness of the muscular tissue can be palpated with the inactivated loop, signaling the termination of the resection.

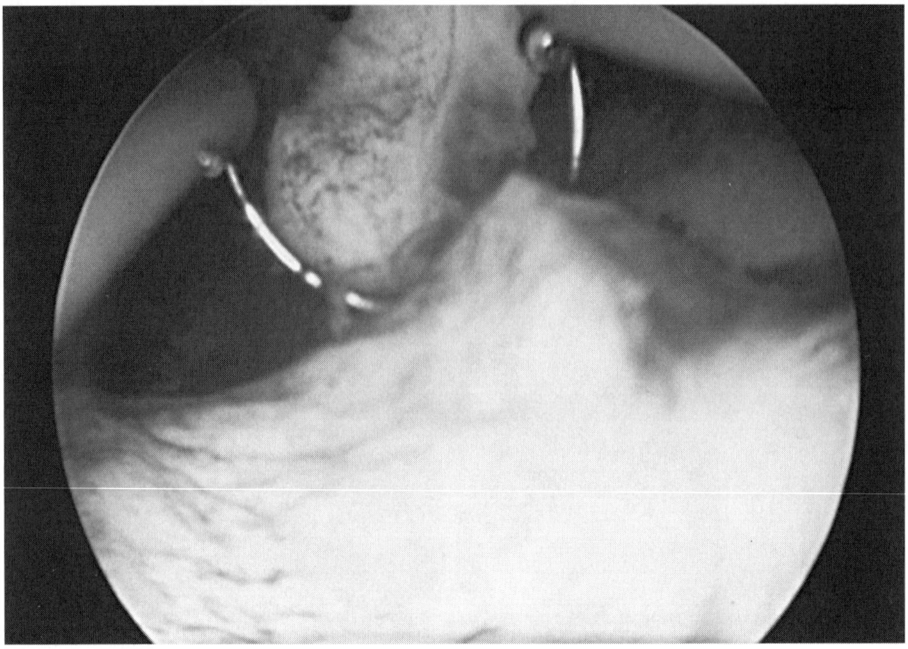

FIG. 6.12.

Resection of large submucous myoma located in posterior uterine wall.

Fiberlasers

The neodymium (Nd):YAG laser can be used for hysteroscopic myomectomy. A bare quartz fiber or sculpted sharp fiber can be utilized to morcellate large fundal myomas when manipulation of the resectoscope may be difficult, and to transect a pedicle of a small submucous leiomyoma (less than 3 cm in diameter) for its removal. The coagulating power of these lasers permits good hemostasis and facilitates morcellations of larger tumors (13,14). Additionally, if a portion of the leiomyoma is left in the uterine wall following resection, a myolysis can be performed by inserting the fiber directly into the tumor and activating the laser at 60 W to 80 W of power, while withdrawing the fiber to cause devitalization of the tumor and permit future protrusion into the uterine cavity (15) (Fig. 6.13).

Donnez et al (15) reported on 60 women with large submucous myomas treated with the Nd:YAG laser in this manner. In 12 cases, the

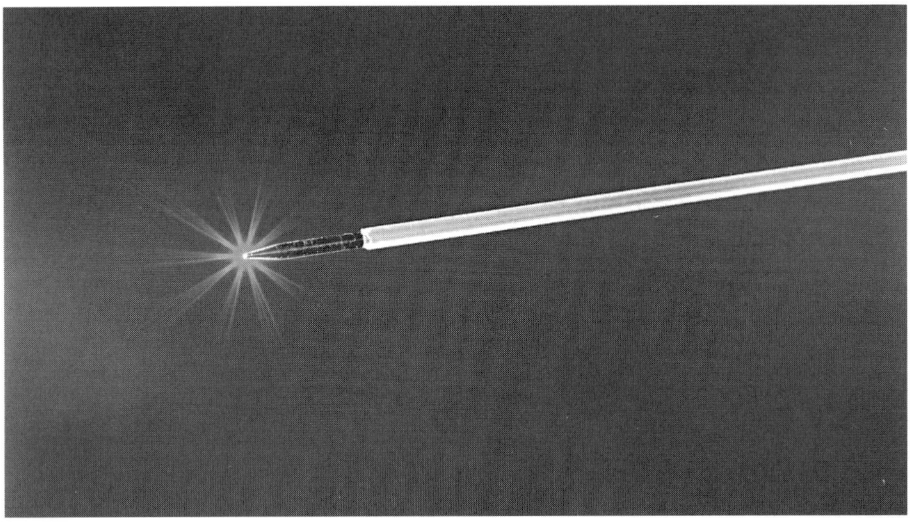

FIG. 6.13.

Sculpted quartz conical fiber for Nd:YAG laser contact use. Tip size 300μ (Laser Sonics, Inc., Milpitas, CA).

largest portion of the myoma was not inside the uterine cavity and myomectomy was carried out by two-step hysteroscopy. Six to 8 weeks after this partial resection, the final removal of the remaining portion of the leiomyoma was successfully accomplished.

Operative hysteroscopy and resectoscopy are best performed under continuous video monitoring. Video cameras today can provide excellent resolution and a wide field of view that enhances visualization and permits not only comfortable performance of hysteroscopic operations, but the sharing of the procedure with the operating room team. The recorded procedure can be reviewed later with the patient and can be stored for future reference. Most video cameras require a potent xenon or halogen light source. The three-chip cameras with a high horizontal resolution with more than 800 lines permit excellent resolution of tissues, surpassing the accuracy of the naked eye view (Fig. 6.14). Light sensitivity is increased, assuring optimal visualization of the surgical field and decreasing the need for potent light sources. Video printers can be used to instantly generate video prints and slides of excellent color repro-

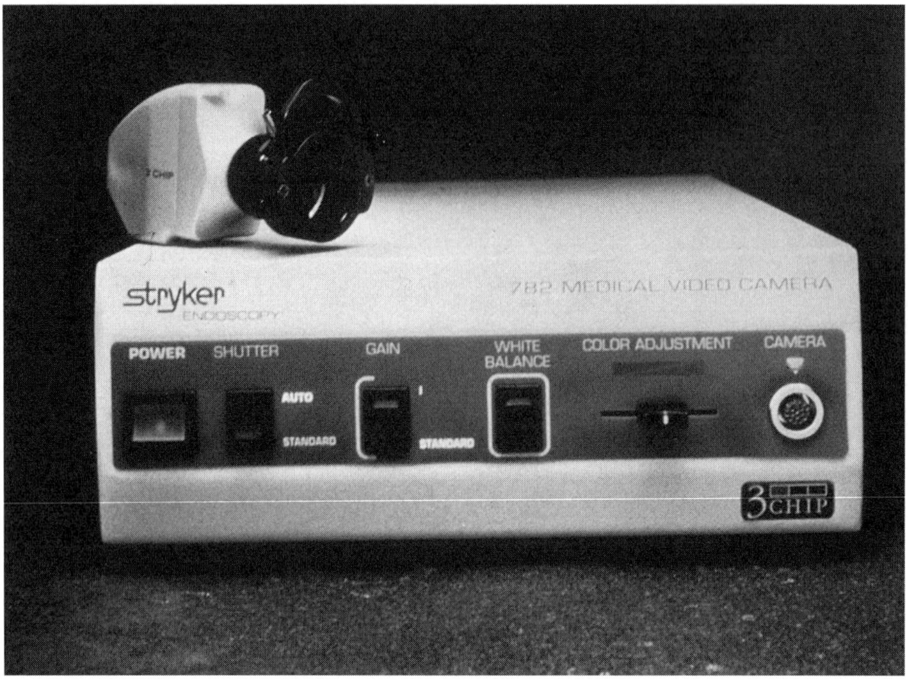

FIG. 6.14.

Three-chip camera for endoscopic surgery (Stryker Endoscopy, Santa Clara, CA).

duction. The addition of methalhalide as an illumination source has enhanced visualization by offering continuous light emission and more accurate color reproduction.

Mechanical Twisting and Avulsion

In the years before endoscopic methods were available to observe the uterine cavity, pedunculated submucous leiomyomas were sometimes seen protruding at the cervical os; by twisting and avulsion, these tumors were removed. Recently, Goldrath (16) used a similar technique, identifying the leiomyoma by hysteroscopy and dilating the cervix with laminaria to permit adequate manipulation and removal. Three to eight or more laminaria were necessary to permit adequate cervical dilatation. This method has been largely supplemented by refined, elegant hysteroscopic and resectoscopic methods that permit more precise dissection and hemostasis.

OTHER ADJUNCTS TO HYSTEROSCOPIC MYOMECTOMY

Vaginal and Abdominal Ultrasound and Fluid-Enhanced Sonography

By endoscopic observation, only the topography of intrauterine lesions can be outlined; other intramural tumors may not be detected. It is important to evaluate the uterine body completely to rule out leiomyomas that are not detectable by endoscopy. This can be accomplished by abdominal or vaginal sonography, or both, depending on the size and location of the tumor (17,18). When intramural myomas are evaluated, vaginal sonography is useful. If the myomas are not large and distort the uterus significantly, the abdominal sonography is useful. When sonography is used to evaluate the uterine walls, the number, size, and location of these leiomyomas should be established along with their relationship to the endometrial sonographic stripe. If submucous myomas penetrate the uterine wall, it is possible to determine myometrial invasion by measuring the thickness of the uterine wall as well as tumor penetration. A useful formula was proposed by Fleischer et al (19), dividing the tumor penetration (A) by the adjacent thickness of the uterine wall (B) and multiplying the result by 100 to obtain a percentage of invasion ($A/B \times 100 = \%$ of invasion) (Fig. 6.15).

Because most leiomyomas are hypo- or isoechogenic, it is sometimes difficult to differentiate the true interface between myometrium and myoma, and several cuts are required at various planes, particularly in lobulated leiomyomas. To obtain contrast and resolution of these tumors, the examination is performed during the secretory phase, when the hyperechogenic endometrium can be best delineated. Sometimes it is difficult to distinguish polyps from myomas, due to the hyperechogenicity of polyps. Then, early follicular phase examination may be helpful (17).

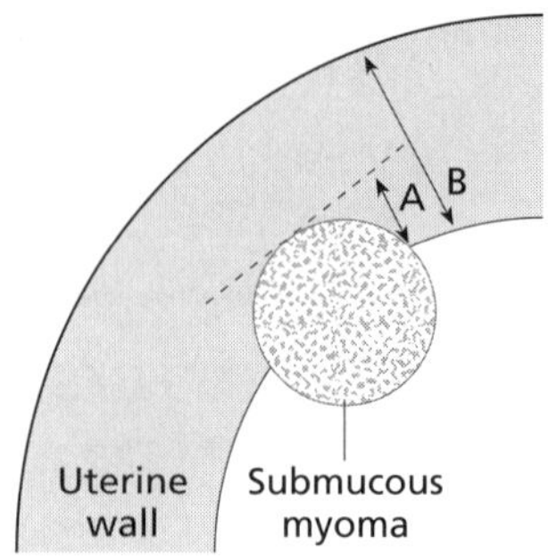

FIG. 6.15.

Diagrammatic representation of submucous myoma's intramural extension (A) and uterine wall thickness (B).

To facilitate these assessments, particularly intramural invasion of a submucous myoma, fluid can be injected into the uterine cavity while sonography is performed, enhancing the configuration of the myoma and helping in its delineation at the junction with the myometrium. Cicinelli et al (20) evaluated 52 premenopausal women before hysterectomy for benign gynecologic conditions by conventional transvaginal sonography, transabdominal sonohysterography, and hysteroscopy. The results of these three techniques in terms of diagnosis, size, intracavitary growth, and location of the submucous myomas were compared with those revealed by direct inspection of the surgical specimens. While conventional transvaginal sonography had a sensitivity of 90% and a specificity of 98%, transabdominal sonohysterography had sensitivity, specificity, and predictive values of 100%, as did hysteroscopy.

Magnetic Resonance Imaging

Magnetic resonance imaging evaluation of the uterus can precisely outline leiomyomas and is most useful in evaluating submucous tumor penetration in the uterine wall, determining depth of penetration with precision. Cost has prohibited its general use in clinical practice, but MRI may be helpful particularly in patients with multiple leiomyomas that significantly distort the uterine cavity and uterine body, and in obese patients who cannot be scanned transabdominally (21).

Hysterosalpingography

Hysterosalpingography (HSG) is a routine screening method of evaluation of the uterine cavity and fallopian tubes in infertile patients. In the presence of a normal hysterosalpingogram, direct intrauterine visualization will seldom discover significant pathology distorting the symmetry and architecture of the uterine cavity. HSG allows evaluation of the symmetric convolutions of the fallopian tubes, revealing sacculations or diverticuli and salpingitis isthmica nodosa, as well as normal tubal folds at the ampullary portion and tubal patency. In evaluating the uterine cavity, HSG shows the symmetry and form of the uterine cavity and when submucous leiomyomas are present, it outlines their contour and location. Distortion of the uterine cavity is clearly shown (22). In conjunction with sonography, hysterosalpingography offers an excellent evaluation when the uterus contains myomatous tumors. Used preoperatively, it can be helpful in delineating the treatment. Once the tumor has been removed, particularly if it is larger than 3 cm, HSG can determine the restoration of normal symmetry if performed 3 months or more following therapy, after the uterine body has returned to normal (23).

Preoperative Medical Treatment

Many patients with symptomatic uterine myomas develop secondary anemia and require treatment to re-establish normal hemoglobin levels before surgical treatment. It is important to prepare these patients before hysteroscopic surgery, to eliminate excessive debris, mucus, and blood clots, which are usually present in the uterine cavity. Medications include progestins, danazol and, of late, gonadotropin-releasing hormone (GnRH) analogs.

Progestins: While progestins in the form of medroxyprogesterone acetate (Provera), 10 to 20 mg per day orally, can be useful in controlling the bleeding and can shrink the tumors, pseudodecidualization of the endometrium can impair visibility during hysteroscopy. Success in controlling the bleeding is unpredictable and the treatment is difficult to adjust to each patient. Significant side effects, particularly fluid retention and depression, can adversely affect compliance (24).

Danazol: This weakly androgenic heterocyclic compound may exhibit anabolic properties. An inhibitory action on gonadotropin-releasing hormone and gonadotropin secretion results in suppression of menstruation, inhibits ovulation, and produces endometrial atrophy (25). Danazol has been used in the treatment of abnormal bleeding caused by uterine leiomyomas, with unpredictable results. Breakthrough bleeding usually occurs, and the growth of leiomyomas cannot be inhibited. Compliance is poor due to its androgenic side effects. For these reasons its use for treatment before hysteroscopic surgery has not been satisfactory.

GnRH Analogs: GnRH analogs can control bleeding once the flare-up phase is completed, when desensitization and downregulation of the pituitary occur. Bleeding can be controlled and some myomas may also decrease in size, particularly those with involvement of myometrium. Blood flow decreases and total atrophy of the endometrium is obtained, facilitating intrauterine visualization and the resection of these myomas (26). Not all submucous leiomyomas require preoperative hormonal treatment. Those that do produce excessive bleeding are usually larger than 3cm. If the patient is anemic, her hemoglobin should be returned to normal levels before surgery. Usually 2 to 3 months' therapy with a leuprolide acetate depot, 3.75mg IM, injected on a monthly basis, is most useful in these situations (27–29).

AVOIDING COMPLICATIONS

Complications of hysteroscopic removal of leiomyomas can derive from use of the resectoscope, scissors, or fiberlasers; the use of different energy sources such as electrosurgery and laser energy; and the fluids used to distend the uterus. Because cervical dilatation usually is required to introduce the operative gynecologic resectoscope at 8- to 9-mm outer diameter, laceration of the cervix by the tenaculum can occur, but these lacerations usually are easily handled and repaired. During cervical dilatation, perforation of the uterus, although unusual, can occur, and is usually related to faulty technique; therefore, dilatation must be carried out with care, bypassing the internal os without attempting to reach the uterine fundus with the dilator. Tapered dilators that increase in size smoothly are most useful such as Pratt dilators or Hegar dilators in half-size increments. The resection of sessile leiomyomas should be done only to the level of the uterine wall, without attempting to dig or scoop out tissue from the uterine wall; this is the best measure to prevent perforation of the uterus with the activated cutting loop (30).

Myoma fragments should be gently removed with instruments or by suction aspiration with soft plastic curets. Under no circumstances should the activated cutting loop be used if it is not controlled by direct viewing. If the view is clouded, the operation should be stopped until a clear view is obtained.

Resection or coagulation at the cornual regions of the uterus should be done with utmost care and precision to avoid perforation, as these tissues are the thinnest areas of the uterine body.

Fluids to distend the uterine cavity should be meticulously monitored to measure the amount of fluid infused and the amount of fluid recovered; when deficits of fluids devoid of electrolytes of 700 to 800 mL are obtained, the operation should be stopped and the patient monitored closely for early signs of fluid overload, not only with vital signs and pulse oximetry, but also urine output. If the operation is resumed, serum sodium should be monitored serially. The decision to stop the operation will depend on the clinical situation and most importantly on the determination of a serum sodium. If fluids with electrolytes or those that contain sodium are used, the same precautions should be taken if a deficit of 1000 to 1500 mL occurs. If the urine output is low, diuretics can be used, in the form of furosemide (Lasix), 10 to 20 mg IV, while urine output is closely monitored (31,32) (Table 6.1).

Concomitant laparoscopy is usually performed during difficult hysteroscopic surgical manipulations. While its use for submucous myomectomy is seldom required, the practitioner should be ready for its liberal use when large tumors, or those situated at the cornual regions, are removed or in any situation in which difficulty is encountered in determining the uterine cavity symmetry. The laparoscope can be used without light or a dimmed light observing the hysteroscopic light for uneven diaphanoscopy or light transillumination. Alternatively, the light of the hysteroscope can be turned off and the laparoscopic light observed

TABLE 6.1

Hysteroscopic myomectomy: avoiding fluid overload

Discuss with anesthesiologist: procedure, IV fluids, vital signs, pulse oximetry, patient's risks
Consider epidural anesthesia in high-risk patients
Have accurate account of fluid deficit (inflow-outflow)
Look for signs of decompensation: vital signs, temperature (esophageal probe), pulse oximetry, electrocardiogram
Evaluate electrolytes (Na), status of procedure, patient's condition, if deficit >700 mL
Stop procedure if deficit >800 mL, electrolytes (Na) decrease, + signs of decompensation

as the laparoscope approaches the uterine surface. This manuever can show the unequal transillumination of tissue and a residual tumor or thin uterine walls caused by resection (33).

Concomitant sonography has been used to monitor intrauterine hysteroscopic operations. This method can delineate the uterine wall thickness while also monitoring the resection of myomas during the operation. This intraoperative ultrasonic guidance is best performed transabdominally to permit a good mobilization of the resectoscope, which could be impaired by a transvaginal approach. The bladder is filled with saline solution to permit a window for ultrasonic imaging (34,35).

The use of prophylactic antibiotics for hysteroscopic myomectomy is controversial. Unless laminaria tents are used to dilate the cervix, infection is most unusual, particularly if the appropriate precautions are taken to avoid contamination. Only those patients with cardiac lesions, prosthetic cardiac valves, or a history of mitral valve prolapse with regurgitation proven by echocardiography are candidates for antibiotic therapy as prophylaxis against bacterial endocarditis (36). The use of estrogens and terminal progesterone following submucous leiomyoma resection to enhance re-epithelialization also remains controversial. Endogenous estrogens have been shown to be sufficient for re-epithelialization of transected uterine septa. The healthy surrounding endometrium is the reservoir for re-epithelialization. This is in contrast to Asherman's syndrome, in which the surrounding endometrium has been traumatized and devitalized. Patients with Asherman's syndrome will benefit from artificial hormonal stimulation after hysteroscopic treatment. Vasopressin (Pitressin) has been used sporadically to cause vasoconstriction and decrease fluid absorption (37). Use of Pitressin remains controversial, as does the use of adrenalin-containing solutions (38). A diluted form of Pitressin must be used to avoid secondary effects of vasopressin that enhance antidiuretic hormone (ADH) production, and can trigger fluid overload.

Should excessive bleeding occur immediately after surgery, tamponade with an indwelling catheter, 20 to 30 mL, can be used for 12 to 24 hours to control bleeding. Prophylactic antibiotics should be prescribed to prevent infection.

RESULTS OF TREATMENT AND FOLLOW-UP

Treatment of abnormal uterine bleeding produced by submucous leiomyomas is successful in over 90% of all cases (39). Leiomyomas that are pedunculated and completely resected respond best to treatment, assuming that the uterus does not harbor other leiomyomas. When sessile leiomyomas are treated hysteroscopically, success depends on the portion of the leiomyoma that invades the uterine wall. In general, when more than 50% of the myoma is intracavitary, the success in removing this type of leiomyoma approaches 90%, as most of the leiomyoma can be resected transcervically. When more than 50% of the leiomyoma invades the uterine wall, if the hysteroscopic approach is used, a second-stage operation is required later in the majority of patients to remove the myoma once it has been pushed into the uterine cavity by the continuous myometrial contractions. Wamsteker et al (40) evaluated 51 patients with abnormal uterine bleeding caused by submucous leiomyomas. The patients were treated hysteroscopically and bleeding was controlled in 48 (94.1%) of all patients after their final resection. With more extensive

TABLE 6.2

Hysteroscopic myomectomy for abnormal bleeding

Author	No. of Patients	Type of Myoma: Pedunculated	Type of Myoma: Sessile	Method	IUD	E/P	Antibiotics	Cure (%)	Recurrence (%)
Haning et al (1980)	1	–	+	Resectoscope	–	+	+	1	–
DeCherney and Polan (1983)	8	+	+	Resectoscope	Foley	+	+	8	–
Neuwirth (1983)	28 (2 lost to follow-up)	+	+	Resectoscope	Foley	+	+	17 (60.7)	9 (32.1)
Lin et al (1986)	13	+	–	Resectoscope (9) Rigid scissors (4)	Foley	+	+	9 (69.2)	4 (30.7)
Hallez and Perino (1988)	300	+	+	Resectoscope	+	+	+	299[a]	–
Baggish (1989)	23	+	–	Nd:YAG laser	Foley (5 patients)	–	+	NR	NR

Valle and Sciarra (1990)	52	+	−	Semirigid scissors	−	−	−	52 (100.0)	NR
Donnez et al (1990)	60	48	12	Nd:YAG laser	−	−	−	48 (80.0)	12 (20.0)
Loffer (1990)	53 (10 were polyps)	18	25 (2 patients had 2 procedures)	Resectoscope	NR	−	−	40 (93.0)	3 (6.9)
Corson and Brooks (1991)	92	92	−	Resectoscope	NR	−	+	65 (81.2)[b]	15 (18.7)[b]
Derman et al (1991)	94	94 (2 intraoperative laparotomies)	−	Resectoscope	Rubber balloon	+	+	71 (75.5)	23 (24.5)
Wamsteker et al (1993)	51	25	26 (several patients had 2–3 procedures)	Resectoscope	−	−	+	48 (94.1)	3 (5.9)
Totals	775							656 (84.6)	68 (8.7)

IUD, intrauterine device; E/P, estrogens/progesterone; NR, not reported; +, yes; −, no.
[a] One patient required laparotomy. [b] From 80 patients.
Source: Adapted from Siegler AM, Valle RF. Therapeutic hysteroscopic procedures. Fertil Steril 1988;50:685.

intramural involvement, the chances of achieving complete resection by one procedure alone decreases, and the mean number of procedures to achieve complete resection increases.

Derman et al (41) reported on the long-term effectiveness of hysteroscopic removal of leiomyomas in 94 patients. Of these patients, 24.5% reported late postoperative bleeding problems and 15.9% required additional surgery. After 9 years of follow-up, 83.9% of the patients had not required further operation.

The immediate success of hysteroscopic myomectomy reaches 90% and the long-term success, while decreased somewhat, approaches 85%. Failures may be related more to selection and complete evaluation of patients in order to detect all uterine myomas, their size, and their location. The incomplete resection of submucous leiomyomas obviously will produce further symptomatology and require additional therapy in the future (42) (Table 6.2).

SUMMARY AND CONCLUSIONS

Uterine leiomyomas are frequently occurring neoplastic disorders that may require surgical therapy because of persistent bothersome symptoms. Of these tumors, the most symptomatic, in terms of abnormal uterine bleeding, are those of the submucous type. For these tumors, in the past only a hysterotomy with its concomitant laparotomy or hysterectomy was available for surgical treatment. With the introduction of hysteroscopy, these tumors can be approached and removed transcervically, sparing the patient a laparotomy or a hysterotomy and its concomitant sequelae.

Three instruments can be used to remove submucous leiomyomas hysteroscopically: scissors, the resectoscope, and fiberlasers. The most common treatment is electrosurgical resection utilizing a cutting loop guided through a gynecologic resectoscope. Scissors are useful for small pedunculated leiomyomas and fiberlasers are helpful for morcellation and removal of these tumors.

Because excessive fluids, while distending the uterine cavity, can be absorbed by the patient, it is important to monitor meticulously the inflow and outflow quantities of these fluids and to derive a deficit to permit estimation of the absorbed fluid and prevent fluid overload.

The short- and long-term follow-up has proved the effectiveness of these operations, not only for patients who desire future fertility but for any patient afflicted with bleeding secondary to these tumors. They are the best alternative, either to abdominal myomectomy by hysterotomy or hysterectomy.

Because the success of hysteroscopic myomectomy follows a complete and meticulous evaluation of not only the uterine cavity but the whole uterine body, it is important to evaluate and rule out other concomitant leiomyomas present, which will determine the best approach to follow in therapy, selecting those patients who will benefit most from hysteroscopic treatment.

REFERENCES

1. Buttram VC Jr, Reiter RC. Uterine leiomyomata: etiology, symptomatology, and management. Fertil Steril 1981;36:433.
2. Garcia CR, Tureck RW. Submucosal leiomyomas and infertility. Fertil Steril 1984;42:16.
3. Vollenhoven BJ, Lawrence AS, Healy DL. Uterine fibroids: a clinical review. Br J Obstet Gynaecol 1990;97:285.
4. Siegler AM. Hysterosalpingography. Fertil Steril 1983;40:139.
5. Hricak H, Tscholakoff D, Heinrichs L, et al. Uterine leiomyomas: conclusion of MR histopathologic findings and symptoms. Radiology 1986; 158:385.
6. Gross BH, Silver TM, Jaffe MH. Sonographic features of uterine leiomyomas. J Ultrasound Med 1983;2:401.
7. Valle RF, Sciarra JJ. Hysteroscopy: a useful diagnostic adjunct in gynecology. Am J Obstet Gynecol 1975;122:230.
8. Baggish MS, Sze EHM, Rosenzweig BA, et al. Direct hysteroscopic observation to document the reasons for abnormal bleeding secondary to submucous myoma. J Gynecol Surg 1989;5:149.
9. Valle RF. Hysteroscopic removal of submucous leiomyomas. J Gynecol Surg 1990;6:89.

10. Loffer FD. Removal of large symptomatic intrauterine growths by the hysteroscopic resectoscope. Obstet Gynecol 1990;76:836.
11. Corson SL, Brooks PG. Resectoscopic myomectomy. Fertil Steril 1991; 55:1041.
12. Lin BL, Iwata Y, Lin KH. Removing a large submucous fibroid hysteroscopically with the two-resectoscope method. J Am Assoc Gynecol Laparosc 1994;1:259.
13. Donnez J, Schurs B, Gillerot S, et al. Treatment of uterine fibroids with implants of gonadotropin-releasing hormone agonists: assessment by hysterography. Fertil Steril 1989;51:947.
14. Baggish MS, Sze EHM, Morgan G. Hysteroscopic treatment of symptomatic submucous myomata uteri with the Nd:YAG laser. J Gynecol Surg 1989;5:27.
15. Donnez J, Gillerot S, Bourgonjon D, et al. Neodymium: YAG laser hysteroscopy in large submucous fibroids. Fertil Steril 1990;54:999.
16. Goldrath MH. Vaginal removal of the pedunculated submucous myoma. Historical observations and development of a new procedure. J Reprod Med 1990;35:921.
17. Fedele L, Bianchi S, Dorta M, et al. Transvaginal ultrasonography versus hysteroscopy in the diagnosis of uterine submucous myomas. Obstet Gynecol 1991;77:745.
18. Dodson MG. Use of transvaginal ultrasound in diagnosing the etiology of menometrorrhagia. J Reprod Med 1994;39:362.
19. Fleischer AC, Dudley BS, Entman SS, et al. Myometrial invasion of endometrial carcinoma: sonographic assessment. Radiology 1987;162:307.
20. Cicinelli E, Romano F, Anastasio PS, et al. Transabdominal sonohysterography, transvaginal sonography, and hysteroscopy in the evaluation of submucous myomas. Obstet Gynecol 1995;85:42.
21. Togashi K, Ozasa H, Konishi I, et al. Enlarged uterus: Differentiation between adenomyosis and leiomyoma with MRI. Radiology 1989;171:531.
22. Green WJ, Fendley SM, Wintzell EC, et al. Cystic degeneration of a large uterine leiomyoma: radiologic and surgical analyses. Invest Radiol 1989; 24:626.
23. Weinstein D, Aviad Y, Polishuk WZ. Hysterography before and after myomectomy. AJR 1977;129:899.
24. Goldzieher J, Maqueo M, Ricaud L, et al. Induction of degenerative changes in uterine myomas by high-dosage progestin therapy. Am J Obstet Gynecol 1966;96:1078.

25. Greenblatt RB, Dmowski WP, Makesh VB, Schesler HFL. Clinical studies with an antigonadotropin—danazol. Fertil Steril 1971;22:102.
26. Matta WHM, Stabile I, Shaw RW, Campbell S. Doppler assessment of uterine blood flow changes in patients with fibroids receiving the gonadotropin-releasing hormone agonist buserelin. Fertil Steril 1988; 49:1083.
27. Friedman AJ, Rein MS, Harrison-Atlas D, et al. A randomized, placebo-controlled, double-blind study evaluating leuprolide acetate depot treatment before myomectomy. Fertil Steril 1989;52:728.
28. Friedman AJ, Hoffman DI, Comite F. Treatment of leiomyomata uteri with leuprolide acetate depot: a double-blind, placebo-controlled, multi-center study. Obstet Gynecol 1991;77:720.
29. Perino A, Chianchiano N, Petronio M, Cittadini E. The role of leuprolide acetate depot in hysteroscopic surgery: a controlled study. Fertil Steril 1993;59:507.
30. Sullivan B, Kenney P, Seibel M. Hysteroscopic resection of fibroid with thermal injury to sigmoid. Obstet Gynecol 1992;80:546.
31. Witz CA, Silverberg KM, Burns WN, et al. Complications associated with the absorption of hysteroscopic fluid media. Fertil Steril 1993;60: 745.
32. Baggish MS, Brill AI, Rosensweig B, et al. Fatal acute glycine and sorbitol toxicity during operative hysteroscopy. J Gynecol Surg 1993;9:137.
33. Lin BL, Iwata Y. Modified laparoscopy for monitoring transcervical surgery. Am J Obstet Gynecol 1990;163:243. Letter.
34. Lin BL, Iwata Y, Miyamoto N, Hayashi S. Three-contrasts method: an ultrasound technique for monitoring transcervical operations. Am J Obstet Gynecol 1987;156:469.
35. Letterie GS, Kramer DJ. Intraoperative ultrasound guidance for intrauterine endoscopic surgery. Fertil Steril 1994;62:654.
36. Lavie CJ, Khandheria BK, Steward JB, et al. Factors associated with the recommendation for endocarditis prophylaxis in mitral valve prolapse. JAMA 1989;262:3308.
37. Corson SL, Brooks PG, Serden SP, et al. Effects of vasopressin administration during hysteroscopic surgery. J Reprod Med 1994;39:419.
38. Molnar BG, Broadbent JAM, Magos AL. Fluid overload risk score for endometrial resection. Gynaecol Endosc 1992;1:133.
39. Siegler AM, Valle RF. Therapeutic hysteroscopic procedures. Fertil Steril 1988;50:685.

40. Wamsteker K, Emanuel MH, de Kruif JH. Transcervical hysteroscopic resection of submucous fibroids for abnormal uterine bleeding: results regarding the degree of intramural extension. Obstet Gynecol 1993;82:736.
41. Derman SG, Rehnstrom J, Neuwirth RS. The long-term effectiveness of hysteroscopic treatment of menorrhagia and leiomyomas. Obstet Gynecol 1991;77:591.
42. Broadbent JAM, Magos AL. Menstrual blood loss after hysteroscopic myomectomy. Gynaecol Endosc 1995;4:41.

CHAPTER

7

Vaginal Myomectomy

Eric J. Bieber
Samir N. Hajj
Beth A. Plunkett

THE PROLAPSED SUBMUCOSAL FIBROID

The first reported case in the United States of a vaginal myomectomy on a prolapsing submucosal myoma was in 1844 (1). Unfortunately, a limited amount has been written subsequently regarding this clinically relevant entity. Uterine myomas are the most common tumor of the female genital tract, with an incidence that has been estimated at anywhere from 20% to 30% to as high as 75% when small-diameter (3–4 mm) myomas are included. Approximately 5% to 10% of myomas will become submucosal, growing inward toward the uterine cavity rather than growing outward and becoming subserosal. It has been estimated that one in four to one in eight submucosal myomas may present as pedunculated intracavitary masses. In one study of over 1200 hysterectomies performed for symptomatic myomas, 1.3% were noted to contain pedunculated myomas (2). In another large study that covered a 10-year period, 46 of 1785 (2.5%) women who underwent hysterectomy or myomectomy were noted to have pedunculated submucous myomas (3).

Presenting Symptoms

Uterine myomas may present with a wide variety of symptoms ranging from asymptomatic in some individuals to highly symptomatic, depending on the number and location of the myomas within the uterus. Submucosal myomas, and in particular pedunculated myomas, may commonly present with the acute findings seen in Table 7.1. The most common presenting symptoms for prolapsing pedunculated myomas include menometrorrhagia in 74%–88% of patients, uterine contractions (81%), and lower-abdominal pain (20%–65.5%). In reviewing the literature wide variances can be seen in the reported incidence of menorrhagia, pain, and contractions for a control group of patients who presented solely with uterine fibroids. This can well be rationalized by the fact that some of these patients may have had submucous myomas along with multiple other myomas.

The exact mechanism responsible for intracavitary myomas that cause irregular bleeding or menometrorrhagia, or both, is ill defined. Theories have included ulcerations on the surface of the myoma (however, this is rarely seen hysteroscopically), changes in the vascularity of the endometrium overlying the myoma, and a decreased ability of the uterus to contract around myometrial or endometrial vessels thus

TABLE 7.1

Presenting symptoms of uterine myomas

SYMPTOM	PROLAPSED (%)	UTERINE FIBROID (%)
Menometrorrhagia	74–88	63–89
Lower-abdominal pain	20.0–65.5	19.5–74.4
Uterine contractions	81	54.9
Vaginal discharge	44–59	27
Anemia	57	40
Fever	4.2–13	0–3.7
Sensation of vaginal mass	15–20	1
Acute vaginal bleeding	59	10

increasing subsequent bleeding. The evolution of a submucous myoma to a completely intracavitary myoma to a prolapsing myoma has been reported. We recently encountered a case in which office hysteroscopy demonstrated an approximately 30% to 50% intracavitary submucous myoma. Following treatment with a gonadotropin-releasing hormone (GnRH) analog, the patient was brought to the operating room (OR) for submucous myoma resection. At the time of her surgery the cervical os was noted to be dilated with a mass sitting behind the external cervical os at the level of the internal os. The myoma had transformed itself into a completely intracavitary myoma, which was in the process of attempting to deliver itself. At this point, only a small stalk remained (see Plate 4). The entire sequence of events is seen in Figure 7.1.

Completely intracavitary and prolapsed myomas are also associated with increased vaginal discharge and sensation of a vaginal mass as well as acute vaginal bleeding. A prolapsing of intracavitary mass ultimately causes pressure on the internal cervical os, leading to uterine contractions, dilation, effacement, and eventual expulsion of the mass through the cervix into the vagina. In this way it has often been compared symptomatically to labor. Ben-Baruch and colleagues (3) reported that in patients who presented with prolapsing myomas 58.7% were admitted for acute bleeding episodes, compared to 9.8% of a control group of patients with fibroids. In addition, patients were noted to have a much higher rate of anemia (19.6%) compared to the control group (4.4%). Riley (4) reported an average hemoglobin of only 8.6 g/dL in 41 patients presenting with prolapsing myomas, whereas the control group of patients presented with an average hemoglobin in 11.4 g/dL with nonprolapsing fibroids. He also noted an increase in clinically significant anemia, with 7 of 41 (17%) patients presenting with hemoglobins of 6.0 g/dL or less and 1 patient with a hemoglobin of 3.0 g/dL.

The evolution of a submucous myoma to a myoma transiting the cervix on a small stalk may predispose these masses to torsion, necrosis, and subsequent infection. This process would account for as high a number as 1 in 7 patients presenting with fever, as well as the chronic vaginal discharge reported in as many as one half of patients with pedunculated myoma. Ben-Baruch et al (3) reported that 6 of 46 patients presented with elevations in temperature, leukocytosis, or purulent vaginal

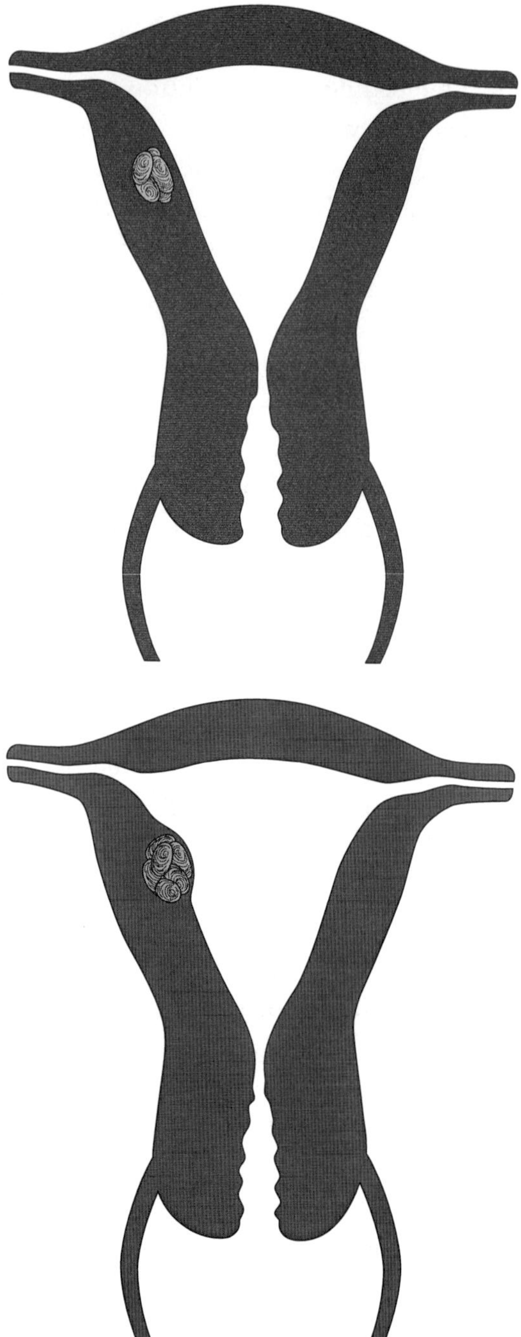

A

B

FIG. 7.1.

Demonstration of the evolution of a myoma from intramural (A), to partly intracavitary (B), to completely intracavitary with a sessile base (C), to pedunculated intracavitary myoma (D), to prolapsing myoma on a thin pedicle (E).

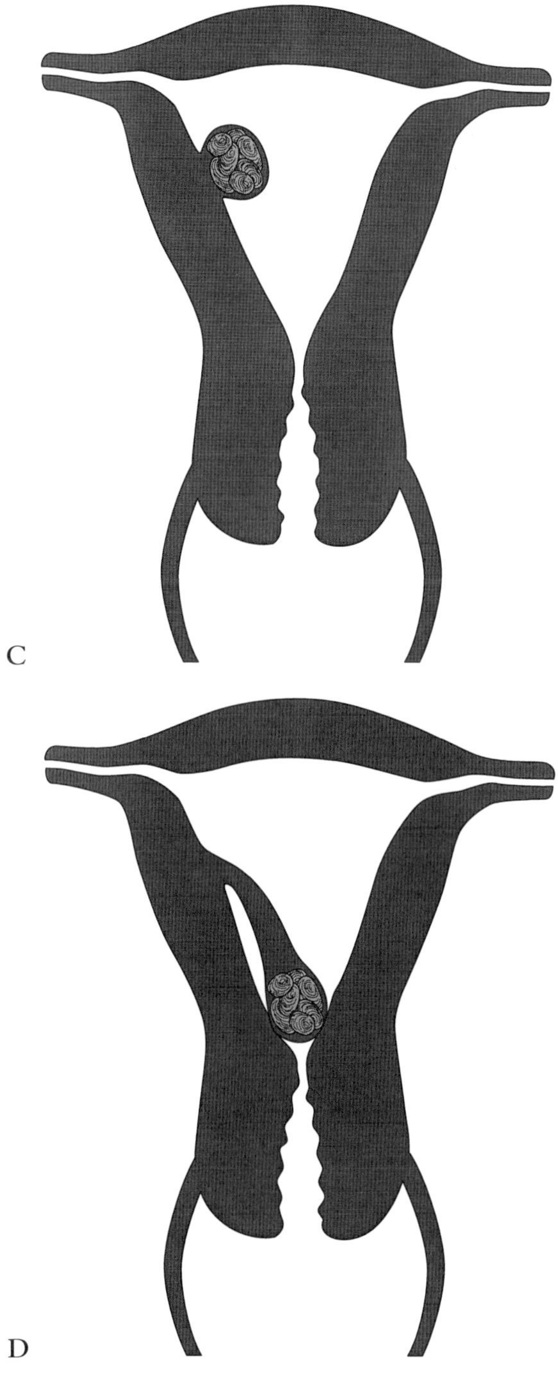

FIG. 7.1

Continued

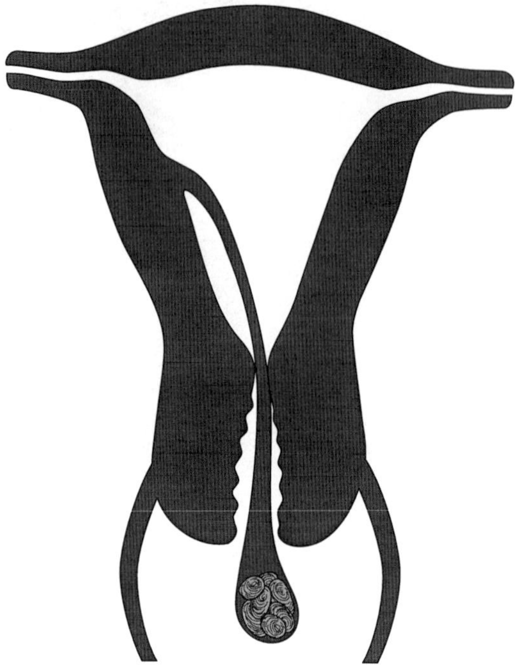

FIG. 7.1

Continued

discharge. In each case, histopathologic examination demonstrated necrotic, infected myomas.

The association of intracavitary submucosal myomas or prolapsing myomas with infertility, spontaneous abortion, and premature labor or other obstetric complications is less well defined. Early authors suggested that such myomas are associated with patients of low parity or nulliparity. However, Riley (4) found a high parity level in his patients.

While myomas that have prolapsed partially or completely through the external cervical os and are visible on vaginal examination are readily identified, the pedunculated, completely intracavitary myoma may be more difficult to diagnose. Ben-Baruch et al (3) noted that in many patients the uterus was not significantly enlarged and no correlation existed between myoma and uterine size. We have similarly noted patients with completely intracavitary myomas who were highly symp-

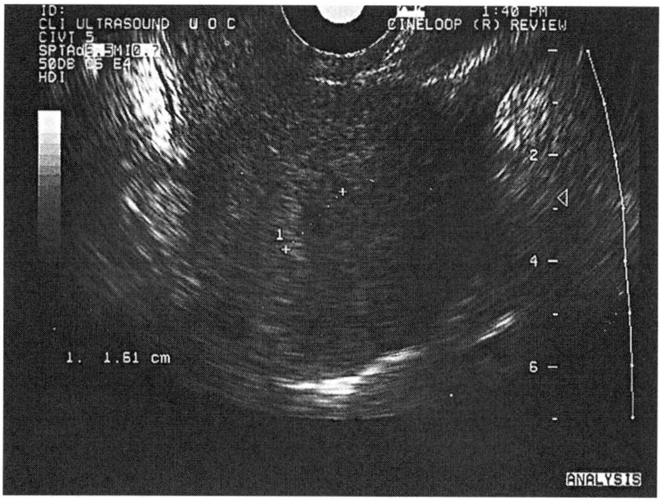

FIG. 7.2.

Ultrasound demonstrates a $1\frac{1}{2}$-cm mass within the uterine cavity. Without a contrasting agent it is difficult to determine if this is thickened endometrium or an intracavitary mass.

tomatic with low hemoglobins, but whose myomas were "camouflaged" by the surrounding myometrium. A 3-cm myoma may be well contained within a normal-sized uterus and may be almost impossible to appreciate on bimanual examination. Often during routine dilation and curettage, the surgeon may follow the curvature of the myoma in the belief that the cavity is ante- or retroverted and may lose the appreciation of an intracavitary mass. Presenting symptoms such as significant abnormal bleeding, vaginal discharge, fever, or contractions should raise clinical suspicions regarding intracavitary disease. Ultrasound can be utilized to define the intracavitary portion of the myoma (Fig. 7.2), as is described in Chapter 2. Hysterosalpingosonography may have even higher sensitivity and specificity for delineating intracavitary lesions as well as the percent intracavitary/intramural involvement (Fig. 7.3; see also Plate 5). Hysteroscopy also provides excellent sensitivity and specificity for such a diagnosis.

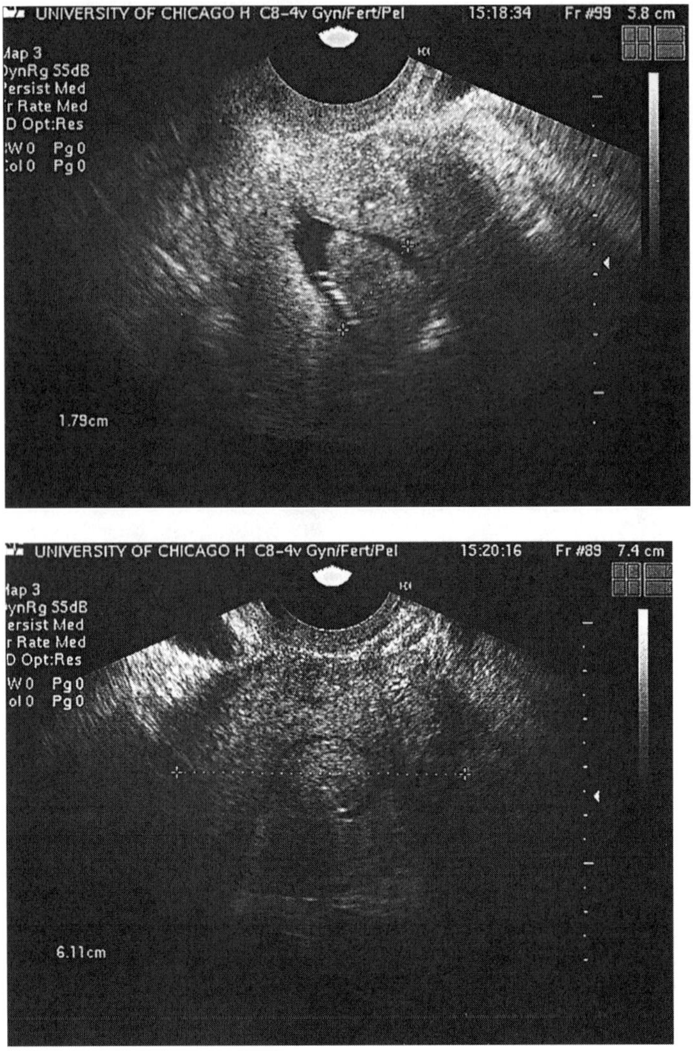

A

B

FIG. 7.3.

In the same patient as in Fig. 7.2, saline is being used as a contrast medium. A. An intracavitary lesion arises from the fundus. B. Transverse imaging below the fundus demonstrates saline surrounding the lesion (see also Plate 5).

SURGICAL MANAGEMENT

Partially Prolapsed or Prolapsed Myomas

Because of the high incidence of anemia in patients who present with intracavitary and prolapsing myomas, a complete blood count (CBC) should be ordered immediately to ascertain the level of anemia. In patients who are profoundly anemic, transfusion and subsequent surgery should be performed. We recently noted a patient who had undergone previous laparotomy myomectomy who presented with a hemoglobin of less than 5 g/dL (see Plate 6). The patient had an almost completely intracavitary myoma that was readily resected following transfusion to an appropriate level to allow surgery (see Plate 7).

If the patient presents with evidence of underlying infection, broad-spectrum parenteral antibiotics should be instituted before surgery. Little information is available regarding the need or outcome of patients treated or not treated with antibiotics who do not have evidence of an underlying infection.

Historically, the surgical treatments have included vaginal myomectomy or hysterectomy. More recently, hysteroscopic techniques have also provided excellent results. Multiple factors must be considered in discussing these treatment options with the patient, including risks of the procedure, patient age, desire for future fertility, the presence or absence of other fibroids, and the size and location of the pedunculated mass. Historically, in patients who have presented with multiple myomas as well as prolapsing myoma, the recommendation has been for a two-stage procedure. The first stage involves removal of the submucous myoma followed by an abdominal or vaginal hysterectomy. The concept was that the prolapsed myoma would predispose patients to a higher level of infectious morbidity. To date, however, there is little evidence to support that this is indeed true.

Brooks and Stage (2) described a methodology for removal of prolapsed, pedunculated submucosal myomas. In their group of patients, they noted 5 of 17 women with hemoglobins of less than 5 g/dL. They reported pedunculated masses that ranged from 2 to 10 cm in diameter with cervical dilation between 1 and 10 cm. They recommended placement of a Mayo renal pedicle clamp across the myoma stalk, removal of the mass with Mayo scissors, and then taping of the clamp handle to the patient's thigh for 24 hours. They performed no suturing and experienced no significant bleeding.

Modern instrumentation, including the widespread use of hysteroscopy, has simplified the management of these cases. If the myoma is small, a variety of instruments can be utilized including a Krause clamp or a standard curved 6. In addition, devices that are available in every operating room, including a ring forceps, Sopher ovum forceps, or tenaculum, can also be utilized. Depending on the size and nature of the lesion, we have performed these surgeries in the office or in the OR under paracervical block with or without intravenous sedation or using general anesthesia as needed. If a small pedicle is present, the lesion can be twisted until it is completely loosened without the need for subsequent suturing. If the pedicle is deemed highly vascular, sutures or endoloops can be placed before removal of the lesion. Electrosurgical devices can also be utilized to coagulate the pedicle while transection is being performed. Suturing or electrosurgical transection can be readily performed if the lesion has delivered itself into the vaginal canal. This is significantly more difficult when the lesion remains intracavitary.

With large myomas, morcellation may need to be performed prior to completed removal. Ranney and Frederick (5) interestingly reported on a large, 12-cm pedunculated myoma. They suggested that size may not be a contraindication if the cervical os is significantly dilated. In this case, morcellation was utilized to deliver the 12-cm myoma through the 7-cm dilated cervix without difficulty. The authors noted that the patient was then followed for 25 years after the time of her initial presentation without the need for subsequent treatment. When a myoma has only partly been delivered through the os and cervical dilation may be limited, it may be possible to replace these myomas within the uterine cavity, allowing them to be treated as intracavitary masses, as is described in the next section. In the past, it had been suggested that such patients have their myoma replaced, the cervix sutured closed, and an abdominal hysterectomy performed. In general, such cases can now be managed in a more conservative fashion.

Nonprolapsed Pedunculated Fibroids

A more difficult situation to manage surgically is the nonprolapsed pedunculated myoma. Often these myomas will be discovered at the time of hysteroscopy in evaluating patients for abnormal uterine bleeding. Similar methods as have been described previously can be utilized, including electrosurgical transection, stalk cauterization, or attempts to suture the pedicles. Historically, an alternative included raising the bladder flap and incising the cervix anteriorly (i.e., a vaginal hysterotomy). In difficult situations this will allow identification of the myoma pedicle and the ability to more directly clamp and suture ligate the base. In general, this type of surgical methodology has been replaced by hysteroscopic directed myoma removal.

Goldrath (6,7) reported on the use of laminaria to aid in surgical dilation and subsequent myoma removal. In his series of 151 symptomatic patients who presented for surgery, 92% successfully underwent myomectomy (6,7). The methodology included use of two to three laminaria placed in the cervix for 5 to 6 hours. Following this, a second insertion was performed, placing eight or more laminaria overnight. This allowed significant dilation, and in some cases an index finger could be placed within the uterine cavity. With such significant dilation the myomas were able to be grasped at the widest diameter using instruments such as ring forceps, tenaculum, or ovum forceps. While this procedure works well for small or medium-sized fibroids, it is difficult to achieve adequate dilatation for larger myomas.

Most recently the gynecologic resectoscope or operative hysteroscope using scissors has been utilized to remove intracavitary masses (as described in Chap. 6). In myomas that have a small pedicle to the uterine wall, it is imperative during hysteroscopic resection (where there may be limited dilation) not to cut the pedicle until the myoma has been almost completely resected. We are aware of case reports of transection of such pedicles with large, completely intracavitary myomas in which it was not possible to effect resection of the myoma once the pedicle was removed.

The pedicles act as an anchor and allow the resection to be performed more easily.

COMPLICATIONS

Complications of vaginal myomectomy include hemorrhage in a small percentage of patients. In Goldrath's series (7) only 7 of 151 patients were noted to have excessive bleeding following myoma removal. The uterus' ability to contract causes arterial and venous tamponade, clot formation, and effective hemostasis in most cases. However, when necessary, a Foley catheter can be placed within the uterine cavity to tamponade blood vessels. We have only rarely found this to be necessary. When this is performed, patients should be watched for 3 to 4 hours, at which time the Foley catheter can be deflated and the patients observed for another several hours. If bleeding persists, the catheter should be inflated overnight. If no further bleeding occurs, the catheter can be removed. It should be remembered that in a normal-sized uterus the cavity may have a volume of only 3 to 4mL, requiring minimal inflation of a Foley balloon. Rarely is it necessary to use the large 30-mL balloon. Several authors have reported on vaginal hemorrhage in patients with submucous myomas who were being treated with GnRH analogs (8,9). In one case the patient had been treated for 8 weeks, reducing the uterine size from 18 to 12 weeks' gestation (8). Histopathology demonstrated no significant necrosis. As in this case, the etiology of episodes of hemorrhage in patients with submucous myoma, on or off GnRHa analog treatment, is unclear.

Additional risks include cervical laceration and a low risk of cervical incompetence as well as uterine perforation or postoperative infection. Interestingly, in Goldrath's series (7), 55 patients underwent subsequent hysteroscopy. In no patients were intrauterine adhesions observed, demonstrating the ability of the endometrium to regenerate in most cases without subsequent scarification (7).

While it is generally appreciated that nonobstetric uterine inversion is a rare event, there have been reports of submucous myomas delivering and inverting the uterus concomitantly (Fig. 7.4). Henderson (10)

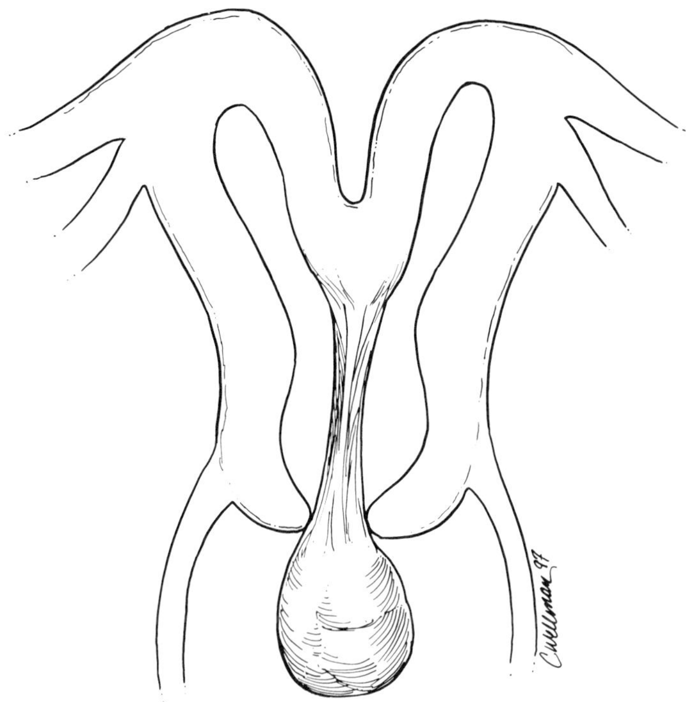

FIG. 7.4.

Graphic demonstration of how an intracavitary myoma can prolapse through the cervix causing subsequent uterine inversion.

reported on a patient presenting with chronic uterine inversion who had a 10-cm submucous myoma with a broad base attached to the fundus of the uterus that was completely inverted. It was noted that both ureters and the bladder were pulled beyond the introitus. It has been suggested that such patients may present with the classic symptoms associated with prolapsing myoma or polyps and a mass that will be readily apparent on examination. However, uterine inversion may not be initially appreciated, and if surgery is performed, the potential exists for significant ureteral, bladder, or rectal injury secondary to the anatomic distortion. It has thus been suggested that the uterine cavity be evaluated by a uterine sound, dilator, or hysteroscope before any interuterine mass is removed in order to have an appreciation of the underlying anatomy (11).

RESULTS

In the limited data that exist in the world literature, vaginal myomectomy regardless of route seems to compare favorably to either vaginal or abdominal hysterectomy.

Ben-Baruch et al (3) found only three cases in which vaginal myomectomy failed and an abdominal operation had to be performed. They noted a hospital stay that was one-third as long as the comparison group (2.4 vs. 7.8 days). In 34 patients followed for an average of 5.5 years, 80% had no subsequent symptomatology, 6% underwent hysterectomy, and 9% had recurrent submucosal myomas. Both Riley (4) and Dicker and colleagues (12) reported substantial reductions in postoperative pyrexia, transfusion, and hospital stays in patients who underwent vaginal procedures versus the control group of patients who underwent total abdominal hysterectomy. It is of interest that Riley found postoperative morbidity to be similiar in patients undergoing hysterectomy with and without prolapsing myomas, suggesting that staged procedures are not necessary.

CONCLUSION

Vaginal myomectomy performed transvaginally or transcervically is a valuable procedure in some patients. These women often present with acute symptomatology. Conservative operations, where appropriate, decrease patient morbidity while seeming to provide good long-term outcome.

REFERENCES

1. Rock JA. Telinde's operative gynecology. 7th ed. Philadelphia: Lippincott, 1992:2.
2. Brooks G, Stage AH. The surgical management of prolapsed pedunculated submucous leiomyomas. Surg Gynecol Obste 1975;141:397–398.

3. Ben-Baruch G, Schiff E, Menashe Y, Menczer J. Immediate and late outcome of vaginal myomectomy for prolapsed pedunculated submucous myoma. Obstet Gynecol 1988;72:858–861.
4. Riley P. Treatment of prolapsed submucous fibroids. SA Med J 1982; 62:22–24.
5. Ranney B, Frederick I. The occasional need for myomectomy. Obstet Gynecol 1979;53:437–441.
6. Goldrath M. Vaginal removal of the pedunculated submucous myoma: the use of laminaria. Obstet Gynecol 1987;70:670–672.
7. Goldrath M. Vaginal removal of the pedunculated submucous myoma: historical observations and development of a new procedure. J Reprod Med 1990;35:921–954.
8. Thorp JM, Katz VL. Submucous myoma treated with gonadotropin releasing hormone agonist and resulting in vaginal hemorrhage. J Reprod Med 1991;36:625–626.
9. Friedman AJ. Vaginal hemorrhage associated with degenerated submucous leiomyomata during leuprolide acetate treatment. Fertil Steril 1989;52:152.
10. Henderson PR. A large submucous fibroid polyp causing inversion of the uterus. Aust NZ J Obstet Gynaecol 1980;20:251–254.
11. Jeffcoate N. Principles of gynaecology. 4th ed. London: Butterworths, 1975:246–275.
12. Dicker D, Feldberg D, Dekel A, et al. The management of prolapsed submucous fibroids. Aust NZ Obstet Gynaecol 1986;26:308–311.

CHAPTER

8

Myomectomy in Infertility Patients

Joseph S. Sanfilippo

Uterine leiomyomas are defined as benign proliferations of smooth-muscle cells and fibrous connective tissue that are thought to arise either from the uterine smooth muscle per se or from the smooth muscle surrounding blood vessels within the uterine musculature. They are located either submucous (protruding into the endometrial cavity), intramural (within the uterine wall), or subserosal (associated with serosal surface of the uterus). In addition, pedunculated subserosal tumors are believed to emanate from the serosa. They may detach and be associated with a secondary blood supply from another organ, at which point they are termed *parasitic* leiomyomas. While uterine leiomyomas are the most common neoplasms of the female pelvis, they also have been identified in secondary locations such as the right atrium (1). Metastatic spread can occur; approximately 100 cases of intraluminal extension of benign smooth-muscle tumors into the uterine and pelvic veins have been reported (2).

Leiomyomas have been identified in 20% to 25% of women of reproductive age (3). Thus, concern exists for leiomyomas in association with infertility.

In the patient who presents with recurrent second trimester spontaneous abortions or preterm labor, the distinct possibility of submucous leiomyomas should always be considered. In addition, primary infertility with an apparent uterine factor, especially if distortion of the endometrial cavity is seen on hysterosalpingography or saline-enhanced ultrasound, should also be considered to have leiomyomas as the underlying etiology (3). To date, there are no controlled data to support a causal association between leiomyomata uteri and adverse reproductive outcome (4). Leiomyomas can be associated with bilateral tubal occlusion, and thus with infertility as well. Careful determination of other possible etiologies of either recurrent spontaneous abortions, preterm labor, or primary infertility is an appropriate prerequisite before myomectomy.

Leiomyosarcoma is a de novo neoplasm and does not represent degenerative change from a benign leiomyoma (5). In the patient who presents with rapid increase in size of a pelvic (i.e., uterine) mass, leiomyosarcoma is a distinct consideration in the differential diagnosis. The diagnosis is established with a histopathologic assessment of greater than 10 mitoses per 10 consecutive high-power fields. The overall incidence of leiomyosarcoma in surgery performed for leiomyomas varies between less than 0.1% and approximately 1% (3,6).

EVALUATION

When a patient presents with infertility, especially recurrent second trimester spontaneous abortions, assessment of the endometrial cavity is appropriate. The more traditional approach has included that of hysterosalpingography (HSG) with the ability to identify a filling defect. When observed at the time of contrast material injection, the medium will be noted to circle around the defect within the cavity. As specific HSG films are obtained, a defect in the dispersion of the contrast material is noted. The procedure enhances the physical examination, the latter being associated with bimanual examination in which an enlarged, firm, nontender, and irregularly contoured uterus is present. Uterine size is estimated in conjunction with gestational size. The clinician often elects to obtain a hemoglobin and hematocrit, especially if an element of abnormal uterine bleeding, as well as cervical cytology, is present. If evidence of a bleeding diathesis is found, a coagulation profile and bleed-

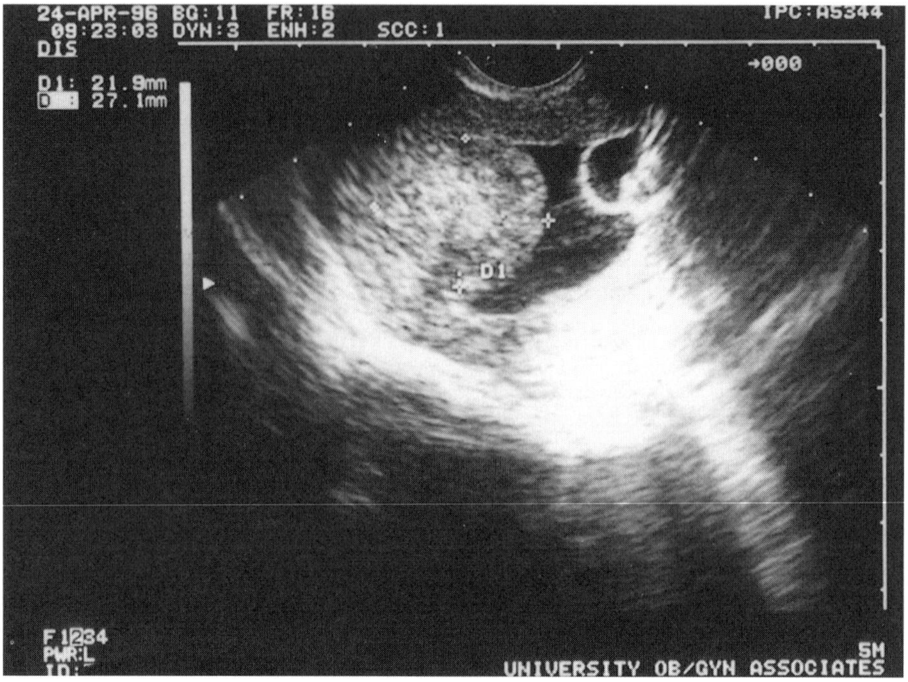

FIG. 8.1.

Saline-enhanced ultrasound showing filling defect consistent with leiomyomas.

ing time are indicated. An endometrial biopsy may be necessary, depending on the specific clinical circumstance, patient age, and so forth.

Ultrasonography has been a hallmark for identifying leiomyomas, especially if the clinician is interested in size and location. More recently, saline-enhanced ultrasonography has been utilized to distend the endometrial cavity and provide ultrasonographic assessment of submucous leiomyomas (Fig. 8.1). This can be easily accomplished with the injection of normal saline or a similar physiologic solution. A number of catheters, including those utilized with assisted reproductive technology, will facilitate the introduction of fluid into the endometrial cavity at the time of ultrasonography.

Magnetic resonance imaging (MRI) has also been utilized to obtain further information regarding leiomyomas, but this remains a point of controversy with respect to the cost-benefit ratio for the imaging procedure.

TREATMENT

The American College of Obstetricians and Gynecologists (ACOG) Committee on Quality Assurance has provided clinicians with the ACOG criteria for myomectomy (5) (Table 8.1).

A conservative approach (myomectomy) becomes indicated in the patient who desires to preserve her childbearing capabilities. Statistics support clinical improvement with myometomy in that approximately 80% of patients have subjective improvement such as correction of pelvic pain and pressure, as well as menstrual abnormalities (hypermenorrhea) (3).

Clinicians often elect to prescribe medical therapy before surgical intervention. This is primarily in the form of gonadotropin-releasing hormone agonist (GnRHag). In general, uterine volume is reduced 30% to 50% with this therapy (5). The physiologic changes appear to be associated with a hypoestrogenemic state, that is, pseudomenopause. Unfortunately, symptoms such as vasomotor symptoms and the potential for decrease in bone mineral density often develop. Each of these entities appears to improve with discontinuation of therapy, although the leiomyomas return to baseline size within approximately 15 weeks after completion of therapy (7).

SURGICAL ALTERNATIVES

Laparotomy

While the traditional laparotomic approach to leiomyomas remains in vogue, it continues to have the potential for significant intraoperative blood loss, adhesion formation, and the morbidity and mortality associated with exploratory laparotomy. Depending on the clinical circumstance, it may not be the procedure of choice.

TABLE 8.1

American College of Obstetricians and Gynecologists (ACOG) criteria for myomectomy

Procedure: Myomectomy*

Indication: Leiomyomas in infertility patients as a probable factor in failure to conceive or in recurrent pregnancy loss

Confirmation of Indication:*

In the presence of failure to conceive or recurrent pregnancy loss:

1. Presence of leiomyomas of sufficient size or specific location to be a probable factor
2. No more likely explanation exists for the failure to conceive or recurrent pregnancy loss

Actions Prior to Procedure:

1. Evaluate other causes of male and female infertility or recurrent pregnancy loss
2. Evaluate the endometrial cavity and fallopian tubes (e.g., hysterosalpingogram)
3. Document discussion that complexity of disease process may require hysterectomy

Unless otherwise stated, each numbered item must be present.

*Evaluation of the quality of care provided with this procedure, when performed for the indication listed, will be possible through assessment of ongoing or repetitive patterns of care ("trending").

Source: Modified from American College of Obstetricians and Gynecologists. Quality assessment and improvement in obstetrics and gynecology. Washington, DC: ACOG, 1994.

Endoscopy

Endoscopic approaches have continued to evolve with technical advances, both from the hysteroscopic and laparoscopic perspectives.

Hysteroscopy: When a leiomyoma is identified in a submucous location and is equated with the appropriate clinical circumstance for removal, hysteroscopic assessment is a viable alternative. Often the patient is first placed on GnRH agonist therapy for approximately 8 weeks before the surgical intervention. A number of approaches to resection include use of a wire loop attached to a resectoscope. The technique includes dilatation of the endocervical canal to 7 to 9 mm. The hysteroscope is attached to a light source and an electrolyte-free distending medium is introduced into the endometrial cavity. A flow-through system within the endometrial cavity provides for adequate distention and evacuation of blood facilitating visualization. Careful monitoring of intake and output, that is, determination approximately every 15 minutes, is important. A cutting or blended (cutting and coagulation) current is utilized for the resection. As "chips of myoma" are created, they are periodically removed from the cavity. Recently, a thermolabile probe that provides vaporization of the myoma and, thus, eliminates the need for removal of myoma chips has become available (Fig. 8.2). The end point of resection is when the myoma has been resected to a level flush with the endometrial cavity. Thus, it is not possible to completely excise the submucous leiomyoma from a hysteroscopic approach.

It is quite important that monitoring of intake and output be continuously observed and when a mismatch of 700 mL or more (i.e., more is taken in than recovered) occurs, the procedure should be aborted and assessment of serum electrolytes obtained immediately. Diuretics such as furosemide can be administered. Depending upon the circumstance (serum sodium level), saline infusion may be necessary. Continued monitoring of serum potassium is of importance, especially with respect to the potential for cardiac problems. With profound hypokalemia, the patient may also require insulin administration. The low-viscosity fluids without electrolytes that are commonly utilized for resection include dextrose and water, 1.5% glycine, 3% sorbitol, and 2.8% sorbitol plus 0.5% mannitol (Cytal).

Laparoscopy: Laparoscopic resection of subserous and intramural leiomyomas is clearly one alternative approach (8). The fundamental principles of this approach include identification of the subserous leiomyoma, injection of a dilute vasopressin solution (1 ampule 20 units vasopressin in a 1:50 to 1:100 dilution with irrigation solution), ideally

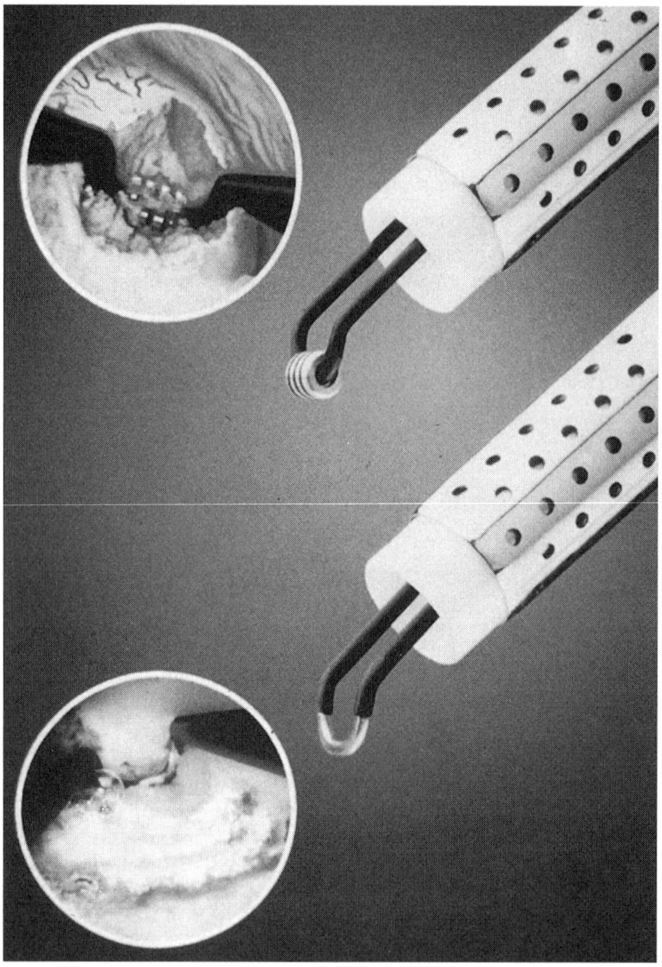

FIG. 8.2.

Vaportrode. (Courtesy of Circon ACMI, Santa Barbara, CA.)

injected via a spinal needle directly into the serosa over the myoma. This is followed by electrosurgical incision (monopolar) coagulation, often used with a needle point applicator, to incise the serosa-capsule over the myoma. The myoma is then enucleated, with an effort being made to remove the capsule-fibroid intact. A myoma screw (Fig. 8.3) is often helpful to serve as a handle to accomplish this goal. Prerequisite placement of several lower-abdominal ports allows introduction of the appropriate instrumentation. Upon completion of this segment, hemostasis is accomplished with use of either bipolar or monopolar coagulation current. Every effort to remove as many myomas from one incision as is feasible should be incorporated into the technique. Reapproximation of the musculature is then accomplished via laparoscopic suturing that utilizes either intracorporeal or extracorporeal knot-tying techniques. Efforts to prevent adhesion formation should

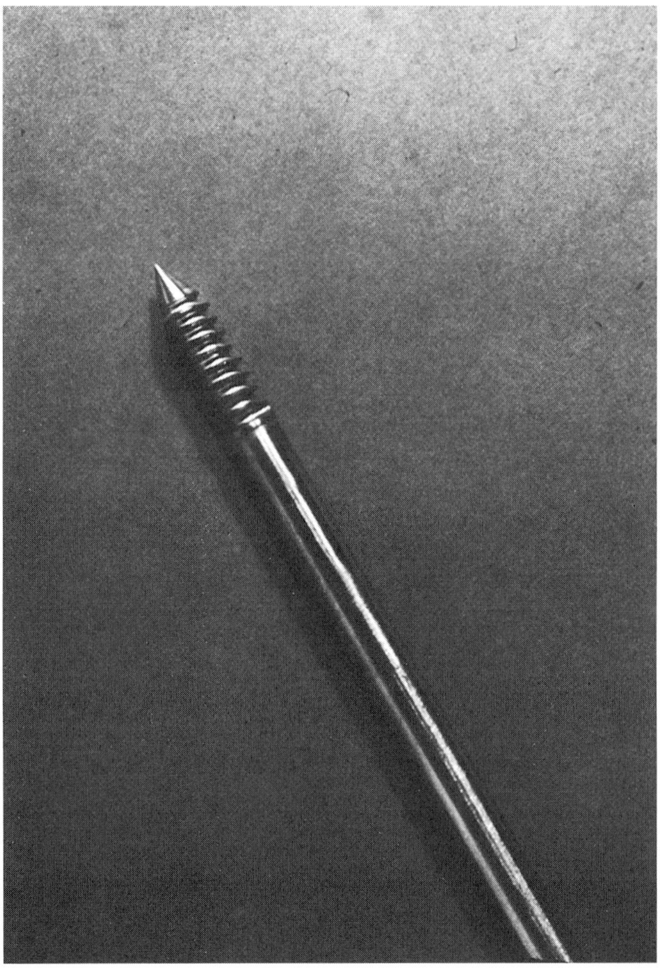

FIG. 8.3.

Myoma screw.

be considered with the use of materials such as absorbable oxidized regenerated cellulose (Interceed; Johnson & Johnson, New Brunswick, NJ) or polytetrafluoroethylene barrier (Gore-Tex Surgical Membrane; W.L. Gore and Associates, Flagstaff, AZ) which can facilitate this objective. The myoma is then removed by either sectioning-morcellation or through a colpotomy incision. A 10-mm or larger port facilitates laparoscopic removal.

Laparoscopic Myolysis

An alternative to elimination of leiomyomas via an endoscopic approach includes coagulation of leiomyomas in an effort to affect the vascularization and shrinkage of the tumors with use of either a laser [neodymium (Nd):YAG laser] or bipolar needles directed into the leiomyoma, which serve to compromise the blood supply and, thus, provide elimination of the leiomyoma (9–11).

Cryomyolysis is a new technique that requires use of a cryothermal unit (CryoMedical Sciences, Inc., Rockville, MD). A dilute vasopressin solution is utilized followed by monopolar coagulation at the site of planned insertion of the cryoprobe (Fig. 8.4). The most commonly utilized size is a 4.8-mm (diameter) probe. The leiomyoma is identified and "sized." In a patient who desires preservation of her childbearing abilities, it is recommended that simultaneous ultrasonographic assessment be utilized; this facilitates identification of the endometrial cavity.

The cryothermal procedure involves freezing of the leiomyoma with insertion of the cryoprobe directly into the leiomyoma. An iceball is then formed that can be monitored sonographically. End point includes expansion of the freeze to within several millimeters of the endometrial cavity. Once the initial freeze occurs at −180°C, it is maintained for several minutes, during which time palpation (laparoscopically) of the leiomyoma is performed with use of a probe or similar device. Irrigation of the probe as ice forms immediately above the leiomyoma is recommended; Ringer's lactate or a similar irrigation solution is utilized for this purpose. Care must be taken not to have adjacent organs touch the probe during the freezing process. Once an end point is reached, there is a thaw down to −20°C followed by a second freeze,

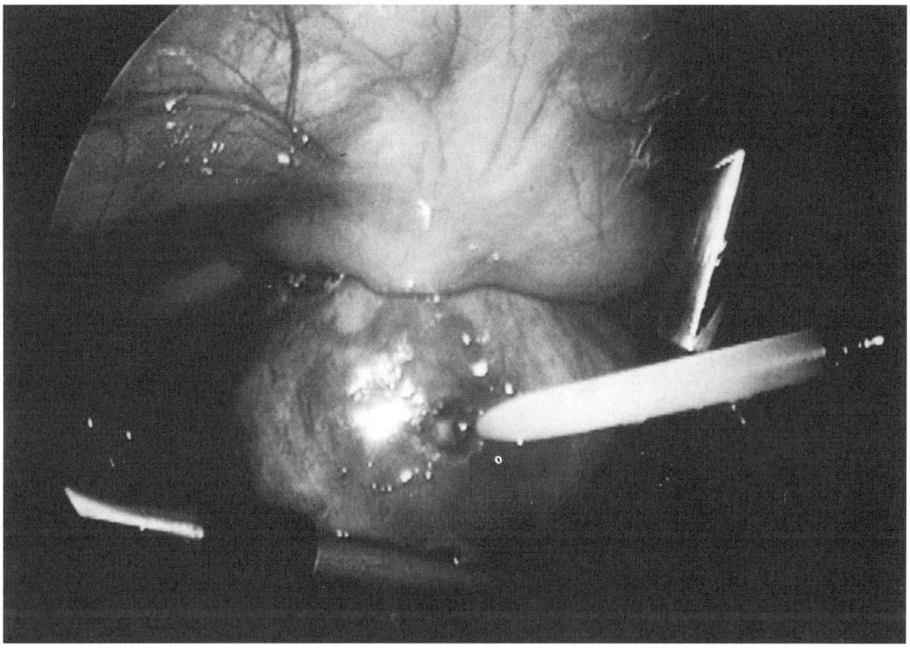

FIG. 8.4.

Technique of cryomyolysis demonstrating cryoprobe.

accomplished in a similar manner. Once this is achieved, thawing occurs and the probe is removed. Any bleeding points are controlled with monopolar coagulation. This is then followed by introduction of a hemostatic agent, such as Topical Thrombin (Parke-Davis, Morris Plains, NJ) followed by placement of Interceed. Preliminary information attests to the cryomyolysis procedure being a most efficacious approach to endoscopic treatment of leiomyomas.

SAFETY AND COMPLICATIONS

Safety concerns, including air embolism, remain of primary importance. Monitoring of vital signs and pulse oximetry including assessment of carbon dioxide levels must be carried out. Identification of a fall in end-tidal CO_2 as well as oxygen saturation, often accompanied by the presence of a mill-wheel murmur, is indicative of air embolization. If this occurs, the procedure should be terminated immediately, with the patient placed in either a left lateral decubitus or deep Trendelenburg's position and given pure oxygen. It may be necessary to introduce a subclavian catheter or direct intracardiac aspiration for removal of the air embolus. Other precautions to prevent air embolization include prevention of air entry through the cannula as the resectoscope is removed, with the surgeon placing his/her finger over the end of the hysteroscopic sheath as the resectoscope is removed. Proper training, including didactic sessions, tutorials, and preceptorships, is most important in acquiring appropriate hysteroscopic skills.

Perhaps the most important advice is to anticipate, and thus prevent, laparoscopic complications associated with myomectomy. Preoperative evaluation for any underlying bleeding diathesis, anemia, pelvic inflammatory disease, or pregnancy should be carried out. Hemorrhagic complications have been reported at myomectomy when degenerating leiomyomas or pregnancy, or both, are present (12,13).

As previously noted, patients must also be informed preoperatively of the potential for adhesion formation following the myomectomy. Concern for the rare, but potential, finding of sarcomatous change (incidence 0.1–1.0%) must also be kept in mind. As deemed necessary, a biopsy should be performed before the myomectomy procedure. Intraoperative bleeding is best controlled with use of coagulation or suture reapproximation, or both. Once again, anticipation and prevention of "potential bleeding" represent the most logical approach. Patients should also be informed of the potential for uterine dehiscence at the site of myoma including when a laparoscopic approach occurs (14).

SUMMARY

Careful patient selection, proper counseling, and obtaining an informed consent provide the appropriate prerequisites for proceeding with myomectomy when indicated through any of a number of approaches.

The most feasible surgical procedure must take into account physician expertise, preoperative medical therapy as indicated, and the understanding on the part of the patient that the potential for recurrence and subsequent surgical intervention is of paramount importance. In general, a recurrence rate of 8% and a reoperation rate of 7% have been reported (15).

REFERENCES

1. Politzer F, Kronzon I, Wieczore R, et al. Intercardiac leiomyomatosis: diagnosis and treatment. J Am Coll Cardiol 1984;4:629.
2. Stancanelli B, Seminari G, Vita A, et al. Extension of a pelvic tumor into the right atrium. N Engl J Med 1995;33:1013–1014.
3. Buttram VC Jr, Reiter RC. Uterine leiomyomata: etiology, symptomatology and management. Fertil Steril 1981;36:433–445.
4. Vollenhoven BJ, Lawrence AS, Healy DL. Uterine fibroids: a clinical review. Br J Obstet Gynaecol 1990;97:285–298.
5. ACOG Technical Bulletin No. 192, May 1994.
6. Parker WH, Fu YS, Berek JS. Uterine sarcoma in patients operated on for presumed leiomyoma and rapidly growing leiomyoma. Obstet Gynecol 1994;83:414–418.
7. Friedman AJ, Hoffman DI, Comite F, et al. Treatment of leiomyomata uteri with leuprolide acetate depot: a double-blind placebo-controlled multicentered study. Obstet Gynecol 1991;77:720–725.
8. Dubuisson JB, Lecuru F, Foulot H, et al. Myomectomy by laparoscopy: a preliminary report of 43 cases. Fertil Steril 1991;56:827–830.
9. Donnez J, Gillerot S, Bourjon D, et al. Neodymium:YAG laser hysteroscopy in large submucous fibroids. Fertil Steril 1990;54:999.
10. Nisolle M, Smets M, Malvaux V, et al. Laparoscopic myolysis with Nd:YAG laser. J Gynecol Surg 1993;9:95.
11. Goldfarb HA. Removing uterine fibroids laparoscopically. Contemp Obstet Gynecol 1994;39:50.
12. Hassan F, Arumugan K, Sivanesaratnan V. Uterine leiomyomata in pregnancy. Int J Gynaecol Obstet 1991;34:45–48.
13. Sanfilippo JS, Lincoln SR. Laparoscopic uterine myomectomy: hemorrhagic complications. In: Corfman R, Diamond M, DeCherney A, eds.

Complications of laparoscopic surgery. Cambridge, MA: Blackwell Science, 1993:98.
14. Harris WJ. Uterine dehiscence following laparoscopic myomectomy. Obstet Gynecol 1992;80:545–546.
15. Verkauf BS. Myomectomy for fertility enhancement and preservation. Fertil Steril 1992;58:1.

CHAPTER

9

Prevention of Adhesions Following Myomectomy

Togas Tulandi

One common cause of postsurgical adhesions is myomectomy (1–3). Adhesions between loops of bowel can cause bowel obstruction and abdominal pain, whereas adnexal adhesions can impair fertility. The purpose of this review is to evaluate factors that may be associated with adhesion formation and methods to minimize adhesion formation.

ADHESION FORMATION AFTER MYOMECTOMY

Site of Myomectomy Incision

Myomectomy is often associated with adhesion formation. Most of the adhesions are found between the uterine incision and omentum and intestine. Adhesions are almost always formed after a myomectomy by laparotomy (3–6). However, laparoscopic myomectomy is also associated with adhesion formation (1,2,7,8) (Table 9.1). Myomectomy with a posterior uterine incision is associated with a higher degree of adnexal adhesions than that with fundal or anterior uterine incision (3). The most favorable incision is one that is located anteriorly.

TABLE 9.1

Adhesions after laparoscopic myomectomy

STUDY	TOTAL NO. OF PATIENTS	SIZE OF MYOMA (CM)	ADHESIONS*
Nezhat et al, 1991 (2)	154	3–15	30/56 sites (53.6%)
Daniell and Gurley, 1991 (7)	17	3–7	1/1 patients (100%)
Dubuisson et al, 1991 (8)	49	1–11	1/6 patients (16.6%)
Hasson et al, 1992 (1)	56	3–16	16/24 patients (66.6%)

*Evaluated at the second-look laparoscopy.
Source: Reproduced by permission from Tulandi T. The role of laparoscopy in the management of leiomyoma uteri. SOGC 1994;16:1903–1908.

Postoperative adhesions are usually found between the bladder and the anterior wall of the uterus, preserving the adnexa. Myomectomy with fundal incision causes intra-abdominal adhesions, but it is associated with a mild degree of adnexal adhesions. Clearly, the worst is posterior uterine incision.

Estrogen and Adhesions

Estrogen has also been associated with increased adhesion formation in animal models (9–13). In a rabbit model, oophorectomized animals had decreased total adhesion scores compared to those of intact animals. In a rat model, fat necrosis and fibrotic changes were found less often in the absence of estrogen. These findings suggest the possible role of estrogen in adhesion formation. In the clinical setting, the hypoestrogenic state can be induced by the administration of luteinizing hormone-releasing hormone (LHRH) analog or antagonist. It also reduces the size of the myoma, leading to a smaller incision, less tissue dissection, less bleeding, and less suture material. Whether the hypoestrogenic state leads to fewer postmyomectomy adhesions remains unknown.

SURGICAL TECHNIQUE TO MINIMIZE ADHESION FORMATION

Myomectomy with anterior uterine incision is associated with the least adhesion formation while posterior incision causes a high degree of adhesions (3). Therefore, anterior incision should be the incision of choice and posterior incision should be avoided. Leiomyoma on the posterior uterine wall can be removed by fundal incision, but this may not always be possible. The site of uterine incision that allows removal of as many myomas as possible should also be selected. Incision can be done with laser, electrocautery, or a regular knife with no difference in clinical results. In order to minimize bleeding, a dilute solution of vasopressin (0.5 units/mL) is first injected into the incision site.

The myomectomy incision is closed in layers. The deep myometrium can be closed with any type of suture material without influencing adhesion formation. However, suture that incorporates the uterine serosa should not be reactive material including catgut. Two layers of 1-0 suture for the deep layers and 4-0 suture for the serosal layer are usually used. The suture materials are either polyglactin (Vicryl), polyglycolic acid (Dexon), or polydioxanone (PDS). However, the braided fibers of polyglactin may produce a sawing effect in tissue leading to more injury and adhesions compared to monofilament suture such as polydioxanone (14).

Adhesion formation can also be reduced by gentle tissue handling, meticulous hemostasis, and avoidance of tissue drying. This can be achieved by constant irrigation of the operative field. Infection can predispose to adhesion formation, and prophylactic antibiotics can be administered. Tissue necrosis and ischemia should be avoided. In a rat model, Ringer's lactate solution decreases adhesion formation (15). Many reproductive surgeons routinely instill 500 to 1000 mL Ringer's lactate solution at the completion of the procedure. This practice is safe and economical, but its efficacy in reducing postmyomectomy adhesions is unclear.

Second-Look Laparoscopy

A second-look laparoscopy to liberate the adhesions should be considered especially after a myomectomy with posterior incision. Among infertile women with a large uterine leiomyoma of at least 16 weeks' size, conception occurs in the majority of patients who undergo a myomectomy and second-look laparoscopy (3) (Fig. 9.1). A second-look laparoscopy should be performed early (within 6 weeks) after the initial surgery. After a reproductive surgery, late second-look laparoscopy is associated with a more difficult lysis of thick, vascular, and organized adhesions, and it does not increase the pregnancy rate. Early second-look

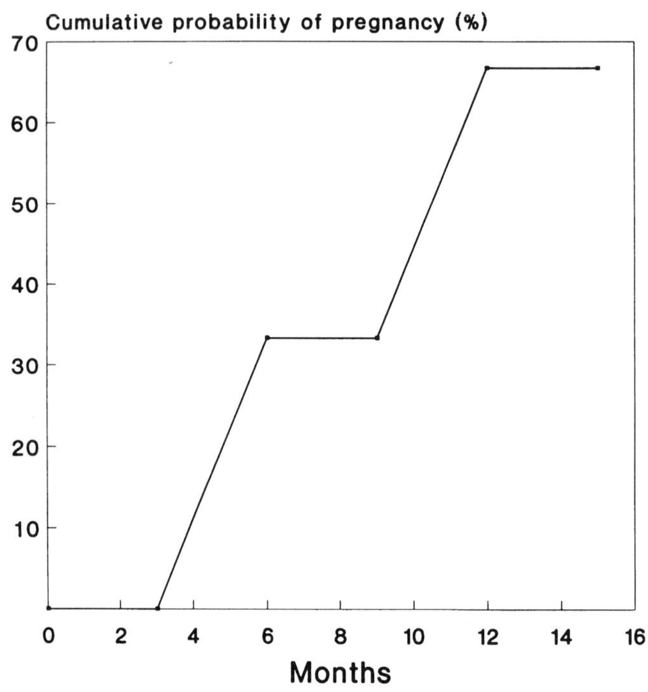

FIG. 9.1.

Cumulative pregnancy rate among women who had a myomectomy and a second-look laparoscopy. Time 0 was the day of myomectomy.
(Reproduced by permission from Tulandi T, Murray C, Guralnick M. Adhesion formation and reproductive outcome after myomectomy and second-look laparoscopy. Obstet Gynecol 1993;82:213.)

laparoscopy has some disadvantages. It requires another anesthesia and is clinically impractical. Furthermore, most insurance companies in the United States do not provide remuneration for this additional surgery. In a monkey model (16), the efficacy of a second-look laparoscopy is similar to that of an adhesion barrier.

Adhesion Barrier and Substances

No adjuvant treatment has been demonstrated to be effective in preventing adhesion formation to the uterine incision sites. Barrier materials, including absorbable oxidized regenerated cellulose (Interceed (TC7), Johnson & Johnson Medical, New Brunswick, NJ) and non-absorbable expanded polytetrafluoroethylene (PTFE; Gore-Tex Surgical Membrane, W.L. Gore and Associates, Flagstaff, AZ) have been used. However, hemostasis at the myomectomy site is rarely complete and it may preclude the use of oxidized regenerated cellulose. In a rat uterine horn model, Poloxamer 407 is effective in reducing adhesion, but the presence of blood also reduces its efficacy (17).

Polytetrafluoroethylene surgical membrane is effective in reducing postmyomectomy adhesion formation (18) (Table 9.2). The mechanism of action of PTFE is based on the principle that surgically injured tissues heal without forming adhesions if the traumatized surfaces in apposition

TABLE 9.2

Adhesion on myomectomy sites covered with expanded polytetrafluoroethylene (PTFE) and those that are uncovered (control)

SITE	PTFE	CONTROL	*p*
Adhesion free	15/27 (55.6%)	2/27 (7.4%)	0.0003
Adhesion score	1.88 ± 0.46	7.55 ± 0.57	0.0001

Source: Reproduced by permission from The Myomectomy Adhesion Study Group. An expanded-polytetrafluoroethylene barrier (Gore-Tex Surgical Membrane) reduces post-myomectomy adhesion formation. Fertil Steril 1995;491:63.

are mechanically separated to allow each surface to heal independently. It has been noted that PTFE prevents adhesion formation and reformation regardless of the type of tissue injury or whether hemostasis is achieved. PTFE can be left in the abdominal cavity. It is among the most inert biomaterials known, resisting chemical and biologic degradation even after several years in vivo. It has been left in the pericardium without clinical sequelae (18). However, the long-term implications of leaving PTFE in the abdominal cavity remain to be seen.

CONCLUSION

Myomectomy, especially with posterior uterine incision, is often associated with intra-abdominal and periadnexal adhesions. In order to minimize the adhesion formation, myomectomy should be done using basic principles of microsurgery, including gentle tissue handling, meticulous hemostasis, and avoidance of tissue drying. Reducing the size of the myoma with LHRH analog leads to a smaller incision, less tissue dissection, and less suture material. The hypoestrogenic state caused by LHRH analog may also promote less adhesion formation. Covering the incision sites with PTFE surgical membrane has been shown to decrease adhesion formation. Alternatively, a second-look laparoscopy to liberate the adhesions can be done.

REFERENCES

1. Hasson HM, Rotman C, Rana N, et al. Laparoscopic myomectomy. Obstet Gynecol 1992;80:884–888.
2. Nezhat C, Nezhat F, Silfen SL, et al. Laparoscopic myomectomy. Int J Fertil 1991;36:275–280.
3. Tulandi T, Murray C, Guralnick M. Adhesion formation and reproductive outcome after myometomy and second-look laparoscopy. Obstet Gynecol 1993;82:213.
4. Starks GC. CO_2 laser myomectomy in an infertile population. J Reprod Med 1988;33:184–186.

5. Jansen RP. Early laparoscopy after pelvic operations to prevent adhesions: safety and efficacy. Fertil Steril 1988;49:26–31.
6. Surrey MW. Postoperative adhesion formation following myomectomy. 41st Annual Meeting of the Pacific Coast Fertility Society, P-006, Indian Wells, CA, April 14–18, 1993.
7. Daniell JF, Gurley LD. Laparoscopic treatment of clinically significant symptomatic fibroids. J Gynecol Surg 1991;7:37–40.
8. Dubuisson JB, Lecuru F, Foulot H, et al. Myomectomy by a laparoscopy: a preliminary report of 43 cases. Fertil Steril 1991;56:827.
9. Metzger DA, Breault DT, Chaffkin L, Luciano AA. The role of estrogen in adhesion formation. 39th Annual Meeting of the Society for Gynecologic Investigations, Abstract P187, San Antonio, TX, March 18–21, 1992.
10. Metzger DA, Breault DT, Chaffkin L, Luciano AA. The role of estrogen suppression versus oophorectomy in adhesion formation. 40th Annual Meeting of the Society for Gynecologic Investigations, Abstract P347, Toronto, Ontario, Canada, March 31–April 3, 1993.
11. LaMorte A, Gutmann JN, Carcangiu ML, et al. The role of estrogen in adhesion formation. 40th Annual Meeting of the Society for Gynecologic Investigations, Abstract P292, Toronto, Ontario, Canada, March 31–April 3, 1993.
12. Grow DR, Coddington CC, Seltman H, Hodgen GD. Role of hypoestrogens in adhesion formation after myometrial surgery in primates. 50th Annual Meeting of the American Fertility Society, San Antonio, TX, November 5–10, 1994.
13. Wright JA, Sharpe KL. Gonadotrophin releasing hormone agonist (GnRHa) therapy reduces postoperative adhesion formation and reformation following adhesiolysis in rat models for adhesion formation and endometriosis. 50th Annual Meeting of the American Fertility Society, San Antonio, TX, November 5–10, 1994.
14. Hurd WW, Himebaugh KS, Cofer KF, et al. Etiology of closure-related adhesion formation after wedge resection of the rabbit ovary. J Reprod Med 1993;38:465–468.
15. Pagidas K, Tulandi T. Effect of Ringer's lactate, Interceed (TC7), and Gore-Tex Surgical Membrane on postsurgical adhesion formation. Fertil Steril 1992;57:199–201.
16. Grow DR, Seltman HJ, Coddington CC, Hodgen GD. The reduction of postoperative adhesions by two different barrier methods versus control in

cynomolgous monkeys: a prospective, randomized, crossover study. Fertil Steril 1994;61:1141–1146.

17. Montgomery Rice V, Shanti A, Moghissi KS, Leach RE. A comparative evaluation of Poloxamer 407 and oxidized regenerated cellulose [(Interceed (TC7)] to reduce postoperative adhesion formation in the rat uterine horn model. Fertil Steril 1993;59;901–906.
18. The Myomectomy Adhesion Study Group. An expanded-polytetrafluoroethylene barrier (Gore-Tex Surgical Membrane) reduces post-myomectomy adhesion formation. Fertil Steril 1995;63:491.

CHAPTER

10

Reproductive and Obstetric Performance in the Postmyomectomy Patient

Lisa A. Hasty

The supreme result of a myomectomy lies in the pregnancy which may follow.
H. A. Kelly

Indications for myomectomy are well documented. These include menorrhagia, metrorrhagia, menometrorrhagia, pelvic pain, or a pelvic mass found at laparotomy in a woman who wishes to maintain her capability to bear children. Myomectomies have been performed for the correction of infertility and recurrent pregnancy loss (1). Myomas may contribute to spontaneous abortion in the first trimester, premature labor in the second and third trimester, placental abruption, fetal malpresentation, dystocia during labor, and postpartum hemorrhage and puerperal infection (2). This operative procedure is intended to preserve childbearing capabilities and eliminate these possible causes of reproductive failure. Therefore, the reproductive and obstetric outcomes for this operative procedure must be examined and understood. In 1958, Rubin (3) reported that 40% of women with multiple fibroid tumors have a history of childlessness. Improvements in reproductive therapies, the difficulty of adoption, and the more frequent occurrence of myomas in the later reproductive years have led to a greater percentage of myomectomies being performed (4). Additionally, no current medical treatment exists to accomplish the permanent resolution of myomas. With the increasing use of this conservative operation to eliminate these tumors, clinicians and investigators should examine the long-term reproductive outcomes for this procedure.

REPRODUCTIVE OUTCOMES

> *Since cure without deformity or loss of function must ever be surgery's highest ideal, the general proposition that myomectomy is a greater surgical achievement than hysterectomy is incontestable.*
>
> Victor Bonney

In 1946, Dr. Bonney was aware of the need for preservation of function. This ideal has been maintained through the years. Investigators continue to identify surgical techniques and various adjunctive therapies to improve subsequent reproductive performance in postmyomectomy patients.

Reproductive outcomes following myomectomy obviously may differ according to the patient population that is studied. As expected, factors such as maternal age, previous pregnancies, and coexistent infertility problems affect outcome. In a study by Ingersoll (5), postmyomectomy reproductive performance was evaluated in two groups of patients: those who had previous pregnancies and those who had been infertile. Of the patients with a previous pregnancy, 60% conceived following the myomectomy procedure. Of the group of patients who had been infertile before their procedure, 20 of 39 conceived postmyomectomy. Myomas have been implicated as a contributory factor to infertility (3,6–10).

The mechanism by which a leiomyoma interferes with conception is dependent upon its location, size, and blood supply. Submucous myomas may interfere with implantation, and myomas involving the cornual portion of the tube may create a physical obstruction leading to infertility. Additionally, large myomas can alter the position of the ovaries in relation to the tubal fimbria (5). The exact way in which some myomas impair fertility is not fully understood. Investigators have speculated that myomas interfere with sperm transport, distort the course of the fallopian tube, compress the cervical canal, or alter the position of the cervix (11).

The interference with implantation may be due to the presence of submucous myomas. Likewise, intramural myomas may disrupt uterine physiology as well as anatomy. Abnormalities of the myometrial venous patterns from compression and obstruction of venous plexi have been demonstrated radiographically (12). Furthermore, histologic abnormalities of the endometrium associated with myomas are often demonstrated (13).

Limited information exists regarding patients who are undergoing myomectomy for infertility isolated to uterine myoma (4). Several reviews have attempted to examine this issue. Of previously infertile women from 18 studies who were undergoing myomectomy, 40% became pregnant postoperatively (14). However, many of these patients had other factors that contributed to their reproductive failure, and the relative importance of myomectomy as a fertility-enhancing operation was difficult to evaluate. Buttram and Reiter's review (14) includes three studies with a total of 76 patients undergoing this procedure with no other apparent cause for infertility, of whom 54% became pregnant postoperatively.

The increased utilization of myomectomy to preserve or enhance fertility requires further evaluation of postmyomectomy outcomes. Verkauf (4) reviewed six large studies of this very issue and reported his own experience (15–19). Studies were performed after 1983 and utilized current microsurgical principles. Furthermore, complete preoperative infertility evaluations were performed to exclude other potential causes of infertility. Thus, 234 patients were similarly evaluated and treated to allow for assessment of future reproductive outcome, treatment of infertility, and/or recurrent pregnancy loss, as well as operative risks (4). All myomectomies were performed for at least one tumor greater than 3 cm in size, and multiple myomectomy was more common than removal of a single myoma.

Table 10.1 represents the reproductive performance of the 234 women involved in the various studies. Of note, 57% of patients with no history of infertility conceived after myomectomy. Most importantly,

TABLE 10.1

Pregnancy in patients attempting conception after myomectomy

		No History of or Evaluation for Infertility			History of Infertility: Recurrent Abortion			History of Infertility: Multifactor			History of Infertility: Myoma Alone			Length of Follow-up with Exposure in All Patients (mo)
Year	Author	No.	Pregnancy (%)	Live Birth	No.	Pregnancy (%)	Live Birth	No.	Pregnancy (%)	Live Birth	No.	Pregnancy (%)	Live Birth	
1983	Berkeley et al (1)	15/22[a]	68.2	59.0	1/3	33.3	33.3	8/19	42.1	26.0	1/6	16.7	16.7	59 (17–127)[b]
1984	Garcia and Tureck (15)										8/13	61.5	46.2‡	At least 10
1986	Rosenfeld (16)										15/23	65.2	56.5	At least 12
1987	Reyniak and Corenthal (17)										7/10	70.0	NS	NS (8–26)[c]
1988	Stark (18)				6/8	75.0	NS				14/24	58.3	NS	20 (12–36)
1990	Smith and Uhlir (19)	16/32	50.0	40.0										NS
1991	Verkauf and Bernhisel (unpublished data)				2/2	100	100	12/21	57.1	47.6	2/3	66.7	66.7	42 (4–112)
	Total	31/54	57.4		9/13	69.2		20/40	50.0		47/79	59.5		

NS, not stated.
[a] Number of pregnancies/total number of patients.
[b] Values are averages or medians with ranges in parentheses.
[c] One termination of pregnancy; one spontaneous abortion followed by subsequent conception in late second trimester doing well.

59% of patients without other apparent causes who underwent this operative procedure for infertility conceived in the follow-up periods. Of note, 69% of those with recurrent pregnancy wastage conceived in the postoperative period.

Tables 10.2 and 10.3 represent the duration of infertility and cumulative pregnancy rates for the various studies. Importantly, the time to conception is short postoperatively. A high percentage conceive within one year despite significant durations of infertility.

Other variables must also be taken into account by investigators including preoperative uterine size and myoma location. Interestingly, investigators Babaknia et al (20) and Ingersoll (5) did not find that preoperative distortion of the uterine cavity affected the likelihood of pregnancy. Malone (21) reported that patients with multiple fibroid tumors were more likely to require future definitive surgery and were less likely to conceive and carry to term than those patients with a single fibroid tumor. In 1981, Buttram and Reiter (14) reported no conceptions following myomectomy in patients with uteri larger than 10 weeks, but subsequent reports have not confirmed this finding (16). Surgical technique and ancillary measures at the time of operation could influence postoperative pregnancy rates. The data collected from the six large studies do not answer these questions conclusively (Tables 10.4 and 10.5). Therefore, the impact of prophylactic antibiotics, tourniquets, vasopressin, and other adjunctive therapies on subsequent pregnancy rates is not known at the present time. The percentage of patients who conceived following myomectomy is clearly highest in the younger age groups, as has been demonstrated by Ingersoll (5) as well as subsequent authors (Table 10.6).

Starks (18) reported improved hemostasis and reproductive performance in myomectomies performed with the carbon dioxide laser versus conventional myomectomy. In the first postoperative year, 75% (15/20) of patients were able to conceive. Larger series are needed to validate this finding. The attention to microsurgical techniques in myomectomies should be emphasized. Berkeley et al (1) and Gehlbach et al (22) concluded that the procedure itself may decrease fertility, probably as a result of adhesion formation. Adhesion formation is a complication of myomectomy, but very few data exist concerning its incidence.

TABLE 10.2

Duration of infertility, cumulative pregnancy rates (PRs), and length of time to conception in women with otherwise unexplained infertility or recurrent abortion undergoing myomectomy and attempting to conceive

				Cumulative PRs[a]								
				0 to 1 Yr		1 to 2 Yr		2 to 3 Yr		Total crude PRs		
Year	Author	No.	Duration of Infertility (mo)	No.	% Cumulative	No.	% Cumulative	No.	% Cumulative	No.	% Cumulative	Time to Conception (mo)[b]
1983	Berkeley et al (1)	9	NS	NS		NS		NS		2/9	22.2	NS
1984	Garcia and Tureck (15)	15	36	5	33.3 (5/15)	2	46.7 (7/15)	0	46.7 (7/15)	8/15	53.3	NS (1–38)
1986	Rosenfeld (16)	23	61 (12–132)[b]	14	60.9 (14/23)	1	65.2 (15/23)	0	65.2 (15/23)	15/23	65.2	NS (3–20)
1987	Reyniak and Corenthal (17)	10	NS	NS		NS				7/10	70.0	NS (8–16)
1988	Starks (18)	32	NS	15	46.9 (15/32)	NS		NS	62.5	20/32	62.5	8.5 (3–36)
1991	Verkauf and Bernhisel (unpublished data)	5	78 (18–108)	1	20 (1/5)	1	40.0 (2/5)	1	60.0 (3/5)	4/5	80.0	39 (9–72)

NS, not stated.

[a] Values are percents with number conceiving/total number in parentheses.

[b] Values are averages or medians with ranges in parentheses.

TABLE 10.3

Proportion of patients conceiving in time subsequent to myomectomy for otherwise unexplained infertility

Year	Author	Time to conception: 0 to 1 Yr				1 to 2 Yr				2 to 3 Yr				Total crude PR
		No.	%	No. Cumulative	%	No.	%	No. Cumulative	%	No.	%	No. Cumulative	%	%
1983	Berkeley et al (1)	NS	NS	NS	NS	NS	NS	NS	NS	NS	NS	NS	NS	16.7 (1/6)*
1984	Garcia and Tureck (15)	5/8	62.5	5/8	62.5	2/8	25.0	7/8	87.5	0/8	0	7/8	87.5	53.3 (8/15)
1986	Rosenfeld (16)	14/15	93.3	14/15	93.3	1/15	6.7	15/15	100					65.2 (15/23)
1987	Reyniak and Corenthal (17)	NS				NS		17/17	100					70.0 (7/10)
1988	Starks (18)	NS				NS						14/14	100	58.3 (14/24)
1991	Verkauf and Bernhisel (unpublished data)	1/2	50	1/2	50	0	0	1/2	50	1/2	50	2/2	100	66.7 (2/3)

NS, not stated.

* Values in parentheses are number conceiving/total number.

TABLE 10.4

Ancillary measures used at surgery

Year	Author	No.	Prophylactic Antibiotics	Corticosteroids	Hyskon*	Clamps or Tourniquet	Vasoconstrictor	Uterine Suspension	Laser
1983	Berkeley et al (1)	50	−	+	+	+	−	18/50	−
1984	Garcia and Tureck (15)	17	+	+	−	+	NS	NS	−
1986	Rosenfeld (16)	23	+	11/23	12/23	−	−	10/23	−
1987	Reyniak and Corenthal (17)	17	+	−	+	−	+	NS	+
1988	Starks (18)	32	+	−	+	NS	NS	+	+
1990	Smith and Uhlir (19)	64	−	−	+	+	+	NS	−
1991	Verkauf and Bernhisel (unpublished data)	31	+	16/31	10/32	−	+	5/31	−

−, not used; +, routinely used; NS, not stated.
*Dextran = 70 in dextrose.

TABLE 10.5

Impact of additional factors potentially affecting conception rates

Year	Author	Entry into Uterine Cavity	Distorted Uterine Cavity Preoperatively	No. of Fibroids Removed	Weight/No. of Myomas or Size of Uterus	No. of Uterine Incisions	Uterine Suspension	Age	Duration of Infertility
1983	Berkeley et al (1)	+	NS	+	+	NS	NS	+	NS
1984	Garcia and Tureck (15)	–	–	NS	NS	NS	NS	NS	NS
1986	Rosenfeld (16)	NS	–	–	–	NS	+	–	+
1987	Reyniak and Corenthal (17)	–	–	NS	NS	NS	NS	NS	NS
1988	Starks (18)	NS	NS	NS	NS	NS	NS	+	+
1990	Smith and Uhlir (19)	NS	NS	NS	–	NS	NS	–	NS
1991	Verkauf and Bernhisel (unpublished data)	–	–	–	–	–	–	–	+

+, positive effect, although not necessarily statistically significant; –, no apparent effect; NS, not stated.

TABLE 10.6

Myomectomy and the age factor

AGE GROUPS (YR)	TOTAL NO.	NO. CONCEIVING	NO. FAILING TO CONCEIVE	% CONCEIVED
21–25	4	3	1	75
26–30	18	14	4	77
31–35	16	8	8	50
36–40	13	3	10	23
41+	5	0	5	0
Total	56	28	28	50

McLaughlin (23) reported only minimal adhesions when second-look laparoscopy was performed 6 to 8 weeks following laser myomectomy, while Starks (18), in a later report of laser myomectomy, noted adhesions in 100% of the 20 women who subsequently underwent laparoscopy or cesarean section. Gehlbach et al (22) reported an adhesion incidence of 68% in patients who underwent subsequent surgery, with the majority of the adhesions involving the uterus and arising de novo. Tulandi et al (24) have demonstrated using second-look laparoscopy that incisions for myomectomy on the posterior uterine wall are associated with more adnexal adhesions than those on the fundus or anterior uterine wall (93.7% vs. 55.5%). The cumulative pregnancy rate in this series of 26 patients was 33.4% at 6 months and 66.7% at 12 months after the procedure. Therefore, these investigations recommend avoiding posterior uterine incision to minimize the incidence of adnexal adhesions, the types of adhesions that are most critical to subsequent fertility.

In addition to de novo adhesions affecting fertility, adhesion reformation is a large factor as well. Several investigations have noted that the presence of even filmy adhesions at the time of myomectomy, which are lysed, is associated with reduced chances of conceiving (22).

The evaluation of second-look laparoscopy and various adjunct therapies should be continued in the hopes of evaluating subsequent pregnancy rates. Many studies have determined that both second-look laparoscopy with adhesiolysis and adjunctive measures are effective in reducing postoperative adhesions. However, postprocedure pregnancy rates have not been evaluated conclusively.

In selected cases, primary laparoscopic removal of myomas may be possible. Several investigations have reported acceptable pregnancy rates following this procedure in a small series of patients. Hasson et al (25) reported 9 of 12 patients conceiving in a 12-month follow-up period. Nezhat et al (26) described a series of 158 patients undergoing laparoscopic myomectomy for a variety of indications. Only six pregnancies were reported, but it is unclear how many patients desired fertility. The authors point out that large prospective studies are necessary to determine the advisability of performing this technique of myomectomy in patients who wish for future fertility.

RECURRENT PREGNANCY LOSS

Myomas may impair the blood supply to the endometrium, causing atrophic changes and interfering with implantation of a blastocyst. Recurrent pregnancy loss may result from the presence of submucous myomas. Furthermore, strategically located intramural myomas may compromise uterine blood flow also leading to early pregnancy wastage (11).

Recurrent pregnancy loss remains an indication for myomectomy. The frequency of recurrent spontaneous abortion following myomectomy is reduced dramatically (6,20). Therefore, this indication remains clear. Garcia and Tureck (15) reported their experience with removal of large (≥5 cm) submucous myomas by the abdominal approach. The subsequent pregnancy rate of patients for the 10-month follow-up period was 61.5%. Broad-based submucous myomas or myomas that deeply invade the myometrium are generally best treated by abdominal myomectomy. In these cases, hysteroscopic removal is unusually incomplete and the risk of intrauterine adhesion formation is increased.

In Buttram and Reiter's (14) review of 1941 patients undergoing myomectomy through a laparotomy incision, fetal wastage was reduced from 41% preoperatively to 19% postoperatively. The combined results of three large series of patients (1,4,18) reveal a 69.2% pregnancy rate in postmyomectomy patients with a history of recurrent abortion. The successful removal of submucous myomas may now be easily accomplished in most cases through hysteroscopic procedures. Corson and Brooks (27) have reported excellent results for hysteroscopic submucous myoma resections in four of six patients with a history of recurrent pregnancy loss who carried to term. Loffer (28) reported similar results. Therefore, removal of myomas in the setting of recurrent miscarriage is frequently rewarding.

OBSTETRIC PERFORMANCE

Uterine leiomyomas are the most common tumor of the uterus, occurring in 20% to 30% of women over age 30 (29). Therefore, myomas are frequently encountered in obstetric patients. Interestingly, multiple studies have evaluated the growth of myomas, revealing that fewer than one third increase in size during pregnancy (30–32). Although most women with uterine myomas have uncomplicated pregnancies, multiple studies have associated leiomyomas in pregnancy with major complications. These include premature labor, abruptio placentae, malpresentation, labor dystocia, intrauterine growth retardation, and pelvic pain (33–35). The location of myomas and uterine size are thought to be critical determinants of these problems (36).

Reports before 1960 found that 57% to 70% of women with leiomyomas had obstetric complications related to the myomas (34,37–40). More recently, Lev-Toaff et al (30) reported that approximately 10% of pregnant patients with leiomyomas had complications related to or caused by the myomas. The discrepancy between the older literature and more recent studies may reflect the fact that earlier studies identified myomas only by physical examination and not by ultrasonographic findings. In two studies using ultrasound to make the diagnosis of a myomatous uterus, it was reported that approximately 30% of women with myomas had pregnancy complications related to the myomas (30,31). Furthermore, the incidence of cesarean delivery is increased in patients with uterine leiomyomas. To prevent the possible complications associated with myomas, many patients are advised to undergo myomectomy before attempting pregnancy. Physicians and patients must be keenly aware of the benefits and risks of this common procedure, especially when future fertility is desired. The potential obstetric risks of not performing the procedure must be compared to the risks of performing a myomectomy. The actual obstetric complications in postmyomectomy patients are reviewed below.

The most serious potential obstetric complication resulting from a previous myomectomy is uterine rupture. The incidence is rare, but several reports exist in the current literature (41–43). Rupture of the uterus is a serious threat to the life of the mother as well as to the fetus. The overall incidence of uterine rupture is 1 in 1500 deliveries (44,45), and most of these cases had predisposing factors such as previous uterine scars, invasive placenta, or a history of instrumented terminations of pregnancy (41). Garnet reports an incidence of 1 in 40 to 60 cases of uterine rupture attributed to myomectomy scars (46,47). These include only ruptures in the third trimester of pregnancy. One case report describes uterine rupture postmyomectomy at 20 weeks' gestation (41).

Georgakopoulos and Berceuse (42) reported a case of sigmoido-uterine rupture during the third trimester. Two years previously, the patient had undergone a myomectomy at 16 weeks' gestation without incident. A myomectomy performed during pregnancy has a high risk of potential uterine dehiscence.

Most recently, Harris (43) reported the first case of uterine dehiscence following a laparoscopic myomectomy. As stated previously, the incidence of uterine rupture is rare; however, practitioners must be aware that this complication exists even remote from term and labor (41). The decision as to route of delivery in a postmyomectomy patient should be based on the complexity of the myomectomy procedure itself. If a myomectomy results in a defect through or immediately adjacent to the endometrium, pregnancies should be delivered by cesarean section (44). This decision is based on the increased likelihood of uterine dehiscence in these patients; however, uterine separation may occur before active labor.

The possibility of placenta accreta exists when a uterine incision has been made for any reason. Fox (45) reported that 25% of patients with placenta accreta had undergone a previous uterine surgery, but the majority of these were cesarean section.

Another risk that concerns future obstetric outcomes in a post-myomectomy patient is that of myoma recurrence. The 10-year cumulative risk for leiomyoma recurrence after myomectomy is approximately 27% (46).

Current counseling recommendations regarding myomectomy include a consideration of all these factors. Recommendations are frequently based on total uterine size as well as the existence of strategically placed myomas. A prior history of pregnancy loss or preterm labor must also be examined.

MYOMECTOMY DURING PREGNANCY

Most clinicians agree that removal of myomas in pregnancy should be reserved for very selective cases. Burton and associates (47) concluded that only myomas with a discrete pedicle that can be easily ligated should be removed. Further dissection may lead to extreme bleeding and possibilities for uterine dehiscence and pregnancy loss (35). Other investigators (48) follow a more aggressive approach and do not believe that pregnancy losses will be increased; however, this remains to be confirmed by others. Furthermore, the removal of myomas at the time of delivery may lead to hemorrhage, and most practitioners agree that removal should be postponed until after pregnancy. This approach is also validated by the fact that myomas tend to regress in size after pregnancy.

CONCLUSION

The decision to proceed with myomectomy must be based on the reproductive and obstetric outcomes if future fertility is desired. The reasons to proceed with this "conservative" procedure continue to be based on the same principles that were outlined by Stevenson in 1964 (6). When a woman with a myomatous uterus becomes pregnant, the pregnancy may go on to term provided that 1) the myomas are not too large or too numerous, 2) the truly large ones are not in the submucous or intramural situations in the uterine wall, 3) the pedunculated subserous myomas do not twist on their pedicles, and 4) necrosis of any of the myomas does not occur.

As physicians we can only attempt to predict each of these situations based on an individual patient's presentation. With improved surgical skills and technology, this surgical procedure of myomectomy is safely and effectively performed in most situations. The development of various adjunctive measures for adhesion prevention may improve the already very acceptable reproductive and obstetric outcomes. In the future, the role of laparoscopic myomectomy must be analyzed in light of reproductive outcomes as well.

REFERENCES

1. Berkeley AS, DeCherney AH, Polan ML. Abdominal myomectomy and subsequent fertility. Surg Gynecol Obstet 1983;156:319–322.
2. Bardeguez AD. Uterine leiomyomas in pregnancy. Clinical consultations. Obstet Gynecol 1990;2:53–57.
3. Rubin IC. Uterine fibroids and sterility. Clin Obstet Gynecol 1958;1: 501–518.
4. Verkauf BS. Myomectomy for fertility enhancement and preservation. Fertil Steril 1992;58:1–15.
5. Ingersoll FM. Fertility following myomectomy. Fertil Steril 1963;14: 596–602.
6. Stevenson CS. Myomectomy for improvement of fertility. Fertil Steril 1964;15:367–384.
7. Malone LJ, Ingersoll FM. Myomectomy and infertility. In: Behrman SJ, Kistner RW, eds. Progress in infertility. Boston: Little, Brown, 1968: 115–122.
8. Brown AB, Chamberlain R, TeLinde R. Myomectomy. Am J Obstet Gynecol 1956;71:759–763.

9. Meyer B, DeCherney AH. Fibroids and fertility. Clinical consultations. Obstet Gynecol 1990;2:24–28.
10. Israel SL, Mutch JC. Myomectomy. Clin Obstet Gynecol 1958;1: 455–466.
11. Hunt JE, Wallach EE. Uterine factors in infertility. An overview. Clin Obstet Gynecol 1974;17:44.
12. Farrer-Brown G, Beilby JOW, Tarbit MH. The vascular patterns in myomatous uteri. J Obstet Gynaecol Br Commonw 1970;77:967.
13. Deligdish L, Lowenthal M. Endometrial changes associated with myomata uterus. J Clin Pathol 1970;23:676.
14. Buttram VC Jr, Reiter RC. Uterine leiomyomata: etiology, symptomatology and management. Fertil Steril 1981;36:433–445.
15. Garcia C-R, Tureck RW. Submucosal leiomyomas and infertility. Fertil Steril 1984;42:16–19.
16. Rosenfeld DL. Abdominal myomectomy for otherwise unexplained infertility. Fertil Steril 1986;46:328–330.
17. Reyniak JV, Corenthal L. Microsurgical laser technique for abdominal myomectomy. Microsurgery 1987;8:92–98.
18. Starks GC. CO_2 laser myomectomy in an infertile population. J Reprod Med 1988;33:184–187.
19. Smith DC, Uhlir JK. Myomectomy as a reproductive procedure. Am J Obstet Gynecol 1990;62:1476–1482.
20. Babaknia A, Rock JA, Jones HW Jr. Pregnancy success following abdominal myomectomy for infertility. Fertil Steril 1978;30:644.
21. Malone LJ. Myomectomy. Obstet Gynecol 1969;34:200–203.
22. Gehlbach DL, Sousa RC, Carpenter SE, Rock JA. Abdominal myomectomy in the treatment of infertility. Int J Gynaecol Obstet 1993;40: 45–50.
23. McLaughlin DS. Micro-laser myomectomy technique to enhance reproductive potential: a preliminary report. Lasers Surg Med 1982;1: 107.
24. Tulandi T, Murray C, Guralnick M. Adhesion formation and reproductive outcome after myomectomy and second-look laparoscopy. Obstet Gynecol 1993;82:213–215.
25. Hasson HM, Rotman C, Rana N, et al. Laparoscopic myomectomy. Obstet Gynecol 1992;80:885–888.
26. Nezhat C, Nezhat F, Silfen SL, et al. Laparoscopic myomectomy. Int J Fertil 1991;36:275–280.

27. Corson SL, Brooks PG. Resectoscopic myomectomy. Fertil Steril 1991; 55:1041–1044.
28. Loffer FD. Removal of large symptomatic intrauterine growths by the hysteroscopic resectoscope. Obstet Gynecol 1990;76:836.
29. Blaustein A. Pathology of the female genital tract. 2nd ed. Berlin: Springer-Verlag, 1982:354.
30. Lev-Toaff AJ, Coleman BG, Aryer PH, et al. Leiomyoma in pregnancy: sonographic study. Radiology 1987;164:375–380.
31. Winer-Muram HT, Muram D, Gillieson MS. Uterine myoma in pregnancy. J Assoc Can Radiol 1984;35:168–170.
32. Bezjian AA. Pelvic masses in pregnancy. In: Sabbagha RE, ed. Diagnostic ultrasound. 2nd ed. Philadelphia: Lippincott, 1987:521–536.
33. Rice JP, Kay HH, Mahony BS. The clinical significance of uterine leiomyomas in pregnancy. Am J Obstet Gynecol 1989;160:1213–1216.
34. Campbell RE. Pregnancy and labor complicated by myomatous tumors of the uterus. Am J Obstet Gynecol 1933;26:1–16.
35. Watson BP. Pregnancy and labor complicated by fibroid tumors. Am J Obstet Gynecol 1932;23:351–360.
36. Exacoustòs C, Rosati P. Ultrasound diagnosis of uterine myomas and complications in pregnancy. Obstet Gynecol 1993;82:97–101.
37. Gainey HL, Keeler JE. Submucous myoma in term pregnancy. Am J Obstet Gynecol 1949;58:727–737.
38. Grandin DJ. A review of 445 pregnancies complicated by fibromyomas. Am J Obstet Gynecol 1949;57:532–540.
39. Lynch FW. Myomas in pregnancy. Am J Obstet Gynecol 1913;68:427–442.
40. Duckering FA. The significance of myoma uteri in pregnancy. Am J Obstet Gynecol 1946;51:819–831.
41. Golan D, Aharoni A, Gonen R, et al. Early spontaneous rupture of the post myomectomy gravid uterus. Int J Gynaecol Obstet 1990;31:167–170.
42. Georgakopoulos PA, Berceuse GR. Sigmoido-uterine rupture in pregnancy after multiple myomectomy. Int Surg 1981;66:367–368.
43. Harris WE. Uterine dehiscence following laparoscopic myomectomy. Obstet Gynecol 1992;80:545–546.
44. Cunningham FG, et al. eds. William's Obstetrics. 19th ed. Norwalk, CT: Appleton & Lange, 1993:537.
45. Fox H. Placenta accreta, 1945–1969. Obstet Gynecol Surv 1972;27:475.

46. Candiani GB, Fedele L, Parazzini F, Villa L. Risk of recurrence after myomectomy. Br J Obstet Gynaecol 1991;98:385.
47. Burton CA, Grimes DA, March CM. Surgical management of leiomyomata during pregnancy. Obstet Gynecol 1989;74:707–709.
48. Glavind K, Palvio DHB, Lauritsen JG. Uterine myoma in pregnancy. Acta Obstet Gynecol Scand 1990;69:617.

CHAPTER

11

Myomectomy in the Nonreproductive Woman

Victoria M. Maclin

Myomectomy is conventionally thought of as a conservative procedure indicated for women with symptomatic leiomyomas who wish to retain their reproductive potential. Customary doctrine dictates that hysterectomy is the treatment of choice for nonreproductive women with symptomatic leiomyomas (1). After all, of what value is a uterus not used for the primary purpose of gestation? Gynecologists are puzzled when a perimenopausal woman insists on avoiding hysterectomy for a benign, yet problematic, condition. This chapter explores some of the psychological, anatomic, and physiologic ramifications of hysterectomy, including but not limited to the uncelebrated role of the uterus and cervix in the female sexual response. The controversy regarding sexual adjustment after hysterectomy is also discussed. After consideration of these factors, myomectomy may prove to be a preferred choice for selected nonreproductive surgical candidates.

PSYCHOLOGICAL FACTORS

Gender identity is determined at birth by the appearance of external genitalia. Sexual self-image is reinforced during puberty with the development of secondary sex characteristics. Yet, for many women, gender identity and sexual self-image are affected by more than their external appearance. The presence of internal reproductive organs carries significant symbolic meaning with major impact on a woman's sense of femininity (2). Indeed, an identity crisis can be precipitated by hysterectomy if a woman believes that the uterus is that which makes her female (3). The uterus is also a symbol of reproduction. For women who value reproduction as a determinant of femininity and self-worth, loss of the uterus can result in a diminished sense of femininity. Women who have devoted most of their lives to childbearing and child rearing may experience diminished self-esteem after uterine loss even if hysterectomy is done after menopause (3,4).

A woman may grieve the loss of her uterus and some of its more familiar functions, either real or misconceived. She may grieve the loss of menstruation even when hysterectomy results in alleviation of significant physical complaints such as pelvic pain and dysmenorrhea (2,4,5). The misconceived notion that the uterus is a source of strength may leave her feeling physically weakened after hysterectomy (2,4).

The stages of incorporating the loss of a body part into one's self-image have been described (4). These four stages are impact, retreat, acknowledgment, and reconstruction. Drummond and Field (4) described these stages as they pertain to hysterectomy. During the *first stage, impact*, the idea that hysterectomy is necessary looms in the consciousness. The woman focuses her attention on the uterus. For a woman with symptomatic leiomyomas, this stage may be facilitated by symptoms such as pain or abnormal patterns of bleeding. During the *second stage, retreat*, the uterus is "depersonalized." The woman may begin a process of figurative separation from her uterus, a contemplative farewell to an "old friend." This is a stage when the health care provider should pay special attention during preoperative counseling. The patient may attempt figurative separation from her uterus by minimizing its symbolic value. Denial that loss of the uterus will have any subsequent effect can lead to unrealistic expectations of the surgical outcome. Unfortunately this denial can be unwittingly fostered by the health care provider. One 42-year-old patient who presented for evaluation of her loss of libido (in spite of estrogen replacement therapy) 2 years after total abdominal hysterectomy with bilateral salpingo-oophorectomy angrily quoted her physician's preoperative counseling: "You won't notice any difference and neither will your husband. Your vagina will remain intact. Sexual relations will be just the same as long as you take your estrogen." This patient had not only lost her libido, but she had not experienced an orgasm since her surgery. Ironically, she and her husband had an active and satisfying sex life before the operation. Her gynecologist failed to fully inform her of the possible consequences of the surgery such as structural changes, altered sensations during sexual relations, or the consequences of losing ovarian hormone production. Unrealistic expectations may also be sustained if the health care provider fails to dispel myths about uterine function. An effective provider should present comprehensive information about the nature and risks of the procedure. All of the patient's concerns should be clarified and addressed in a forthright manner so as to minimize choices based on ignorance or denial.

During the *third stage, acknowledgment*, the well-informed woman contemplates the meaning of her uterus, the nature and impact of the surgery, and the course of illness and recovery. It is during this time that she can affirm a revised self-image and anticipate uterine loss from the perspective of aspiring toward improved health and well-being. During the *final stage, reconstruction*, the woman proceeds with a revised sense of identity and self-worth that are not predicated on reproductive potential or the presence of internal genitalia. This new identity must incorporate the belief that she is a whole person, sexually intact and capable of satisfactory sexual response. It is important that this new identity is affirmed by her sexual partner and others who may be significant in her life. Melody (6) evaluated depressive reactions following hysterectomy and found that patients who developed depression usually did so as a result of "a traumatic social event that the patient perceived as a real, threatened or symbolic act of disapproval. Hysterectomy, to the woman who became depressed postoperatively, came to mean rejection from the social milieu in which she had previously functioned." Affirmation by one's sexual partner is paramount to maintenance of the woman's positive self-image (3) and sexual responsiveness (2,4,7–9). Hysterectomized women whose sexual partners view them as sexually undesirable are more likely to become depressed (10).

ANATOMIC AND PHYSIOLOGIC FACTORS

The human sexual response, as described by Masters and Johnson in 1966, is divided into four phases: excitement, plateau, orgasm, and resolution (Fig. 11.1). In the female, the uterus is involved in each of these phases. During the excitement phase blood flow to the entire pelvic area is increased, with engorgement of the perivaginal vasculature effecting a transudate across the vaginal epithelium, which creates lubrication (Fig. 11.2A). There is also increased blood flow to the uterus, which causes slight uterine enlargement and elevation of the uterus out of the true pelvis. This elevation produces a tenting effect, which, during the plateau phases, is characterized by ballooning of the upper two thirds of the vagina (Fig. 11.2B). According to Williamson (2) this tenting effect is manifested in many women as a feeling of "needing to be filled up or vaginal achiness, an intense desire for intercourse and for internal pressure." During orgasm, the uterus contracts rhythmically

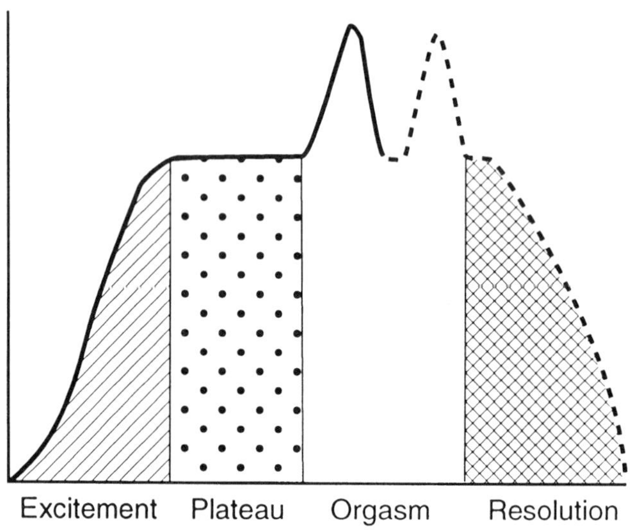

FIG. 11.1.

The four phases of the female human sexual response. The second peak shown with dotted lines during the orgasm phase depicts a woman's ability to achieve multiple orgasm before resolution.

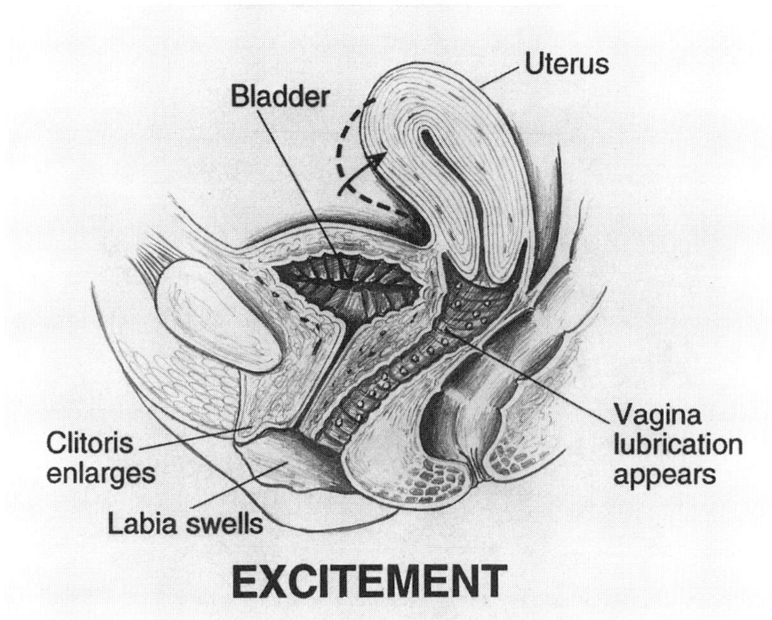

A

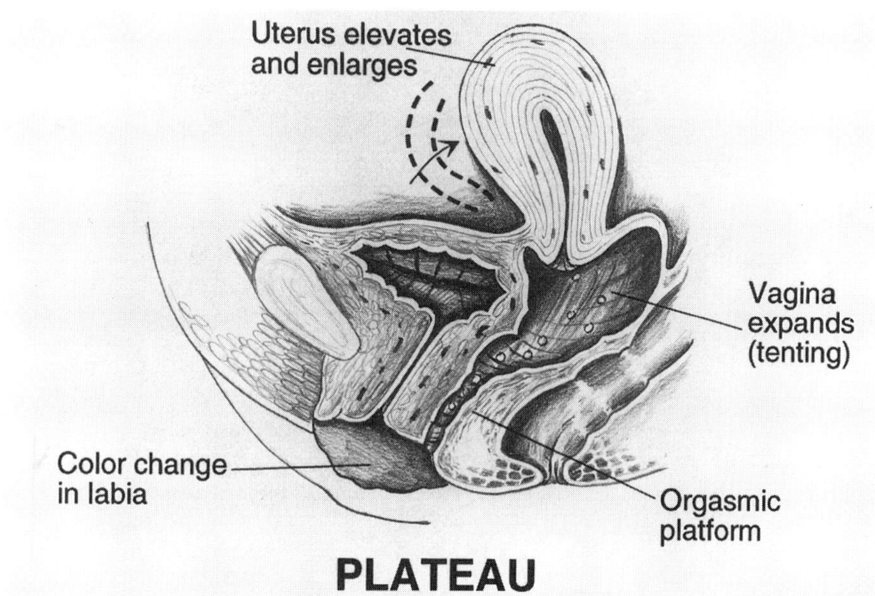

B

FIG. 11.2.

Normal anatomic and physiologic changes of the clitoris, labia, vagina, and uterus during the four phases of female human sexual response: excitement (A), plateau (B), orgasm (C), and resolution (D).

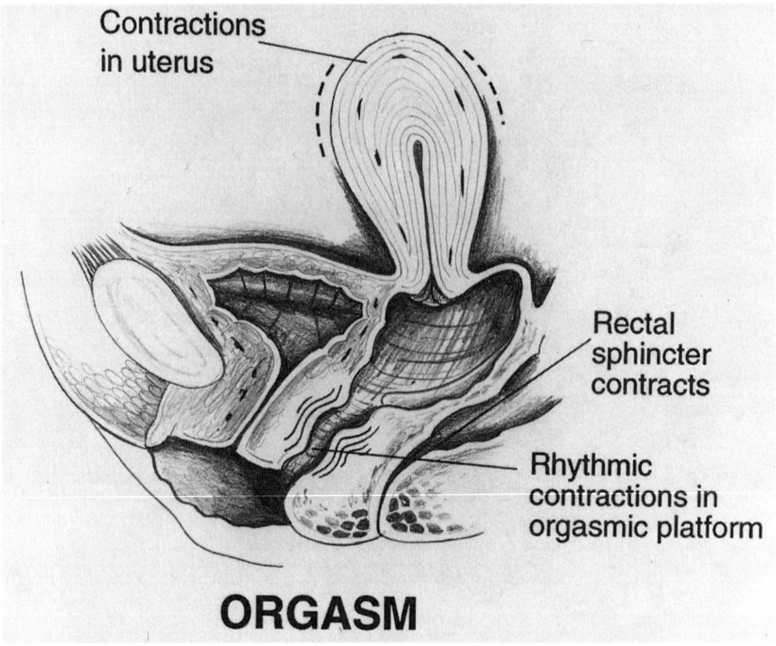

C

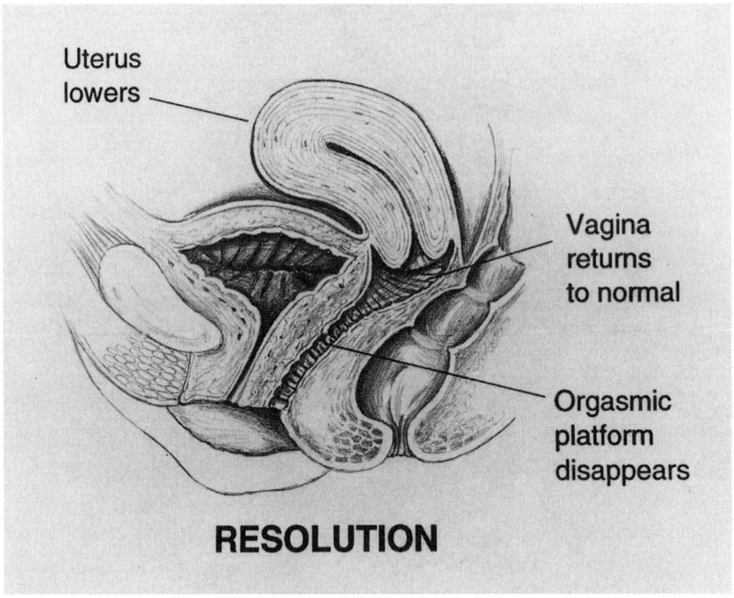

D

FIG. 11.2.

Continued

(Fig. 11.2C). During resolution, the uterus returns to the true pelvis (Fig. 11.2D).

In addition to the above mentioned changes, an intact vaginal apex and cervix may play a specific role in enhancement of arousal and induction of orgasm. Deep penile thrusting with pressure on the inner vagina and cervix may stimulate pressure-sensitive nerves of the Frankenhäuser uterovaginal plexus, which may contribute to enhanced sexual arousal and orgasmic frequency (11).

Vaginal or abdominal hysterectomy without oophorectomy has been shown to result in both acute (12,13) and chronic (14) diminishment of ovarian steroid production. Janson and Jansson (13) demonstrated that acute changes were due to transient reductions in ovarian blood flow. They argued that this ovarian functional impairment was of short duration and of little clinical significance since complete functional restitution of the posthysterectomy ovary usually occurs. This is in contrast to the findings of other investigators who reported an accelerated loss of ovarian function (14,15). Reidel et al (14) retrospectively studied 164 women between the ages of 27 and 42. Only patients under age 42 at the time of the investigation were included in the study. Signs of ovarian failure were reported in 39%. Seidenschnur et al (15) observed hot flushes in one third of women who underwent abdominal or vaginal hysterectomy without bilateral salpingo-oophorectomy. Siddel et al (16) studied 90 women who had undergone abdominal hysterectomy with bilateral ovarian conservation and compared them to 226 women who had undergone spontaneous menopause. The mean age of ovarian failure in the hysterectomized group was 45.4 +/− 4.0 years and was significantly lower than the mean age of 49.5 +/− 4.04 years in the nonhysterectomized group. This premature loss of ovarian function in premenopausal women undergoing simple hysterectomy is attributed to permanent compromise of blood flow to the ovary. The ovary receives its blood supply in part from the tubal branch of the uterine artery and in part from the ovarian artery. Compromise of the uterine arterial blood flow might result in damage of the ovarian microcirculation even if the ovarian artery is unaffected by the surgery.

Premenopausal hysterectomy might have another physiologic consequence that is unrelated to psychosexual changes. It has been suggested that the uterus or uterine secretory factors may play a role in prevention of cardiovascular disease. Centerwall (17) reported that premenopausal simple hysterectomy, even with the preservation of one or both ovaries, is associated with a threefold increase in the subsequent incidence and prevalence of coronary heart disease during the remaining premenopausal years. This increased rate of cardiovascular disease in hysterectomized premenopausal women has not been attributable to estrogen use or cigarette smoking. Centerwall postulated that the uterus may have an unrecognized hormonal function, such as prostaglandin secretion, which prevents atherosclerosis in premenopausal women. Shelton (18) proposed that prostacyclin emanating from the uterus may be a major contributor to the reduced risk of coronary artery disease among women. His hypothesis is supported by 1) epidemiologic evidence that the risk of myocardial infarction increases markedly following hysterectomy whether or not the ovaries are removed, 2) evidence that premenopausal women may have higher circulating levels of prostacyclin than do men of comparable ages, 3) production of prostacyclin by uterine tissue homogenate, 4) preliminary data showing high levels of prostacyclin's stable end product metabolite in the venous drainage of the uterus, and 5) plausible mechanisms through which prostacyclin could mitigate coronary disease. These mechanisms include a direct vasodilatory effect, inhibition of platelet aggregation, or inhibition of atherosclerosis. According to Centerwall, to be sure that premenopausal hysterectomy does not cause more deaths from cardiovascular disease than are saved by prevention of uterine cancer, a prospective study of 20,000 women observed until death is needed. He recommends that, pending further elucidation of this phenomenon, women should be advised of the risk of coronary artery disease following hysterectomy.

The anatomic and physiologic changes effected by simple hysterectomy have a direct effect on all phases of the female sexual response. Diminished ovarian function can result in decreased estrogen and androgen production. Normal circulating levels of estrogen maintain vaginal mucosal suppleness and enhance perivaginal circulation thereby having a direct effect on lubrication during arousal. Conversely, hypoestrogenism leads to vaginal mucosal atrophy and decreased perivaginal circulation resulting in decreased lubrication during arousal and dyspareunia.

Dennerstein et al (19) reported that exogenous estrogen administration may be necessary to prevent dyspareunia, but has no primary effects on sexual desire or enjoyment. Utian (20) reported similar findings. Libido is affected primarily by circulating androgens, particularly testosterone. Testosterone is the androgen that increases sexual desire and response to sexual stimuli in both men and women (21). In 1985, Sherwin et al (22) reported that exogenous androgen enhanced intensity of sexual desire, arousal, and frequency of sexual fantasies in hysterectomized and oophorectomized women. More recently Sherwin (21) reported that testosterone is the hormone most critically implicated in the maintenance of libido in the physiologically menopausal woman and that testosterone replacement should be included in their hormone replacement regimens when they are found to be deficient. Testosterone-deficient women with ovarian failure after simple hysterectomy should be similarly treated. This opinion is further supported by Gelfand (23).

While diminished ovarian steroids may decrease arousal and lubrication during the excitement phase, the tenting effect described previously is impaired after hysterectomy because of absence of the uterus and scarring of the vaginal apex (Fig. 11.3). The physical urge for penetration is noticeably missed by some women (2). Shortening of the vagina and the presence of scar tissue at the vaginal apex may cause pain with thrusting, requiring adjustments of depth of penetration or coital positions. Absence of the cervix and uterus may cause significant changes in orgasmic capacity due to impairment of the nerves of the Frankenhäuser uterovaginal plexus (11). Pleasure that might have been previously perceived because of movement of abdominal organs with the motion of the cervix and uterus during intercourse might also be absent after hysterectomy. Zussman et al (24) included in their 1981 clinical opinion a letter from a patient applying for sex therapy after simple hysterectomy with ovarian preservation. She wrote, "The greatest change since the surgery is this. Before, each time the penis is pushed hard against the cervix, I would feel intense excitement deep inside me, huge waves of pleasure going from the area of my cervix all through my torso. This was by far the most exciting part of sex for me, the real climax. I've tried to be satisfied with the orgasms I get from stimulation of the

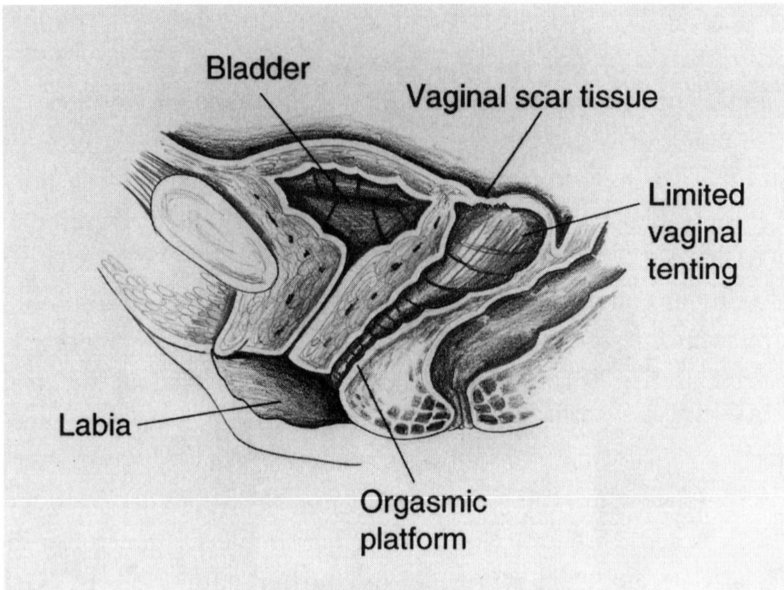

FIG. 11.3.

Structural changes after hysterectomy. Vaginal scarring and shortening result in limited vaginal tenting.

clitoris, that is, mildly pleasurable contractions in the muscles in the front part of the vagina. Maybe I'll get used to it in time, but it isn't nearly as good, and I feel very sad."

In 1953, Kinsey (25) described the importance of internal stimulation. He stated that many women reported that deep vaginal penetration provided satisfaction that was different from that provided by stimulation of the labia and clitoris alone. They identified the cervix as the area that must be stimulated by deep penetration before they could achieve full and complete satisfaction and orgasm. Masters, who maintains that female orgasmic response depends primarily on direct or indirect clitoral stimulation, admitted in a personal communication to Zussman et al (24) that "many women certainly describe cervical pressure as a trigger mechanism for coital responsivity. Such women . . . occasionally are handicapped sexually when such a trigger mechanism is removed surgically." Rhythmic contractions of the uterus may also be missed by women who previously had enhanced uterine sensitivity. During resolution, vasocongestion resolves and the uterus descends back into the true pelvis. It is uncertain whether or not the absence of this phenomenon after hysterectomy contributes to diminishment of sexual enjoyment.

THE CONTROVERSY REGARDING SEXUAL ADJUSTMENT AFTER HYSTERECTOMY

The major point of controversy regarding sexual adjustment after hysterectomy is whether or not diminished sexual response/satisfaction is the result of psychogenic factors or anatomic/physiologic changes. The answer is that both play a significant role in the quality of sexual response.

Current literature suggests that the overall quality of posthysterectomy sexual adjustment is enhanced for most women by a clear understanding of what to expect. The most important factors affecting positive sexual adjustment are support from the woman's sexual partner (2,4,5,7–9,26) and thorough informed consent (2,4,5,8,9,24,26). The woman should have a realistic understanding of the nature of the operation and the structural changes that it will cause. The quality of the relationship with her sexual partner as well as preoperative level of satisfaction should be explored since preoperative sexual activity usually predicts postoperative sexual activity (27) as long as partner support is maintained. Helstrom et al (7) reported on the influence of the partner relationship on sexuality after supracervical hysterectomy (Fig. 11.4). They found that improved sexuality one year after hysterectomy was experienced by 61% of women with a good partner relationship and by 17% of those with a poor relationship (Table 11.1). They also found that no improvement was seen in women with no regular partner relationship. Women with no partner or an ambivalent partner relationship are more at risk for deterioration of sexuality after hysterectomy (Table 11.2). A good partner relationship was found to be even more important than preoperative orgasmic capacity. Helstrom et al evaluated the influence of preoperative sexual dysfunction (27), psychiatric history, and

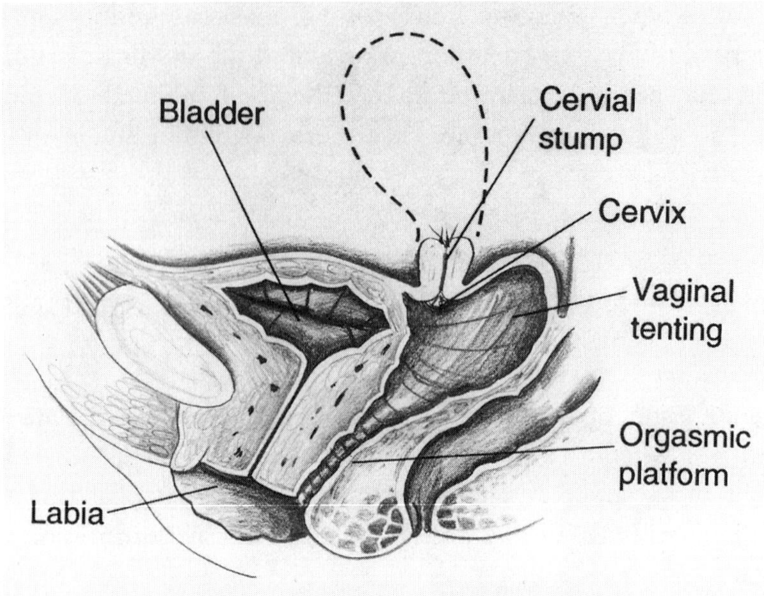

FIG. 11.4.

Structural changes after supracervical hysterectomy. The cervix is left in situ, therefore avoiding vaginal scarring and shortening. Normal vaginal tenting is preserved.

genital pain (28) as predictors of postoperative sexuality. They found that preoperative sexual dysfunction was usually predictive of postoperative sexual dysfunction unless the preoperative deterioration of desire and coital activity was related to pelvic pain. Those who had relief of their preoperative discomfort by the operation had improved sexuality postoperatively. Other investigators agree (29). Psychiatric problems had, in general, little influence on sexuality (28).

As a part of informed consent, the patient should be questioned preoperatively as to her personal perception of body image and femininity, as well as how she believes that uterine loss may affect this. A frank discussion of sexuality should include an explanation of the phases of female sexual response. The patient's personal experience should then be discussed in detail with respect to desire, arousal, and ability to lubricate and achieve orgasm. She should be given an opportunity to con-

TABLE 11.1

Sexuality in women who rated their sexual partnership as "good" before and after hysterectomy and women with a "bad" partner relationship

Type of Sexual Response		Before Hysterectomy (%) Good (n = 63)	Bad (n = 12)	*p*	After Hysterectomy (%) Good (n = 63)	Bad (n = 12)	*p*
Frequency of desire	≥1–2/wk	70	50	NS	76	25	<.01
Desire less frequent	Yes	24	33	NS	13	58	<.05
Coital frequency	≥1–2/wk	48	17	NS	70	17	<.001
Coitus less frequent	Yes	32	50	NS	16	67	<.001
Orgasm frequency	Always/ mostly	94	66	NS	92	66	NS
Multiple orgasm	Yes	33	17	NS	22	25	NS
Masturbation frequency	≥1–2/wk	6	8	NS	5	0	NS
Deep dyspareunia	Yes	56	67	NS	14	17	NS

NS, not significant.
Source: Reproduced by permission from Helstrom L, Sorbom D, Backstrom MT. Influence of partner relationship on sexuality after subtotal hysterectomy. Acta Obstet Gynecol Scand 1995;74:142–146.

sider to what extent uterine loss may affect her own pattern of sexual response, that is, the extent to which she perceives the cervix and uterus contribute to arousal and orgasm. Sakai et al (30) reported on the impact of perception of femininity and uterine sensation. They studied 171 patients who had undergone simple hysterectomy with ovarian preservation. Of the women who felt a loss of femininity, 70% complained of a decrease in vaginal lubrication. In contrast, among women who felt no loss of femininity, only 35.2% reported decreased lubrication (Table

TABLE 11.2

Sexuality in 104 women before and after subtotal hysterectomy for nonmalignant disease*

Type of Sexual Response		Before Hysterectomy (%)			After Hysterectomy (%)		
		With Partner (n = 94)	No Partner (n = 10)	*p*	With Partner (n = 94)	No Partner (n = 10)	*p*
Frequency of desire	≥1–2/wk	66	30	<.05	67	10	<.001
Desire less frequent	Yes	20	10	NS	21	50	<.05
Coital frequency	≥1–2/wk	47	0	<.01	58	0	<.001
Coitus less frequent	Yes	30	10	NS	28	40	NS
Orgasm frequency	Always/ mostly	91	50	<.01	88	30	<.001
Multiple orgasm	Yes	32	10	NS	27	10	NS
Masturbation frequency	≥1–2/wk	8.5	10	NS	5.3	10	NS
Deep dyspareunia	Yes	59	30	NS	14.9	0	NS

NS, not significant.
*The women are divided into the group of women with regular sexual partnership and women without a partner.
Source: Reproduced by permission from Helstrom L, Sorbom D, Backstrom MT. Influence of partner relationship on sexuality after subtotal hysterectomy. Acta Obstet Gynecol Scand 1995;74:142–146.

11.3). Among women who felt a loss of uterine sensation, 69.2% reported decreased ability to climax, while 81.9% of those who felt no loss of uterine sensation were able to achieve orgasm without difficulty (Table 11.4). These authors show clearly how both psychogenic and structural changes can impact the quality of sexual satisfaction after hysterectomy.

TABLE 11.3

Relation between the feeling of lost femininity and postoperative vaginal lubrication

Type of Sexual Response	Feeling of Lost Femininity		Total	X^2	Significance Level
	None	Present			
Vaginal lubrication					
Increased or no change	46	23	69		
Decreased	25	54	79	18.11	$p < .001$
Total	71	77	148		

Source: Reproduced by permission from Sakai K, Yamamoto T, Kamiya H. Female sexual response after hysterectomy. Nippon Sanka Fujinka Gakkai Zasshi 1983;35:757–763.

Because some women experience diminished sexual satisfaction after loss of uterine sensation, several investigators have advocated supracervical hysterectomy (11,31,32) (see Fig. 11.4). Hasson (11) argues that the shift from subtotal to total hysterectomy occurred before cytologic screening was accepted. With the advent of cytology, colposcopy, and the ability to treat with cone biopsy or even less extirpating procedures, he argues that the cervix should not be removed without proper indication. Edvardsen and Madsen (31) share the same opinion and offer a similar argument. Kilkku et al (32) compared the results of total abdominal hysterectomy to those of supracervical hysterectomy in patients interviewed and examined preoperatively and 6 weeks, 6 months, and 12 months postoperatively (Table 11.5). They found no significant change in libido pre- versus postoperatively within either group or between groups. In other words, libido was not affected pre- or postoperatively by either operation. On the other hand, frequency of orgasm was significantly decreased postoperatively in the total hysterectomy group when compared to preoperative frequency of orgasm. No postoperative change in frequency of orgasm occurred in women who had

Table 11.4

Relation between the loss of uterine sensation during coitus and postoperative ability to climax

Type of Sexual Response	Loss of Uterine Sensation: None	Loss of Uterine Sensation: Present	Total	X^2	Significance Level
Ability to climax					
Increased or on change	86	12	98		
Decreased	19	27	46	34.20	$p < .001$
Total	105	39	144		

Source: Reproduced by permission from Sakai K, Yamamoto T, Kamiya H. Female sexual response after hysterectomy. Nippon Sanka Fujinka Gakkai Zasshi 1983;35:757–763.

undergone supracervical hysterectomy. There was no difference in preoperative frequency of orgasm between the groups, but 12 months postoperatively the difference between them was almost significant ($p < .05$). The authors attributed the decreased frequency of orgasm in the total hysterectomy group to damage to the autonomous innervation of the proximal vagina and vaginal scar tissue.

A woman's accurate preoperative perception of cervicouterine sensation during her sexual response may be the only indication of whether or not total hysterectomy will have a deleterious effect. Helstrom et al (33) reported that preoperative objective assessment of somatic variables was not useful in predicting sexuality after supracervical hysterectomy. They performed genital examination and assessments of sacral nervous function, including vibrotactility of the clitoris, the external anal reflex, and levator muscle strength. No correlation was found between tests for sacral nervous function and a latent factor for sexuality before and after the operation. Preoperative uterine size and pain during pelvic examination did not show any correlation with pre- or postoperative sexual parameters.

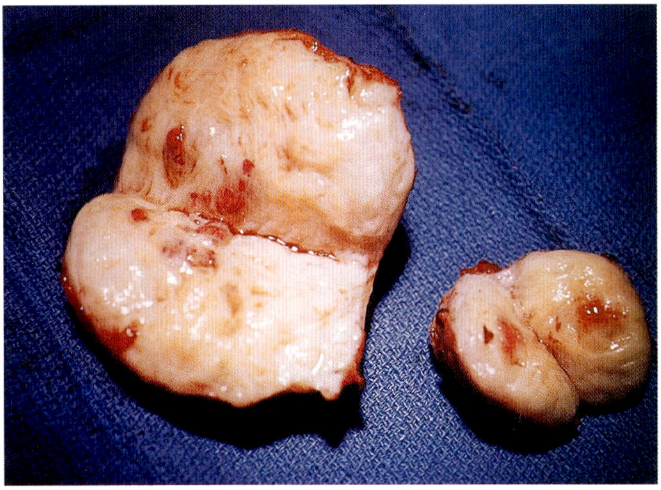

PLATE 1

Leiomyomas bisected to note white and tan cut surface.

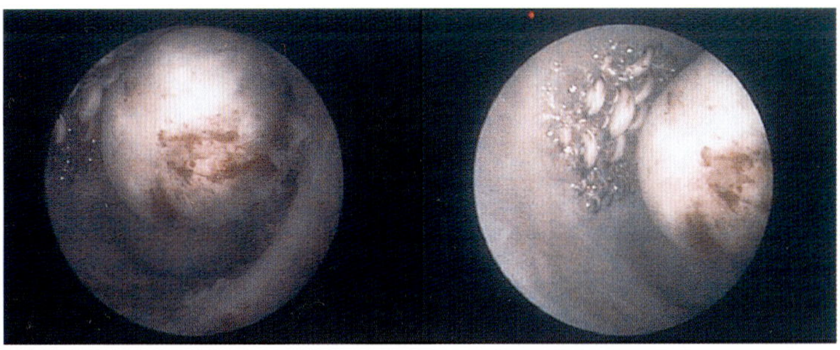

PLATE 2

Left: Hysteroscopic view of submucous myoma. Right: Close-up view of myoma and bubbles from distending fluid.

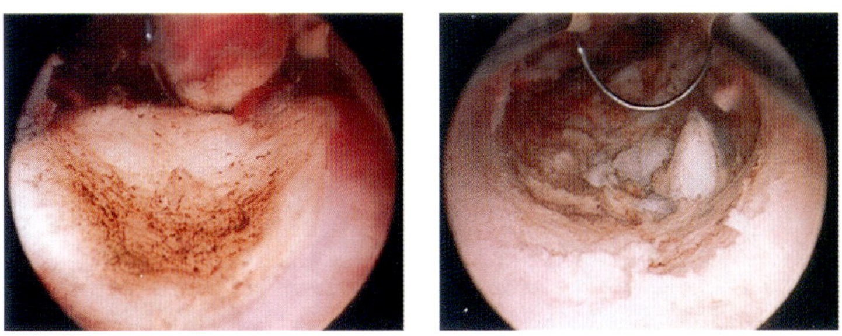

PLATE 3

A. Resectoscopic removal of submucous myoma from posterior lower uterine segment. B. Final resection of remaining myoma fragments.

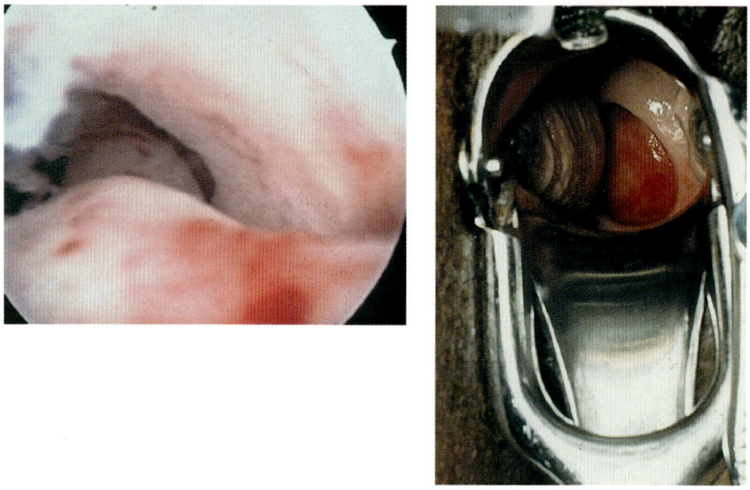

A

B

PLATE 4

A. Hysteroscopic visualization of the pedicle of a myoma located within the cervical canal. Interestingly, this myoma was noted to be partly intramural several months earlier during office hysteroscopy. B. Prolapsing submucosal myoma dilating the cervical os.

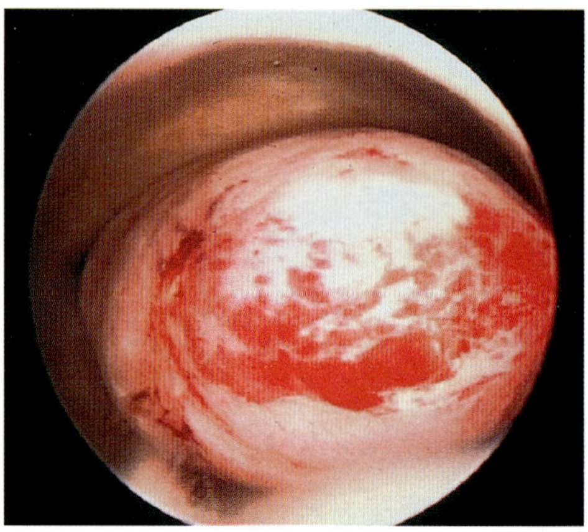

PLATE 5

Hysteroscopic visualization confirms a completely intracavitary myoma. (Same patient as Fig. 7.3, p. 154.)

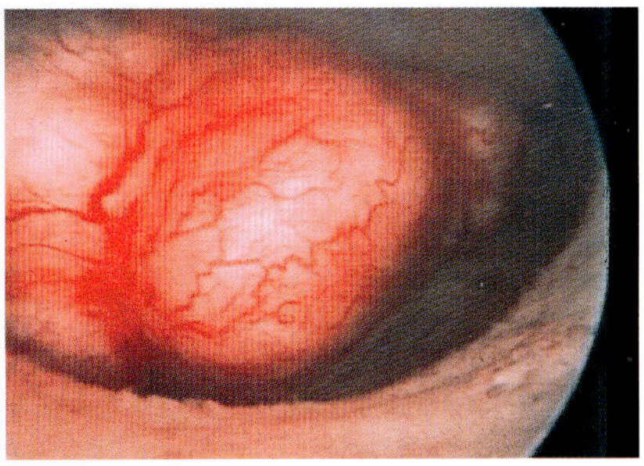

PLATE 6

An isolated intracavitary myoma seen in a patient who presented with severe menorrhagia and life-threatening anemia.

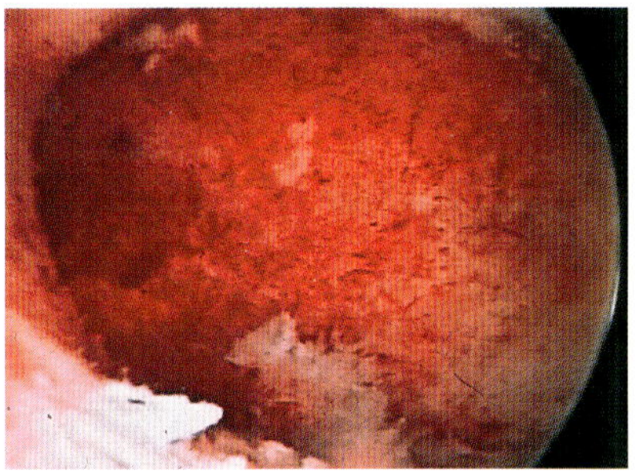

PLATE 7

The patient from Plate 6 following resection of the intracavitary myoma and restoration of the normal intrauterine architecture.

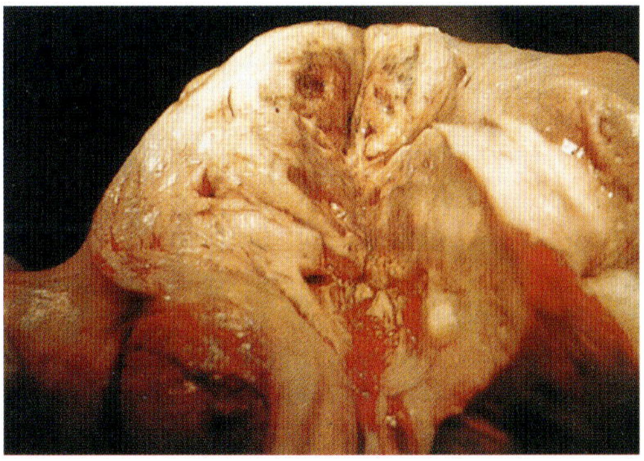

PLATE 8

Gross pathology of a leiomyosarcoma (LMS). It is characterized by a large, pale, unencapsulated, poorly circumscribed soft tissue involving the uterine fundus.

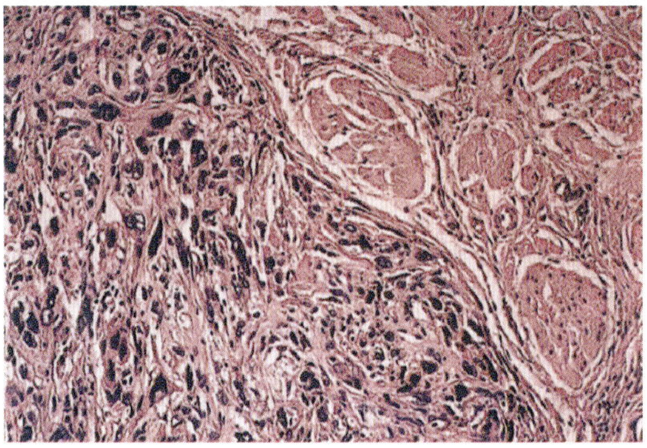

PLATE 9

Microscopic pathology of the gross specimen in Plate 8. There are no well-defined margins between the LMS and myometrium. The tumor was found growing into lymphatics and in continuity between bundles of smooth muscle.

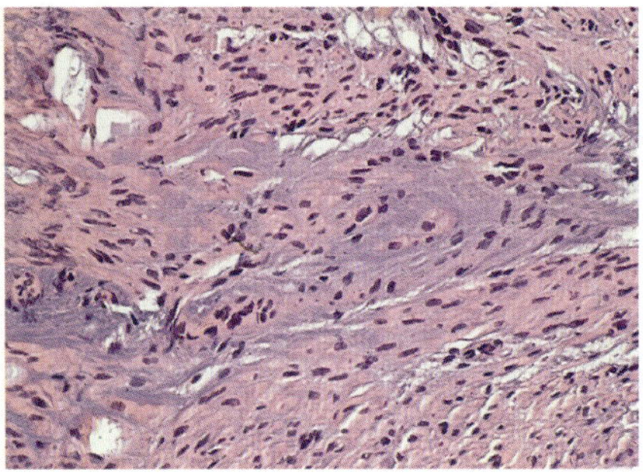

PLATE 10

Thermal injury created by bipolar needle within a submucous myoma. The muscle fibers are indistinct; grayish areas are outright necrotic. The nuclei are irregular and smudged.

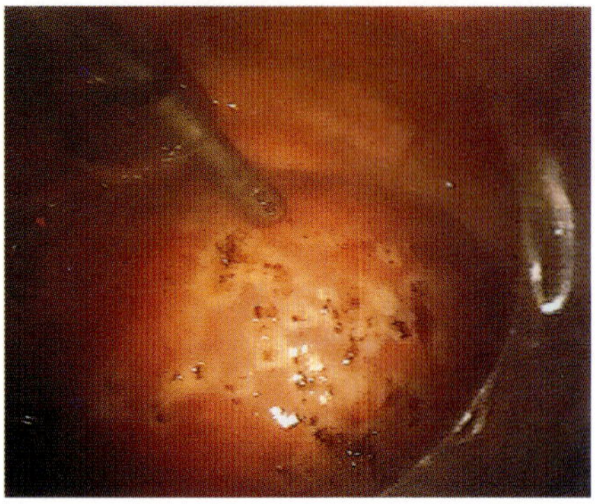

PLATE 11

Multiple punctures have been made into this large posterior myoma. An irrigating cannula is noted on the upper left. Normal saline irrigant enhances bipolar action and conduction. (Digital photograph from video).

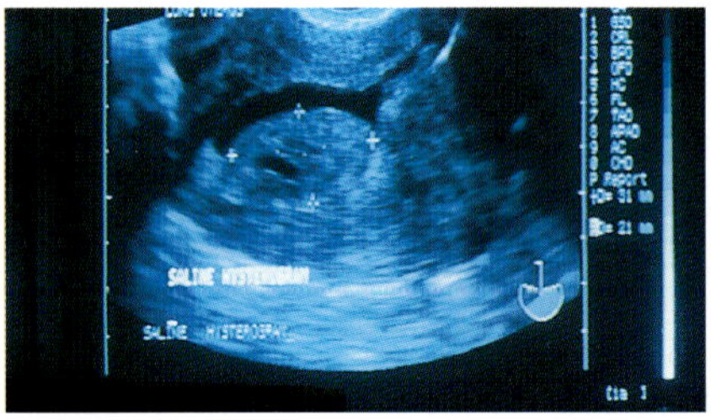

PLATE 12

Saline sonohysterography demonstrates submucosal myoma.

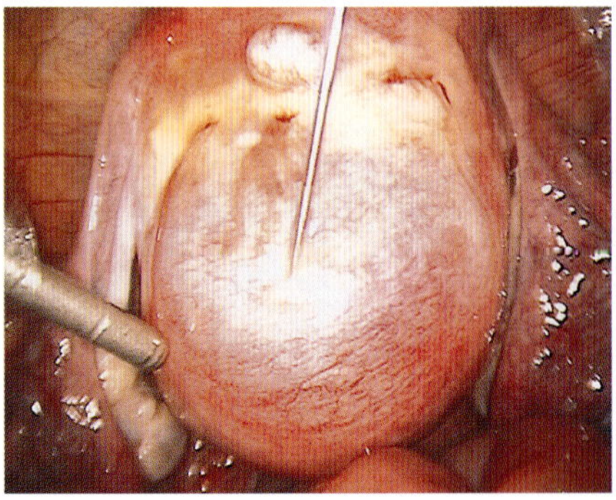

PLATE 13

Vasopressin injected in base of myoma.

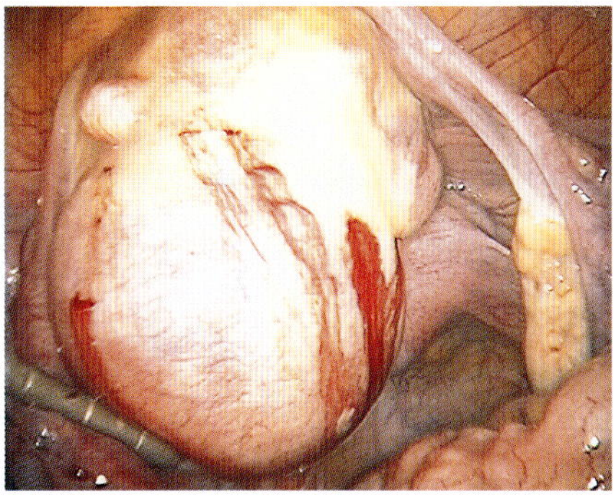

PLATE 14

Intense vasoconstriction of uterine wall helps to define myoma borders.

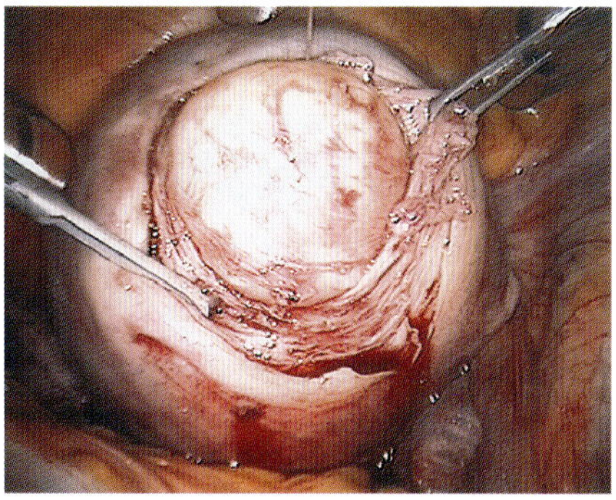

PLATE 15

Uterine serosa incised down to pseudocapsular plane.

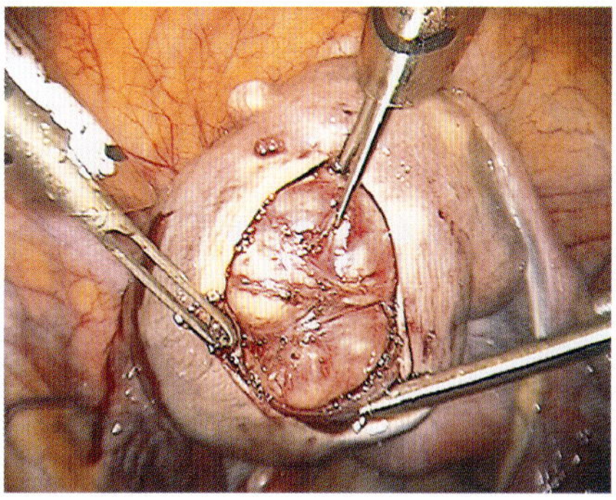

PLATE 16

Dissecting of pseudocapsular plane with endocoagulation.

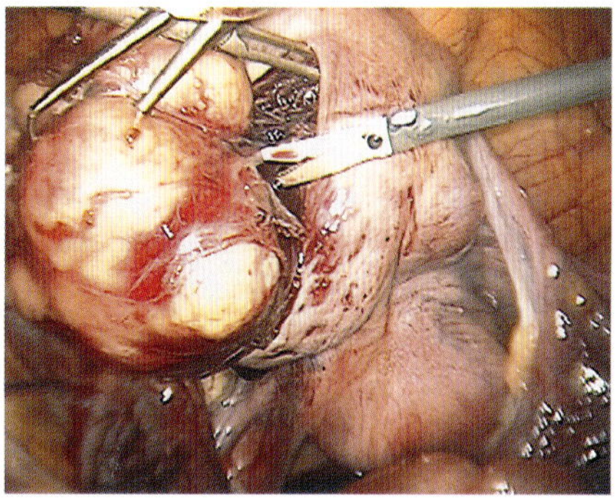

PLATE 17

Traction on myoma as myometrial bed is dissected with bipolar scissors.

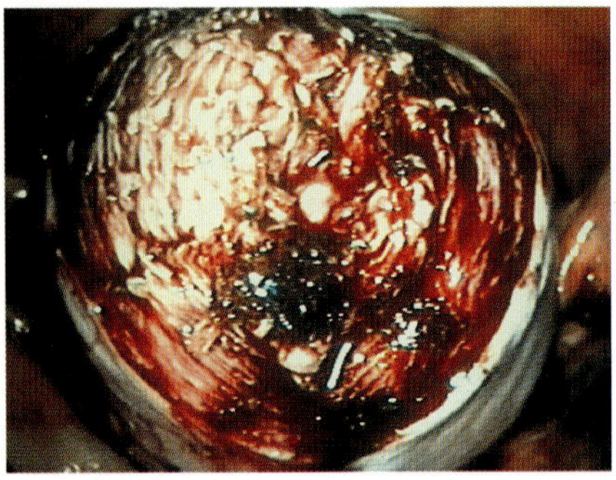

PLATE 18

Hemostatic myoma bed following enucleation.

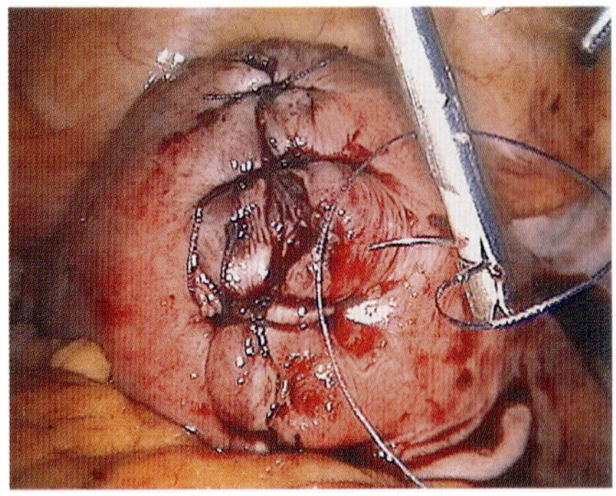

PLATE 19

Curved-needle suture reconstruction of uterus.

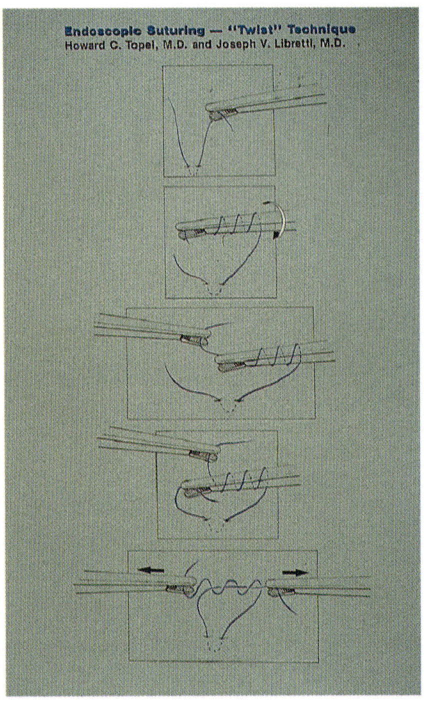

PLATE 20

Square "surgeon" knot formed with a twist knot-tying technique.

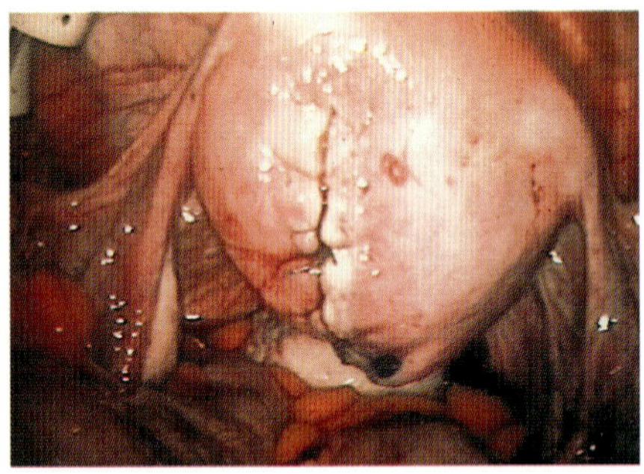

PLATE 21

Posterior uterine wall incision closed with deep interrupted stitches and a continuous locking serosal suture.

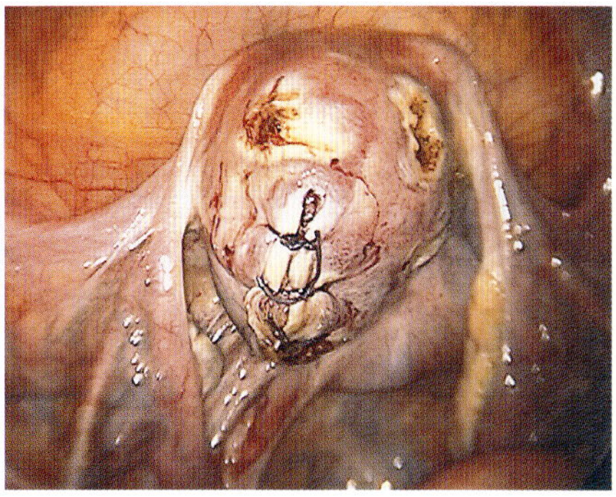

PLATE 22

Completed laparoscopic myomectomy with suture reconstruction.

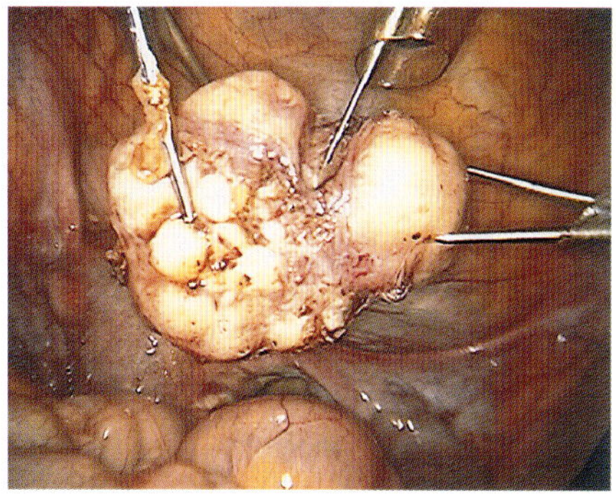

PLATE 23

Endoknife morcellation of large myoma.

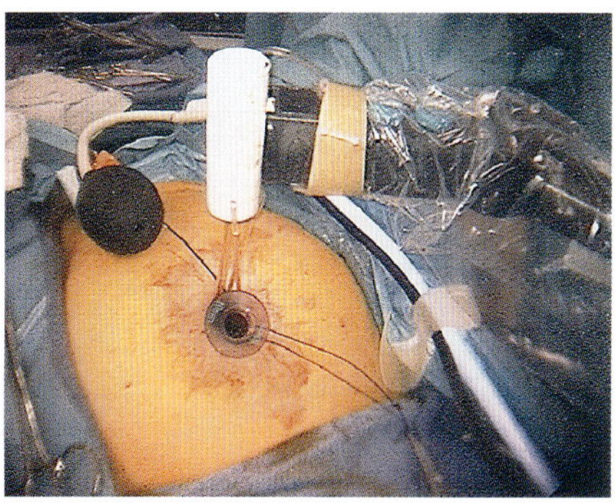

PLATE 24

Gasless laparoscopy with balloon and mechanical abdominal wall elevator.

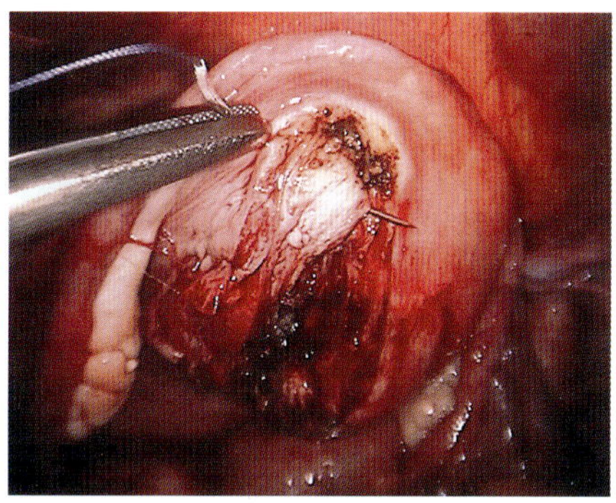

PLATE 25

Gasless suturing technique with laparotomy needle holder and CT-1 curved needle.

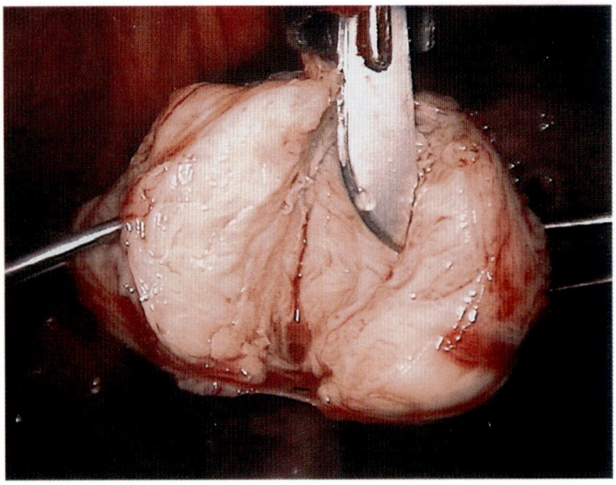

PLATE 26

Rapid morcellation of large myoma with standard scalpel.

A 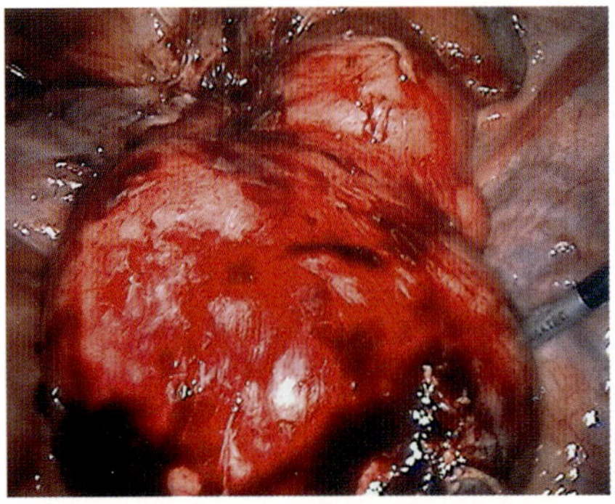

C 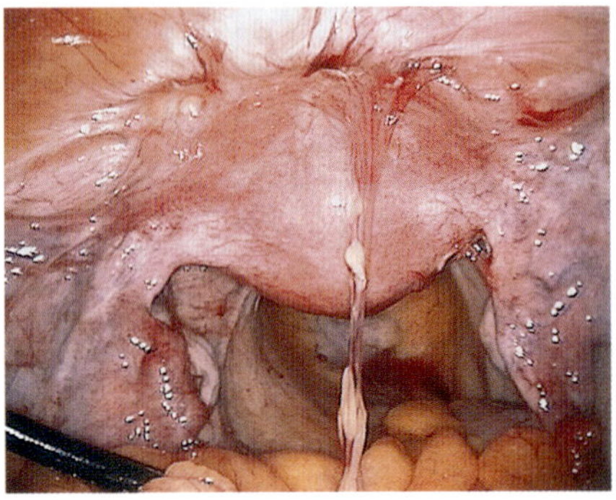

B 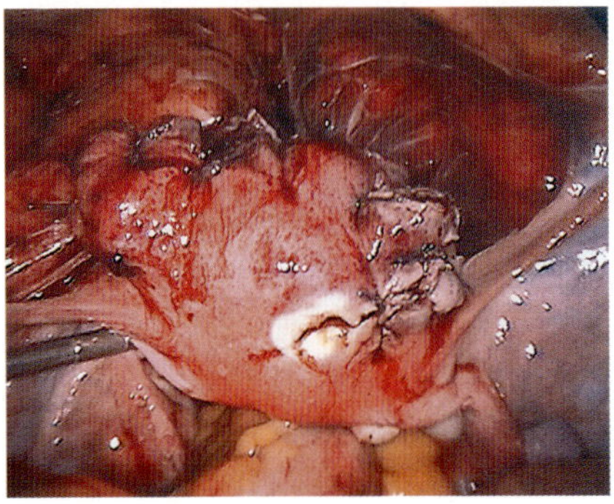

PLATE 27

A. Large fundal myoma (first operation). B. Myomectomy with uterine reconstruction (first operation). C. Second look, 6 months later (second operation). Excellent anatomic and functional outcome.

TABLE 11.5

Orgasmic coituses experienced less than one time out of four (%)

	HYSTERECTOMY (91)	SUPRAVAGINAL AMPUTATION (98)	
Preoperatively	29.7	28.6	↔ NS
6 mo postoperatively	38.5[a]	31.6 NS ↓	↔ NS
12 mo postoperatively	46.7[b]	32.0 NS ↓	↔ [a]

↓, longitudinal comparison within one group; ↔, comparison between the groups; NS, not significant.

[a] Almost significant ($p < .05$).

[b] Highly significant ($p < .001$).

Source: Reproduced by permission from Kilkku P, Gronroos M, Hirvonen T, Rauramo L. Supravaginal uterine amputation vs. hysterectomy. Effects on libido and orgasm. Acta Obstet Gynecol Scand 1983;62:147–152.

Interestingly, Eicher (26) reports that it makes no difference whether a woman has a total hysterectomy or a supracervical hysterectomy as long as she has thorough informed consent with emphasis on discussion of sexual function. He found that lasting or chronic sexual disturbances can largely be avoided and psychosomatic disturbances that influence sexual behavior can be reduced to less than 10% if frank discussion of sexual function is pursued preoperatively, at the time of discharge, and during follow-up examination. He contends that "an all too local/genital approach deflects us from our understanding of the orgasm, as the latter is a central experience on which extra-genital and above all psychological factors also play an important part."

A retrospective study by Sievers and Kohler (5) suggests that *patience* may be required to give postoperative sexual recovery the full benefit of the doubt. These authors studied psychological and sexual sequelae of hysterectomy in 1007 cases between 1½ and 8 years following the operation and reported that a latency of improvement in sexuality can occur after hysterectomy. Of these patients, 78% thought that they had been fully informed about the operation. In 57% of cases, improvement of libido and frequency of orgasm occurred 1 year later and in 10% of cases, improvement occurred 2 years later. In view of these findings, the patient must be informed that restoration of satisfactory sexual functioning may take as much as 2 years, so that she can anticipate this and avert false expectations. Indeed, some women who are contemplating possible hysterectomy may consider this latency of improvement an undesirable outcome.

Detailed informed consent with *emphasis on frank and in-depth discussion of sexuality* as described in this chapter is strongly recommended, but unfortunately is not a standard of contemporary care in the United States. Indeed such counseling is time consuming and may seem impractical within a busy obstetrics and gynecology practice. Yet one should consider that time spent with thorough preoperative counseling will save time postoperatively because of improved outcome and patient satisfaction. The current literature, largely advanced by international investigators, fully supports these factors. The lack of research conducted in the United States dealing with sexual issues reflects our societal discomfort with an open approach to sexual concerns. Our reticence regarding this sensitive subject perpetuates suboptimal care for the patient and impairs the quality of education provided to our students and future health care professionals. It is imperative that we expand our comfort zones and frankly address sexual issues during informed consent before hysterectomy. With the growing body of supportive literature, it will surely become a US standard of care in the future.

In summary, several issues have an impact on how well a woman can achieve sexual adjustment after hysterectomy.

1. The woman should feel that her femininity and sense of self-worth are not threatened by loss of her uterus.
2. The woman who perceives cervical and uterine sensation/pressure as a substantial component of her sexual response and orgasmic capacity should be warned that this can be impaired by total hysterectomy and can be preserved by supracervical hysterectomy.
3. She must understand that structural changes that result from hysterectomy can alter all phases of her sexual response cycle.

4. She should understand that ovarian failure can be accelerated in spite of ovarian conservation, necessitating hormone replacement therapy.
5. The premenopausal woman should be warned that there is a three-fold risk for cardiovascular disease after hysterectomy.
6. The patient should have a supportive partner relationship.
7. Both patient and partner should be informed about the possible consequences of the operation and express understanding of the possible outcome.

In view of the above discussion, the women who are likely to have diminished sexuality after hysterectomy in spite of adequate informed consent include 1) those who are unable to positively incorporate uterine loss into their self-image, that is, those who feel diminished femininity because of their inability to achieve self-validation or validation by their sexual partner, and 2) those who are focused on the cervicouterine contribution to arousal and orgasm and are unable to satisfactorily incorporate clitoral orgasm into their sexual repertoire. Nonreproductive women with symptomatic leiomyomas who fall into either of these two categories will likely be better served by myomectomy.

REFERENCES

1. Boyd ME. Myomectomy. Can J Surg 1986;29:61–63.
2. Williamson ML. Sexual adjustment after hysterectomy. JOGNN 1991; 21:42–47.
3. Poettgen H. Clinical contribution to female identity crisis after loss of the uterus. Psychother Psychosom Med Psychol 1993;43:428–431.
4. Drummond J, Field PA. Emotional and sexual sequela following hysterectomy. Health Care for Women International 1984;5:261–271.
5. Sievers S, Kohler CO. Psychological and sexual acceptance of vaginal hysterectomy for sterilization. Geburtshilfe Frauenheilkd 1977;37:115–123.
6. Melody GF. Depressive reactions following hysterectomy. Am J Obstet Gynecol 1962;83:410–413.

7. Helstrom L, Sorbom D, Backstrom MT. Influence of partner relationship on sexuality after subtotal hysterectomy. Acta Obstet Gynecol Scand 1995; 74:142–146.
8. Chang SB. Factors influencing sexual satisfaction in women who have had a hysterectomy: a comparative group study. Kanho Hakoe Chi 1990;3: 357–367.
9. Ananth J. Hysterectomy and sexual counseling. Psychiatr J Univ Ottawa 1983;8:213–217.
10. Newman G, Newman LE. Coping with the stress of hysterectomy. J Sex Education and Therapy 1985;11:65–68.
11. Hasson HM. Cervical removal at hysterectomy for benign disease. Risks and benefits. J Reprod Med 1993;38:781–790.
12. Stone SC, Dickey RP, Mickal A. The acute effect of hysterectomy on ovarian function. Am J Obstet Gynecol 1974;121:193–196.
13. Janson PO, Jansson I. The acute effect of hysterectomy on ovarian blood flow. Am J Obstet Gynecol 1997;127:349–352.
14. Riedel HH, Lehmann-Willenbrock E, Semm K. Ovarian failure phenomena after hysterectomy. J Reprod Med 1986;31:597–600.
15. Seidenschnur G, Beck H, Uplegger H, et al. Attitude and sex behavior following hysterectomy. Zentralbl Gynakol 1989;111:53–59.
16. Siddel N, Sarrel P, Whitehead M. The effect of hysterectomy on the age of ovarian failure: identification of a subgroup of women with premature loss of ovarian function and literature review. Fertil Steril 1986;47:94–100.
17. Centerwall BS. Premenopausal hysterectomy and cardiovascular disease. Am J Obstet Gynecol 1981;139:58–61.
18. Shelton JD. Prostaglandin from the uterus and woman's cardiovascular advantage. Prostaglandins Leukotrienes Med 1982;8:459–466.
19. Dennerstein L, Wood C, Burrows GD. Sexual response following hysterectomy and oophorectomy. Obstet Gynecol 1976;49;92–96.
20. Utian WH. Effect of hysterectomy, oophrectomy and estrogen therapy on libido. Int J Obstet Gynaecol 1975;13:97–100.
21. Sherwin BB. Sex hormones and psychological functioning in postmenopausal women. Exp Gerontol 1994;29:423–430.
22. Sherwin BB, Gelfand MM, Brender W. Androgen enhances sexual motivation in females: a prospective, crossover study of sex steroid administration in the surgical menopause. Psychosom Med 1985;47:339–351.
23. Gelfand MM. Hormone replacement therapy. Eur Menopause J 1995;2: 22–26.

24. Zussman L, Zussman S, Sunley R, Bjornson E. Sexual response after hysterectomy-oophorectomy: recent studies and reconsideration of psychogenesis. Am J Obstet Gynecol 1981;140:725–729.
25. Kinsey A. Sexual behavior in the human female. Philadelphia: Saunders, 1953.
26. Eicher W. Total and subtotal hysterectomy: psychosexual aspects. Arch Gynecol Obstet 1994;255:S359–S366.
27. Helstrom L, Lundberg PO, Sorbom D, Backstrom T. Sexuality after hysterectomy: a factor analysis of women's sexual lives before and after subtotal hysterectomy. Obstet Gynecol 1993;81:357–362.
28. Helstrom L, Weiner E, Sorbom D, Backstrom T. Predictive value of psychiatric history, genital pain and menstrual symptoms for sexuality after hysterectomy. Acta Obstet Gynecol Scand 1994;73:575–580.
29. Virtanen H, Makinen J, Tenho T, et al. Effects of abdominal hysterectomy on urinary and sexual symptoms. Br J Urol 1993;72:868–872.
30. Sakai K, Yamamoto T, Kamiya H. Female sexual response after hysterectomy. Nippon Sanka Fujinka Gakkai Zasshi 1983;35:757–763.
31. Edvardsen L, Madsen EM. Supravaginal or total hysterectomy? Ugeskr Laeger 1994;156:4694–4699.
32. Kilkku P, Gronroos M, Hirvonen T, Rauramo L. Supravaginal uterine amputation vs. hysterectomy. Effects on libido and orgasm. Acta Obstet Gynecol Scand 1983;62:147–152.
33. Helstrom L, Backstrom T, Sorbom D, Lundberg PO. Sacral nervous function, hormonal levels and sexuality in premenopausal women before and after hysterectomy. Acta Obstet Gynecol Scand 1994;73;570–574.

CHAPTER

12

Leiomyosarcoma of the Uterus

Barbara A. Soltes

Leiomyosarcoma (LMS) is the most common sarcoma of the uterus, comprising nearly 50% of all sarcomas in various series (1). Although LMS represents only about 6% of all gynecologic malignancies, it can be considered one of the most lethal of all uterine malignancies (2). The 5-year survival ranges from 5.5% to 63.6% (3).

PATHOGENESIS

Leiomyosarcomas originate from smooth muscle while endometrial stromal sarcomas originate from endometrial smooth muscle. The majority of LMS arise de novo with very few from preexisting leiomyomas. Much confusion arises when sarcomas develop from tissue that is foreign to the uterus, that is, cartilage, bone, fat, or skeletal muscle. This confusion stems back to as early as 1860, when over 119 different terms were used to describe one variety of sarcoma. By 1864, Zenker devised a classification system based on homologous and heterologous elements within a sarcoma. *Homologous* refers to tissue normally found in the

TABLE 12.1

Classification of uterine sarcomas

- I. Pure sarcomas
  - A. Pure homologous
    1. Leiomyosarcoma
    2. Stromal sarcoma
    3. Endolymphatic stromal sarcoma
    4. Angiosarcoma
    5. Fibrosarcoma
  - B. Pure heterologous
    1. Rhabdomyosarcoma
    2. Chondrosarcoma
    3. Osteosarcoma
    4. Liposarcoma
- II. Mixed sarcomas
  - A. Mixed homologous
  - B. Mixed heterologous
- III. Mixed mesodermal tumors
  - A. Mixed malignant müllerian tumor, homologous
  - B. Mixed malignant müllerian tumor, heterologous
- IV. Unclassified sarcoma
- V. Malignant lymphoma

uterus, whereas *heterologous* refers to tissue that is foreign to the uterus (4). Ober further modified this classification system based on number and type of sarcomatous and carcinomatous tissues present. Kempson and Bari simplified Ober's classification into pure and mixed elements. Pure sarcomas contain only one sarcomatous element, whereas mixed sarcomas are made up of two or more sarcomatous elements. These elements may be either homologous or heterologous. The carcinomatous elements may be either adenocarcinoma or squamous cell (5). The currently

Table 12.2

Staging of uterine sarcomas

Stage	Description
I	Sarcoma limited to the corpus
II	Sarcoma involving the corpus and cervix but not outside the uterus
III	Sarcoma extended outside the uterus but not outside the true pelvis
IV	Sarcoma extended outside the true pelvis and involving the bladder and/or rectum
IVA	Spread to the mucosa of the bladder/rectum
IVB	Distant metastasis

acceptable classification and staging of uterine sarcomas are listed in Tables 12.1 and 12.2.

CLINICAL FINDINGS

Several studies have found that LMS occur more commonly in multiparous women in their fifth decade of life. Leiomyosarcoma tumors have been found to occur in women 10 years younger than women with other uterine sarcomas. There is no racial predilection for this tumor. Norris and Taylor (6) noted a history of prior pelvic irradiation in 12% of 144 patients with uterine sarcomas; however, most of these sarcomas were mixed mesodermal tumors or carcinosarcomas and none were leiomyosarcomas.

The most common presenting symptoms are listed in Table 12.3 (7). Abnormal vaginal bleeding is the presenting symptom seen most frequently. A diagnosis of sarcoma must be entertained when the presenting symptom is a large, friable polypoid mass that extends through a dilated cervix into the vagina. Associated clinical findings include hypertension and obesity in one third of patients (8). The average duration of symptoms is 6 months (7,8).

TABLE 12.3

Presenting symptoms in patients with leiomyosarcoma*

Symptom	Initial Presenting (%)	Recurrent (%)
Abnormal vaginal bleeding	59	6
Pelvic pain	38	34
Enlarged uterus	38	31
Weight loss	13	0
Shortness of breath	9	41
Urinary symptoms	6	3
Bowel obstruction	6	9
Fever	6	0
Leg edema	6	13
Leg paralysis	6	3

*Some patients presented with more than 1 symptom.

PATHOLOGY

Clinical Pathology

The uterus is frequently enlarged and of a variable shape. ALMS is a poorly circumscribed mass that ranges from 4 to 40 cm, often protruding through the cervical os. It is pale, soft, and often mushy in comparison to a benign, firm, solid leiomyoma (see Plate 8).

Microscopic Pathology

Leiomyosarcomas are composed of malignant uterine smooth cells that are elongated with tapered ends. Histologically, they may resemble normal uterine musculature, but as they become less differentiated, the whorling pattern of muscle fibers characteristic of a leiomyoma is not seen (see Plate 9).

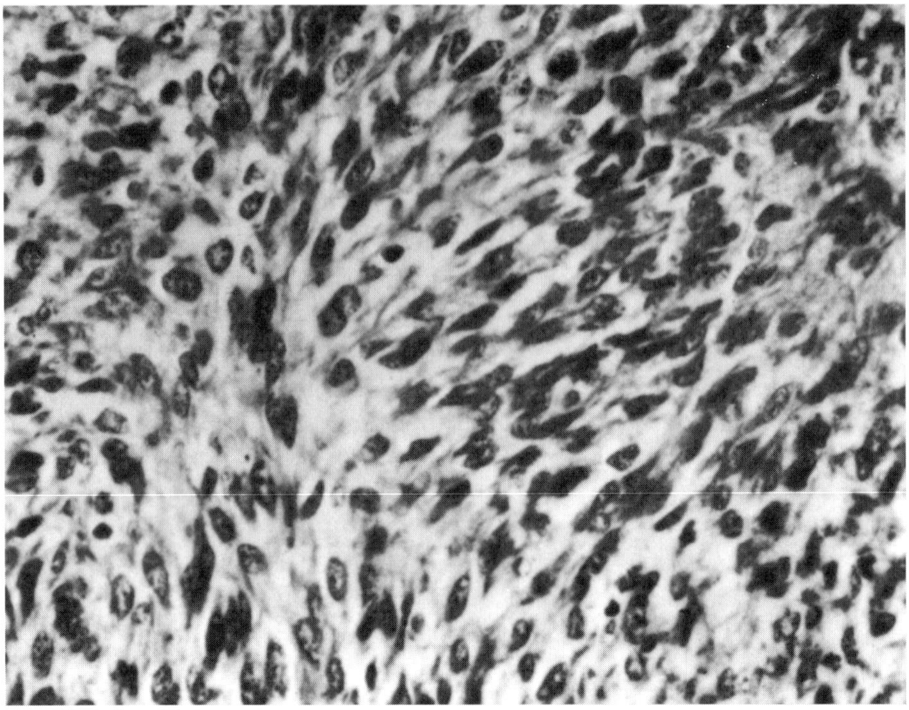

FIG. 12.1.

Tumor with atypical and hyperchromatic nuclei. The variation from a leiomyoma is only slight.

The LMS is generally found growing into large lymphatics or blood vessels with poorly defined margins. It has been found that as the tumor advances, the number of mitotic figures and the likelihood of vasculature invasion increase (9,10) (Figs. 12.1 and 12.2; see also Plate 9).

A number of authors have defined the number of mitotic figures and degree of atypia to differentiate between leiomyoma and LMS (Table 12.4). Most agree that 10 mitotic figures per 10 high-power fields (HPF) with cellular atypia are diagnostic of sarcomas. Other factors include hypercellularity, presence of giant cells, and blood vessel invasion (10,11). Figure 12.3 demonstrates a tumor with 10 mitotic figures per 10 HPF with atypical hyperchromatic nuclei.

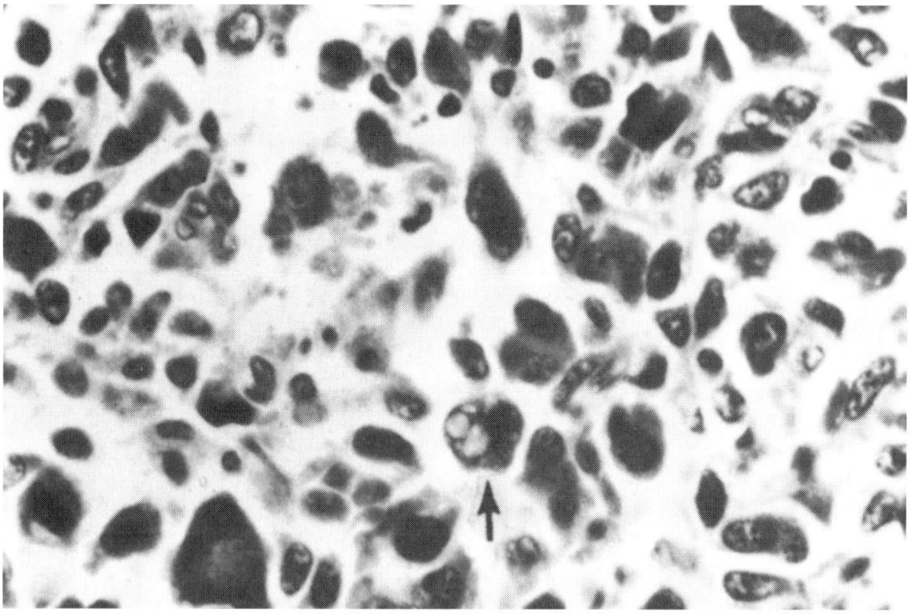

FIG. 12.2.

The most prominent elements of this tumor are multinucleated giant cells with nuclear inclusions, as indicated by the *arrow*.

TABLE 12.4

Histologic classification of smooth-muscle tumors

Mitotic Figures/10 HPF	Atypia	Classification
1–4	Any degree	Leiomyoma
5–9	None	Leiomyoma with high mitotic rate
5–9	Grade I	Low malignant potential
5–9	Grades II/III	Leiomyosarcoma
>10	Grades I–III	Leiomyosarcoma

HPF, high-power fields.

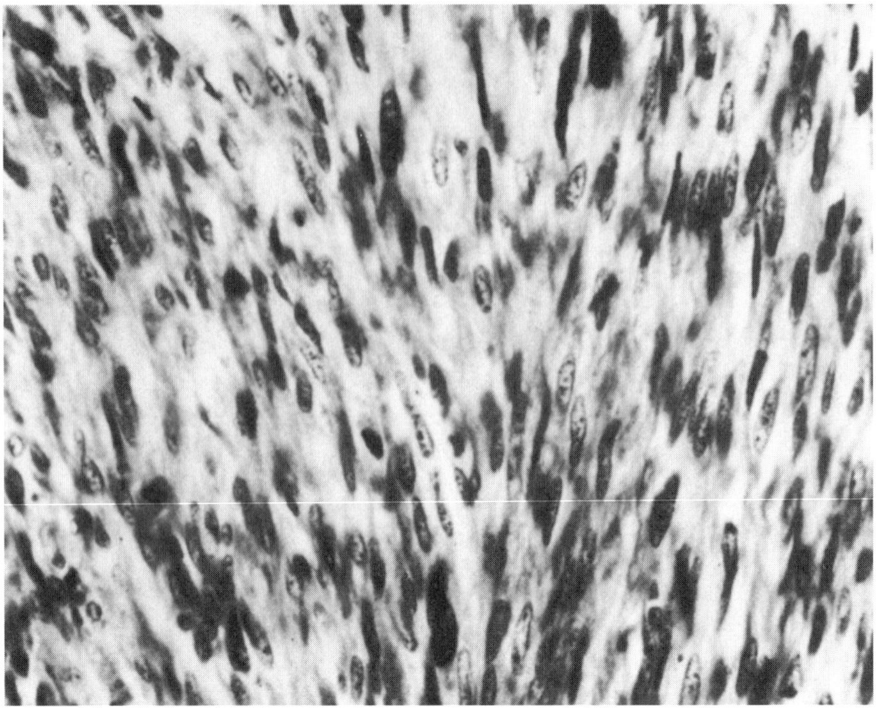

FIG. 12.3.

Grade II LMS with enlarged and hyperchromatic nuclei and 10 mitotic figures per 10 high-power field.

DIAGNOSIS

The majority of patients present with an enlarging uterus over a relatively short period of time, and peri- or postmenopausal bleeding. A histologic diagnosis based on endometrial sampling may not necessarily differentiate an early-stage LMS from a benign leiomyoma (11). Magnetic resonance imaging (MRI) is perhaps the best imaging technique available to characterize benign from invasive disease (12,13). It has multidimensional imaging capacity, which offers a detailed image of complex pelvic anatomy. MRI utilizes signal intensities that are determined by pulse sequences. T-1 and T-2 relaxation times are two parameters inherent to tissue within the pelvis. Signal intensities increase as T-1 time decreases, and they increase as T-2 time increases. Soft tissue and fluids exhibit a hypointense signal on T-1–weighted images, and a hyperintense signal on T-2–weighted images. Muscle and fat exhibit a hyperintense signal on T-1 and an intermediate signal on T-2–weighted images.

Leiomyomas are well-circumscribed masses sharply demarcated from surrounding myometrium. They are of low intensity on both T-1– and T-2–weighted images. On occasion, leiomyomas may display high intensity on T-2 images, indicating a well-vascularized tumor. Calcified or degenerating tumors may exhibit low intensity on T-2 images (Fig. 12.4).

Leiomyosarcomas are not usually sharply demarcated from the myometrium or adjacent vasculature. They may be high- or low-intensity masses with or without speckled high-intensity areas on T-

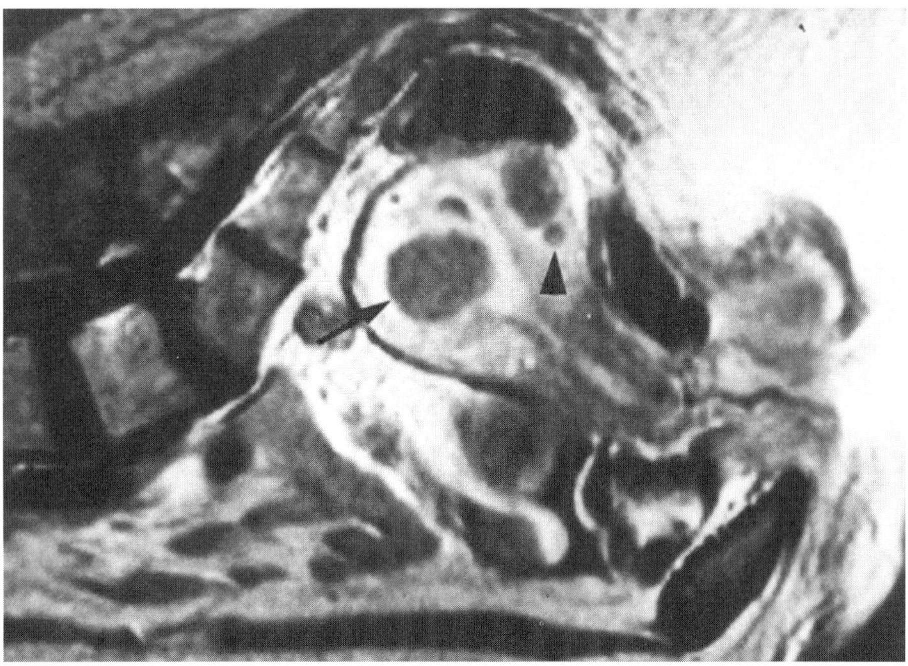

FIG. 12.4.

MRI with a T-2–weighted image of a typical homogeneous leiomyoma. Non-degenerating leiomyomas emit a low intensity on this T-2 image identified by the *arrows*.

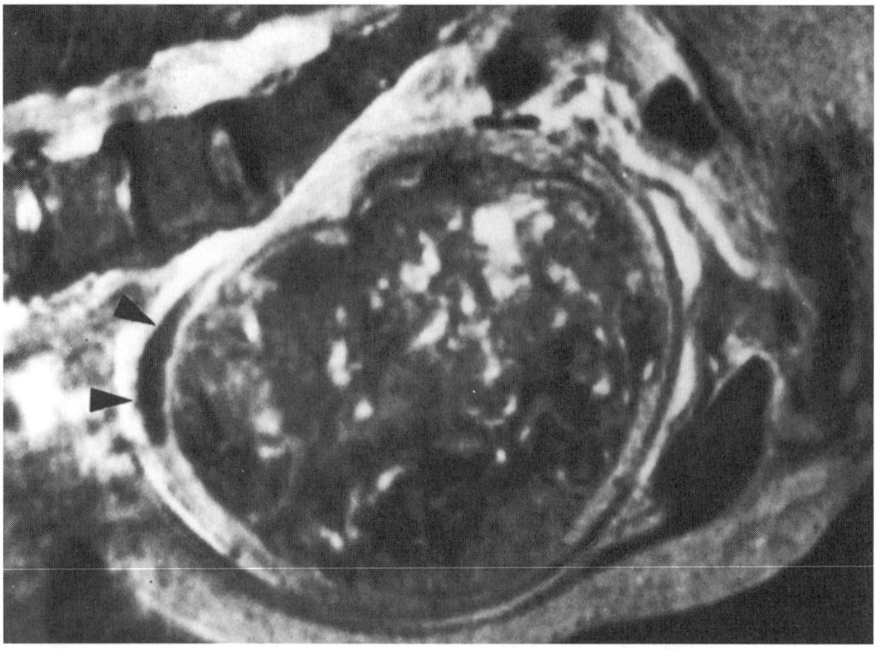

A

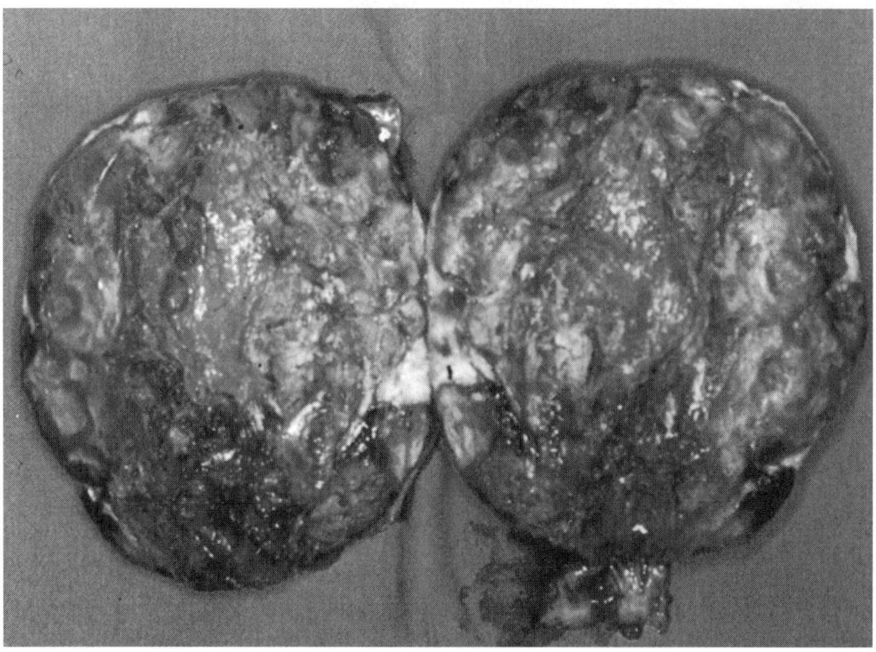

B

FIG. 12.5.

An LMS in a postmenopausal woman with vaginal bleeding. A. A T-2–weighted image reveals a sharply marginated low-intensity mass mixed with speckled areas signifying blood (*arrows*). B. A gross section of the corresponding image indicates a necrotic hemorrhagic mass.

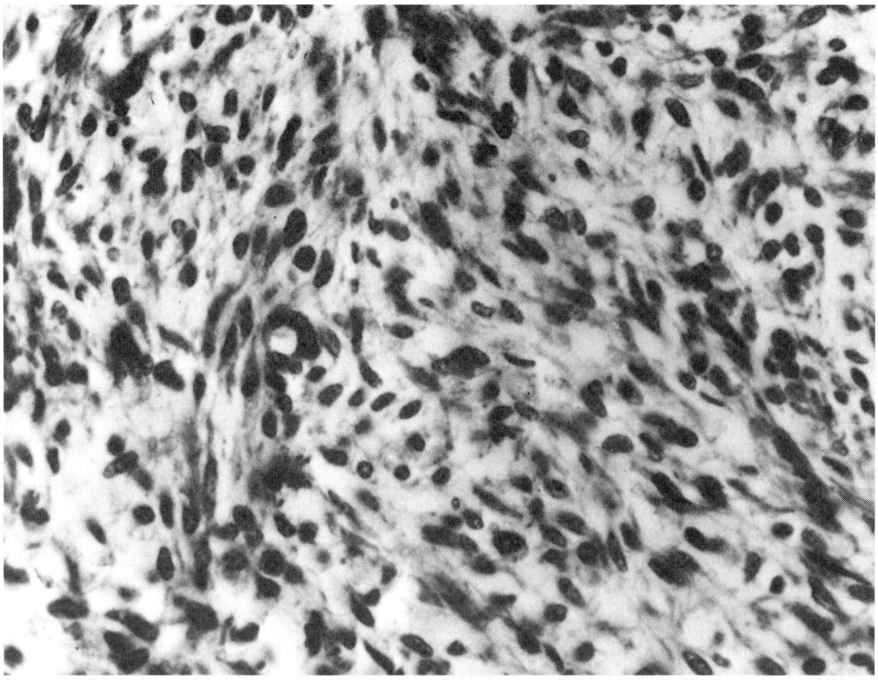

FIG. 12.6.

Grade I LMS, which varies only slightly from a leiomyoma. Basic architecture under low power is a typical leiomyoma with bundles of spindle fibers arranged in an orderly manner. There are occasional foci of necrosis and hemorrhage. The cells are enlarged with few atypical nuclei. The number of mitotic figures averages five to seven per 10HPF.

2–weighted images (Fig. 12.5). In early stages, the tumor may appear similar to the leiomyoma and may be distinguished histologically only on the basis of number of mitotic figures per 10 HPF (Fig. 12.6).

TREATMENT

About 50% of all women with sarcomas have stage I disease. Total abdominal hysterectomy and bilateral salpingo-oopherectomy are standard therapy in the treatment of uterine sarcomas. Several authors advocate bilateral pelvic lymphadenectomy in low-grade tumors in which local spread is common (8).

Pre- or postoperative radiation is of questionable efficacy, as adjunctive therapy in women treated with radiation and surgery had a greater degree of local tumor control, although the degree of recurrence and survival rates have not been significantly different from those in patients who had received no such therapy (14,15). Some studies indicate that doxorubicin is the best single chemotherapeutic agent for adjuvant treatment of these tumors. However, in randomized trials by the Gynecologic Oncology Group that compared treatment with doxorubicin with no further treatment after surgery, no statistically significant difference was seen in recurrence or survival rates between the groups.

PROGNOSIS

Some controversy surrounds the most important prognostic indicator for LMS. One author suggests the menopausal status while others consider the localization of the tumor as the most important factor to affect the prognosis (14–16). Women who are premenopausal when the diagnosis of LMS is made tend to have a better prognosis than postmenopausal women even if evidence of blood vessel invasion, advanced grade, or high mitotic counts is present. Leiomyosarcomas in the younger patient tend to have slower tumor growth patterns and remain more localized within the pelvis (5). LMS confined to the uterus, especially the subserosa, have the best survival.

Overall, women with LMS have a poorer survival rate compared with women with other uterine sarcomas. The overall 5-year survival rate is between 5% in postmenopausal women and 64% in premenopausal women. Sarcomas that are well differentiated and limited to the endometrium without vascular lymph involvement and with mitotic counts of less than 20 per 10 HPF had the best prognosis.

Women with LMS had a recurrence of 63%, with the progression-free interval averaging 20.6 months (16,17). The most common symptoms of recurrence are shortness of breath and pelvic pain (see Table

12.3). The treatment for recurrent disease is chemotherapy, doxorubicin, or a combination of ifosfamide and Mesna. The response rate varies from 10.3% to 17%, with no complete responders (17).

SUMMARY

Fortunately, uterine sarcomas are rare since they carry such a poor prognosis. Leiomysarcomas are the most common uterine sarcoma in the pre- and perimenopausal woman. In any woman with a pelvic mass associated with abnormal vaginal bleeding an evaluation with an endometrial biopsy or curettage is warranted. The diagnosis of LMS is often difficult since many of these tumors may be found in an early stage or with a benign leiomyoma. MRI imaging with a T-2–weighted image is a useful adjunct to the evaluation. Although a large majority of LMS are stage I disease, they still have the poorest prognosis and survival rate of all uterine sarcomas.

REFERENCES

1. Ober W. Uterine sarcomas: histogenesis and taxonomy. Ann NY Acad Sci 1959;74:568.
2. Dinh T, Woodruff JD. Leiomyosarcoma of the uterus. Am J Obstet Gynecol 1982;144:817.
3. Christopherson W, Williamson E, Gray L. Leiomyosarcoma of the uterus. Cancer 1972;29:1512.
4. Blaustein A. Pathology of the female genital tract. New York: Springer-Verlag, 1977:322.
5. Kempson R, Bari W. Uterine sarcomas: classification, diagnosis and prognosis. Hum Pathol 1970;1:331.
6. Norris H, Taylor H. Postirradiation sarcomas of the uterus. Obstet Gynecol 1965;26:689.
7. Vardi J, Tovell H. Leiomyosarcoma of the uterus: clinicopathologic study. Obstet Gynecol 1980;56:428.
8. Disaia P, Creasman W. Clinical gynecologic oncology. St. Louis: Mosby–Year Book, 1993:194.

9. Silverberg S. Leiomyosarcoma of the uterus: a clinicopathologic study. Obstet Gynecol 1971;38:613.
10. Ferenzy A, Richart R, Okagaki T. A comparative ultrastructural study of leiomyosarcoma, cellular leiomyoma, and leiomyoma of the uterus. Cancer 1971;28:1004.
11. O'Connor D, Norris H. Mitotically active leiomyomas of the uterus. Hum Pathol 1990;21:223.
12. Takemori M, Nishimura R, Sugimura K. Magnetic resonance imaging of uterine leiomyosarcoma. Arch Gynecol Obstet 1992;251:215.
13. Pattani S, Kier R, Deal R, Luchansky E. MRI of uterine leiomyosarcoma. Magnetic Resonance Imaging 1995;13:331.
14. Burns B, Curry R, Bell A. Morphologic features of prognostic significance in uterine smooth muscle tumors: a review of eighty-four cases. Am J Obstet Gynecol 1979;135:109.
15. Gilbert H, Kagan A, Lagasse L, et al. The value of radiation therapy in uterine sarcoma. Obstet Gynecol 1975;45:84.
16. Kahanpaa K, Wahlstrom T, Grohn P, et al. Sarcomas of the uterus: a clinicopathologic study of 119 patients. Obstet Gynecol 1986;67:417.
17. Gallup D, Hobbs L, Ross W. Recurrence of uterine leiomyosarcoma 25 years after therapy. Gynecol Oncol 1982;13:293.

CHAPTER

13

Gonadotropin-Releasing Hormone Add-Back Therapy as an Alternative to Myomectomy

Elizabeth A. Stewart

Uterine leiomyomas or fibroids are benign uterine neoplasms that are found in 25% to 75% of all women. Symptoms including abnormal uterine bleeding, particularly menorrhagia, and pelvic pressure and pain can be caused by these neoplasms. Surgical therapy has always been the mainstay of therapy for leiomyomas. Hysterectomy or myomectomy, which removes only the neoplastic tissue, is widely employed. However, interest exists for a nonsurgical method of controlling myoma symptoms. Gonadotropin-releasing hormone (GnRH) agonists can provide dramatic relief from symptoms of leiomyomas. However, the side effects of these medications limit their long-term use.

Gonadotropin-releasing hormone agonists have also been widely used in the preoperative management of patients who are undergoing myomectomy. Does GnRH agonist therapy have a role as an alternative to myomectomy, however? We believe that this is an appropriate alternative in selected patients. Most long-term regimens have utilized steroid hormones to limit the side effects experienced with GnRH agonists alone. In the future we believe that multiple regimens will be available to provide relief of symptoms while limiting side effects.

GOALS OF MEDICAL THERAPY

Medical therapy can be used to relieve a number of leiomyoma-related symptoms. Two broad categories of action of GnRH agonists are useful in obtaining symptomatic relief for patients: reduction in uterine volume and induction of amenorrhea. GnRH agonists are useful in decreasing uterine volume from 34% to 61% (1). This reduction can alleviate non-specific pelvic pressure or pain and specific impingement of leiomyomas on other pelvic structures such as the bowel, bladder, or specific nerves, and perhaps may be useful in decreasing bleeding. The mechanism of this effect is not well understood. The induction of amenorrhea is more clearly related to the profound hypoestrogenism induced by the use of GnRH agonists. Without estrogen to build up the endometrial lining atrophy will ensue. These two end points need to be clearly kept in mind when treatment is initiated.

For certain groups of patients medical therapy can have clear advantages over myomectomy. The most obvious case is the perimenopausal woman who has symptoms related to her leiomyomas. Women with symptoms related to bleeding and to uterine volume may benefit from this approach. The aim of therapy would be relief of symptoms that would not tend to recur after discontinuation of the medication since menopause would bring about resolution of leiomyoma symptoms. However, because of the variability of onset of age of menopause in some women symptoms may recur.

Medical therapy may also be the treatment of choice in women with severe medical illnesses that would contraindicate surgery. Examples include leukemia, aplastic anemia, and severe cardiac or pulmonary complications. In addition some women may have important reasons for postponing surgery to a more convenient time. Examples might include teachers who wish to time their operation during vacation, and medical students or residents for whom surgery at a particular time would mean loss of approximately a year's work.

LIMITATIONS OF THERAPY

Gonadotropin-releasing hormone agonists have been associated with some side effects. Hot flushes are most commonly seen, with 80% to 100% of patients experiencing flushes, often within the first month of therapy (2). Other symptoms that limit the use of therapy less commonly include irregular vaginal bleeding, headaches, mood changes, vaginal dryness and dyspareunia, hair loss, and arthralgias/myalgias (2). The most serious potential side effect of GnRH agonist is the potential for an accelerated rate of bone resorption, which can lead to osteoporosis with long-term therapy. This has been the factor that has limited the use of GnRH agonists to 3 to 6 months of therapy. Multiple studies have been done to assess bone loss over short-term therapy and the results have been conflicting. Some studies suggest that the short-term bone loss is reversible whereas others indicate permanent decrements in bone (3). One technical issue is germane to this issue: The precision of measure of bone densitometry may be close to the percentage of bone lost during these short-term treatments. Therefore, large studies may be needed to address this issue. In addition, there may be significant differences between studies that assess bone density in patients with endometriosis who are undergoing GnRH agonist therapy and those that assess patients with leiomyomas who are undergoing the same therapy. Women with leiomyomas tend to be older and often in perimenopausal transition and to have greater body mass index, which can affect estrogen metabolism (3).

ADD-BACK THERAPY: RATIONALE

For many women, 3 to 6 months of symptomatic relief from leiomyomas will not allow them to avoid surgery but only to optimally prepare themselves for an operation. Therefore, the concept of adding additional therapy to minimize the side effects of prolonged therapy was developed, the so-called add-back regimens. Several theories may be useful in understanding add-back regimens.

Estrogen Threshold Hypothesis

Studies have demonstrated that there is a hierarchy of responsiveness of tissues to the effects of estrogens (4). Thus, since the same dose of estrogen may protect against loss of bone density but not change leiomyoma metabolism a "window" of estrogen dose might be found that would alleviate symptoms of GnRH agonist therapy yet not permit the regrowth of leiomyomas (5).

This hypothesis is illustrated in Figure 13.1. Zone A is the level of estradiol seen in normal cycling premenopausal women. This is the level of estradiol that may be causing leiomyoma-related symptoms as well as supporting normal tissues including bone and vaginal mucosa. Zone C represents postmenopausal or castrate levels of estradiol. These levels are similar to those seen in most women after GnRH agonist treatment. Thus, a reduction in myoma-related symptoms may occur with GnRH agonist treatment but at the expense of bone loss, vaginal dryness, and other hypoestrogenic symptoms. Zone B represents the target range for GnRH add-back therapy under the estrogen window hypothesis. These levels are consistent with early follicular phase estradiol levels and are adequate to maintain certain estrogen-dependent tissues including bone, but to maintain myoma regression. The exact threshhold where these effects are seen is not defined.

Molecular Rearrangement Hypothesis

While the estrogen window hypothesis is applicable to many diseases and symptoms, the molecular rearrangement hypothesis is specific to leimyomas and their regrowth after hormonal therapy. It states that there is a rearrangement of the underlying molecular structure that occurs in leiomyomas or normal myometrium, or both, while GnRH agonist treatment is ongoing. The exact nature of this rearrangement is not yet known; however, studies have indicated that GnRH agonist treatment has specific effects on components of the extracellular matrix (6) and receptors for steroid hormones (7) that may prove to be important in these changes. Once these changes have occurred, low levels of steroid hormones can be added without the rapid regrowth of myomas. Thus, the sequence of administration of hormones may be as important as the levels of the hormones.

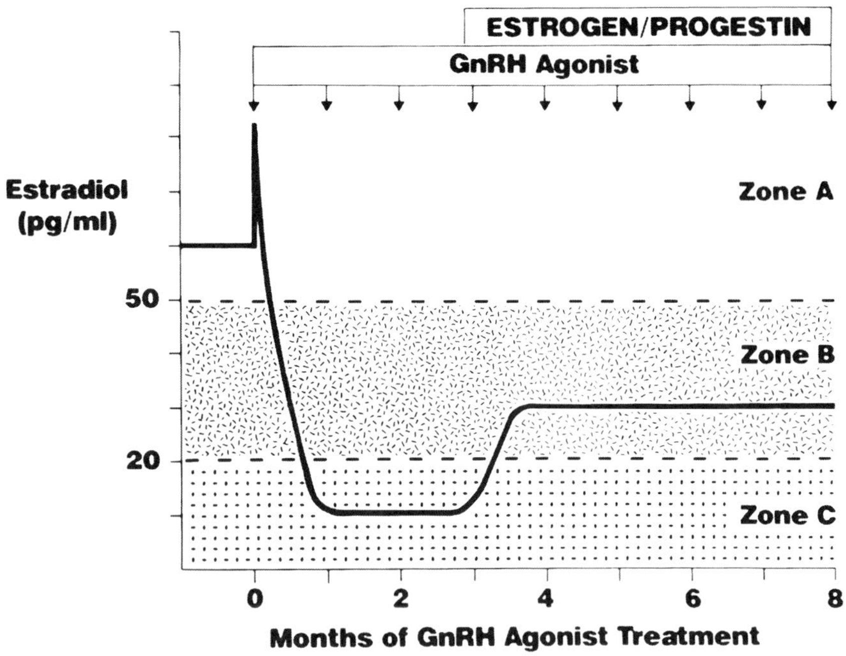

FIG. 13.1.

Estrogen threshold hypothesis. Zone A: Typical circulating estradiol concentrations in premenopausal women are able to support myometrial-fibroid growth and prevent rapid bone resorption. Zone B: Therapeutic window. Myometrial and fibroid volume may decrease at these estradiol levels, but bone resorption is not accelerated. Zone C: Hypoestrogenism, often attained during GnRH agonist therapy, can lead to myometrial-fibroid shrinkage and rapid bone resorption. Note: Estradiol values for each zone may differ among patients. (Reproduced by permission from Friedman AJ, Lobel SM, Rein MS, Barbieri RL. Efficacy and safety considerations in women with uterine leiomyomas treated with gonadotropin-releasing hormone agonists: the estrogen threshold hypothesis. Am J Obstet Gynecol 1990;163:1114–1119.)

This hypothesis would account for differences in response to simultaneous GnRH agonist and hormone administration versus the sequential administration of GnRH agonist first followed by hormonal therapy (Fig. 13.2). A variety of studies have employed the sequential administration of hormones with 3 to 6 months of agonist treatment preceding

TABLE 13.1

Studies of GnRH-agonists with steroidal add-back regimens

Reference	No. of Patients	Length of Treatment (mo)	Design	Agonist	Steroid Components	Initial Reduction (%)	Final Reduction (%)
Friedman et al, 1988 (11)	16	6	Simultaneous	Leuprolide acetate	MPA, 20 mg	86	—
Friedman, 1989 (14)	5	3 + 24	Sequential	Leuprolide acetate	CEE, 625 mg (days 1–25) MPA, 10 mg (days 16–25)	51	55
Maheux et al, 1991 (15)	10	3 + 9	Sequential	Goserelin	CEE, 0.3 mg MPA, 5 mg	50.7	56–70
Lumsden et al, 1989 (16)	6	6	Simultaneous	Goserelin	Tamoxifen, 20 mg	5–27	—

Lumsden et al, 1989 (16)	1	3 + 3	Sequential	Goserelin	Tamoxifen, 20 mg	59	62
Friedman et al, 1993 (18)	51	3 + 9	Sequential	Leuprolide acetate	1. Estropipate, 0.75 mg, + norethindrone, 0.7 mg	64	75
					2. Norethindrone, 10 mg	64	92
Carr et al, 1993 (17)	16	3 + 3	Crossover				
			Protocol A: Steroid 1st	Leuprolide acetate	MPA	A: 100	74
			Protocol B: Steroid 2nd	Leuprolide acetate	MPA	B: 73	78
Friedman et al, 1994 (19)	51	3 + 21	Sequential	Leuprolide acetate	1. Estropipate, 0.75 mg, + norethindrone, 0.7 mg	60	55
					2. Norethindrone, 10 mg	60	95

MPA, medroxyprogesterone acetate; CEE, conjugated equine estrogens.

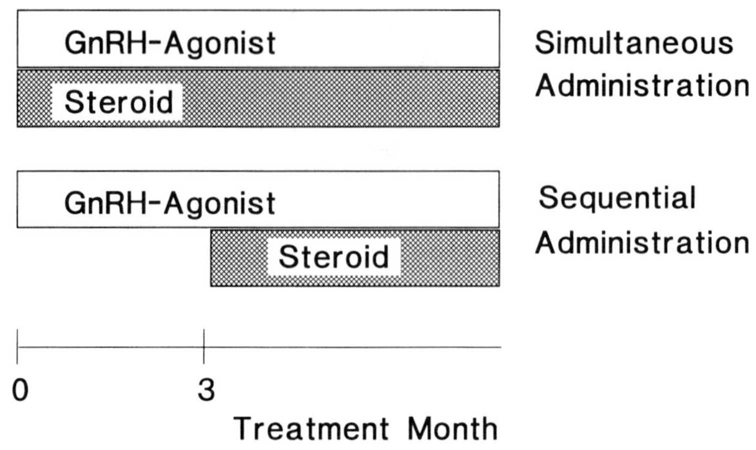

FIG. 13.2.

Two general treatment strategies can be employed during GnRH agonist therapy with steroid hormone add-back. In the simultaneous regimen GnRH agonist and steroidal therapy are started at the same time. In the sequential regimen GnRH agonist is given alone for approximately 3 months and, after the effects of maximal hypoestrogenism have been obtained, steroid replacement is begun. (Reproduced by permission from Stewart EA, Friedman AJ. Steroidal treatment of myomas. Semin Reprod Endocrinol 1992;10: 344–357.)

hormonal replacement. These findings are discussed in detail later (Table 13.1).

STEROID DEPENDENCE OF LEIOMYOMAS

For a long time, leiomyomas have been believed to be steroid-dependent neoplasms. Estrogen has long been implicated as the primary hormone that governs leiomyoma growth. Both clinical observations and biochemical data support this contention. Fibroids develop during the reproductive years and growth can take place in relatively high estrogen states (pregnancy, ovulation induction). In contrast, hypoestrogenic states induce fibroid and myometrial regression (menopause, GnRH agonist therapy). Additionally, there appear to be increased concentrations of estrogens, increased levels of estrogen receptors, and more potent estrogens in leiomyomas than in adjacent normal myometrium (1). All of these factors suggest that leiomyomas are estrogen-dependent neoplasms.

Progesterone may also play a role in the pathogenesis of leiomyomas. Early studies that lacked adequate controls suggested that pharmacologic levels of progesterone caused shrinkage of uterine leiomyomas (1). More recently this issue has been re-examined in light of data that show that the progesterone and glucocorticoid antagonist RU 486 can cause dramatic shrinkage of uterine leiomyomas (8). In addition, a number of recent studies have shown that genes relevant to leiomyoma growth are differentially expressed in the proliferative versus the secretory phase of the menstrual cycle including collagens type I and III (9) and epidermal growth factor (10). However, this has not been demonstrated to be due to the effect of progesterone. A number of studies of add-back therapy in leiomyomas have used progestin add-back alone in the belief that progestin would not influence myoma regrowth but at the same time would be sufficient to prevent bone loss and treat vasomotor flushes.

STEROIDAL ADD-BACK

An initial randomized, placebo-controlled study investigating the use of steroidal add-back therapy employed the simultaneous administration of leuprolide acetate (LA; 0.5 mg/day) plus medroxyprogesterone acetate (MPA; 20 mg/day) (11). This dose of MPA had previously been demonstrated to decrease both the symptomatology of vasomotor flushes (12) and to decrease indices of bone resorption (13). Although this therapy was effective in reducing the hot flashes, it inhibited the decrease in uterine volume seen with agonist therapy alone. Patients who received the MPA/LA combination had a mean reduction in uterine volume of 14% compared to 51% for patients who received LA plus placebo (11).

Alternatively, a second pilot study of five women utilized a sequential regimen with daily LA (0.5 mg/day) for 3 months, at which time conjugated equine estrogens (0.625 mg, days 1–25) and MPA (10 mg, days 16–25) were added for an additional 2 years (14). This regimen allowed the maintenance of the 49% reduction in uterine volume while providing symptomatic relief of vasomotor flushes without measurable decrement in bone density.

Goserelin as a depot formulation of GnRH agonist (3.6 mg every 28 days) was utilized with a lower dose of conjugated equine estrogens (0.3 mg, days 1–25) and MPA (5 mg, days 16–25) in a sequential regimen in 10 women (15). Again a 49% decrease in mean myoma volume was seen and was maintained when steroid hormones were added (15). This regimen was less effective in maintaining relief of hypoestrogenic symptoms, however, and changes in bone density were not assessed.

Insight into the mechanisms of uterine shrinkage is gained through a study that utilized the drug tamoxifen, which has actions as both an estrogen agonist and antagonist. This study utilized depot goserelin (3.6 mg every 28 days) with the simultaneous addition of tamoxifen (20 mg/day) (16). Estradiol concentrations were significantly suppressed in the group given tamoxifen; however, no reduction in uterine volume was seen. A single patient was treated with a sequential regimen, however, receiving goserelin alone for 12 weeks followed by the addition of tamoxifen for 12 weeks. In this patient a reduction in uterine volume of 59% was seen at 12 weeks and maintained throughout the 12 weeks of tamoxifen therapy.

A study of 16 patients used MPA add-back in a randomized, prospective, placebo-controlled, double-blind crossover trial design and assessed changes using magnetic resonance imaging (MRI) (17). All patients received LA (1 mg/day) for the entire 6-month treatment period. Patients on protocol A received MPA (20 mg/day) for the first 3 months and placebo for the last 3 months, and patients on protocol B received placebo for the first 3 months, then crossed over to receive the same dose of MPA for the last 3 months. Magnetic resonance imaging of the uterus was done at the time of entry into the study and at 3 and 6 months.

Uterine volume did not change at 3 months in women who received LA plus MPA for the first 3 months and was reduced to 73% of baseline volume in women who received LA plus placebo (17). After the crossover the women in protocol A who were now taking LA plus placebo experienced an equivalent decrease in uterine volume to 74% of baseline. The patients in protocol B experienced an increase in uterine size with the addition of MPA to 78% of baseline. MRI showed no significant changes in myoma volume at any time in the study, with non-myomatous uterine volume showing changes that paralleled those of total uterine volume. No significant differences were seen in hormonal or lipid parameters between the treatment groups. Measures of bone turnover were not assessed.

A prospective randomized trial following 51 women with either estrogen or estrogen/progestin add-back therapy has reported results at both 1 and 2 years of follow-up (18,19). All patients received LA treatment for 3 months and then were randomized to receive either daily estropipate (0.75 mg) plus norethindrone (0.7 mg) for 14 days each month or norethindrone, 10 mg per day, with no estrogen therapy. Both groups had a mean decrease in uterine volume of 64% at 3 months (18).

At 1 year of follow-up, all patients had an increase in uterine size with steroidal add-back; however, the magnitude of this change was different depending on the steroidal regimen (18). The regrowth in the estrogen/progestin group was not significant (75% of pretreatment), whereas the progestin-only group had a significant increase to 92% of pretreatment volume (18). In addition, the progestin-only group had a significant decrease in high-density lipoprotein (HDL) levels that was not seen in the estrogen/progestin group. The menstrual cycle control was also worse for the progestin-only group, in which significantly more patients experienced bleeding or spotting at 52 weeks compared to those in the estrogen/progestin regimen. Both regimens were successful in increasing the hemoglobin concentration and hematocrit. In addition, both patient groups experienced a significant 3% loss of bone during the LA treatment period that was stabilized by both hormonal add-back regimens. These changes continued to be present after 2 years of follow-up (19). Thus, the estrogen/progestin add-back regimen appears superior to the progestin-only regimen in both safety and efficacy.

NONSTEROIDAL ADD-BACK

Although studies to date have concentrated on combining GnRH agonist therapy with estrogens or progestins, or both, nonsteroidal agents present another avenue of therapy. The treatment of postmenopausal women who are symptomatic with hot flashes provides a useful analogy. Although women with vasomotor flushes are generally prescribed low doses of estrogen and progestin, for those with contraindications or intolerance of this regimen, progestin alone (12), clonidine (20), and Bellergal (21) have all been advocated as therapy.

Although use of nonsteroidal medications to limit vasomotor flushes may have a small role in the treatment of women with GnRH therapy, by far the most important side effect that limits therapy is bone loss, which can potentially lead to osteoporosis. Thus, nonsteroidal agents aimed at preventing bone loss may be important in extending the treatment duration of GnRH agonists. To date studies have not been published using such agents in women with leiomyomas. However, studies are available from other fields that provide insight into their usefulness.

BISPHOSPHONATES

Bisphosphonates act by inhibiting osteoclast-mediated bone reabsorption. Etidronate and pamidronate are commercially available first generation bisphosphonates. Etidronate has proved to be an effective regimen for preventing postmenopausal osteoporosis in women when given in an intermittent, cyclic regimen with calcium supplementation during intervals when etidronate is not given (22,23). Etidronate has also been combined with low-dose norethindrone (2.5 mg/day) in a pilot study of 11 women who underwent GnRH agonist therapy for endometriosis (3). A control group received norethindrone, 10 mg per day. Both regimens decreased pelvic pain and minimized bone loss and vasomotor symptoms compared to those of historic controls (24). However, only the patients treated with high-dose progestin had decreased HDL cholesterol levels. The same regimen with a prospectively monitored, no-treatment control group was recently reported after 48 months of follow-up (25). Again both regimens were successful in maintaining bone density and decreasing symptoms. However, the patients in the high-dose progestin arm of the study showed adverse changes in low-density lipoprotein (LDL) and HDL cholesterol as well as apolipoprotein A1 (25). Thus, the low-dose norethindrone/etidronate arm appeared to be a superior treatment.

A second generation of bisphosphonates is now becoming commercially available, with alendronate as the first member of this class. Alendronate has been demonstrated to decrease the risk of nonvertebral fractures in postmenopausal women and lead to increased bone density (26). No studies to date have been reported that employ these newer agents as add-back therapy.

PARATHYROID HORMONE

Parathyroid hormone (PTH) is an 84-amino-acid polypeptide hormone, the primary function of which is to control extracellular fluid calcium concentrations. It acts on the kidney to increase reabsorption of calcium, enhances calcium reabsorption from bone, and influences calcium absorption from the gastrointestinal tract. The N-terminal fragment is crucial for receptor binding and thus this fragment (hPTH-[1-34]) is often used clinically. When administered intermittently PTH increases bone formation. A recent study examined the use of PTH (40 mg/day) in a prospective study of 40 women who were receiving the GnRH agonist nafarelin (200 μg twice a day) for 6 months for the treatment of endometriosis (27). Women treated with nafarelin plus PTH showed significantly more maintenance of bone density when measured by dual energy x-ray absorptiometry and an increase in biochemical markers for bone formation compared to women who received nafarelin alone (27). Nausea was the major side effect and occurred more commonly in patients who received PTH.

CALCITONIN

Calcitonin is another peptide hormone that may have utility as an agent useful for nonsteroidal add-back. Physiologically, it decreases serum calcium by reducing osteoclast-mediated bone reabsorption. It has been useful in preventing postmenopausal osteoporosis (28,29). Human calcitonin caused significant nausea and flushing; however, a synthetic salmon calcitonin that is available as a nasal spray minimizes these side effects. There have been no studies to date investigating calcitonin in combination with GnRH agonist therapy.

CONCLUSION

Gonadotropin-releasing hormone agonist therapy, when combined with steroidal therapy, can be a safe and effective treatment for uterine leiomyomas. Studies are needed to examine the role of nonsteroidal add-back therapy for women with leiomyomas. The chemical nature of add-back therapy, the sequence of administration of medications, and the dose chosen can all be important considerations of therapy. In addition, the clinician must have clear therapeutic goals in mind and know whether a reduction in uterine volume or the induction of amenorrhea, or both, will achieve those goals.

Current studies have defined the end points of therapy after 2 years of treatment. Continued study is required not only to obtain further data on safety and efficacy but also to explore issues that relate to compliance with and cost-effectiveness of these therapies.

REFERENCES

1. Stewart EA, Friedman AJ. Steroidal treatment of myomas. In: Barbieri RL, Speroff L, eds. Seminars in reproductive endocrinology. vol. 10(4). New York: Thieme Medical, 1992:344–357.
2. Friedman AJ. GnRH agonists: patient selection, drug information, monitoring and side effects. In: Barbieri RL, Friedman AJ, eds. Gonadotropin releasing hormone analogs: applications in gynecology. New York: Elsevier, 1991:17–38.
3. Lemay A, Surrey ES, Friedman AJ. Extending the use of gonadotropin-releasing hormone agonists: the emerging role of steroidal and nonsteroidal agents. Fertil Steril 1994;61:21–34.
4. Chetkowski RJ, Meldrum DR, Steingold KA, et al. Biological effects of transdermal estradiol. N Engl J Med 1986;314:1615–1620.
5. Friedman AJ, Lobel SM, Rein MS, Barbieri RL. Efficacy and safety considerations in women with uterine leiomyomas treated with gonadotropin-releasing hormone agonists: the estrogen threshold hypothesis. Am J Obstet Gynecol 1990;163:1114–1119.
6. Stewart EA, Rhoades AR, Nowak RA. Leuprolide acetate treated leiomyomas retain relative overexpression of collagen type I and collagen type III messenger RNAs. J Soc Gynecol Invest 1995;2:278.
7. Rein MS, Friedman AJ, Stuart JM, MacLaughlin DT. Fibroid and myometrial steroid receptors in women treated with the gonadotropin-releasing hormone agonist leuprolide acetate. Fertil Steril 1990;53: 1018–1023.
8. Murphy AA, Kettel LM, Morales AJ, et al. Regression of uterine leiomyomata in response to the antiprogesterone RU486. J Clin Endocrinol Metab 1993;76:513–517.
9. Stewart EA, Peck K, Friedman AJ, Nowak RA. Relative overexpression of collagen type I and collagen type III messenger RNAs by uterine leiomyomas during the follicular phase of the menstrual cycle. J Clin Endocrinol Metab 1994;79:900–906.
10. Harrison-Woolrych ML, Charnock-Jones DS, Smith SK. Quantification of messenger ribonucleic acid for epidermal growth factor in human myometrium and leiomyomata using reverse transcriptase polymerase chain reaction. J Clin Endocrinol Metab 1994;78:1179–1184.
11. Friedman AJ, Barbieri RL, Doubilet PM, et al. A randomized double-blind trial of a gonadotropin releasing hormone agonist (leuprolide) with or

without medroxyprogesterone acetate in the treatment of leiomyomata uteri. Fertil Steril 1988;49:404–409.

12. Schiff I, Tulchinsky D, Cramer D, Ryan KJ. Oral medroxyprogesterone in the treament of postmenopausal symptoms. JAMA 1980;244:1443–1445.
13. Mandel FP, Davidson BJ, Erlik Y, et al. Effects of progestins on bone metabolism in postmenopausal women. J Reprod Med 1982;27:511–514.
14. Friedman AJ. Treatment of leiomyomata uteri with short-term leuprolide followed by leuprolide plus estrogen-progestin hormone replacement therapy for 2 years: a pilot study. 1989;51:526–528.
15. Maheux R, Lemay A, Blanchet P, et al. Maintained reduction of uterine leiomyoma following addition of hormonal replacement therapy to a monthly luteinizing hormone-releasing agonist implant: a pilot study. Hum Reprod 1991;6:500–505.
16. Lumsden MA, West CP, Hillier H, et al. Estrogenic action of tamoxifen in women treated with luteinizing hormone-releasing hormone agonists (goserelin)—lack of shrinkage of uterine fibroids. Fertil Steril 1989;52: 924–929.
17. Carr BR, Marshburn PB, Weatherall PT, et al. An evaluation of the effect of gonadotropin-releasing hormone analogs and medroxyprogesterone acetate on uterine leiomyomata volume by magnetic resonance imaging: a prospective, randomized, double-blind placebo-controlled crossover trial. J Clin Endocrinol Metab 1993;76:1217–1223.
18. Friedman AJ, Daly M, Juneau-Norcross M, et al. A prospective, randomized trial of gonadotropin releasing-hormone agonist plus estrogen-progestin or progestin "add-back" regimens for women with leiomyomata uteri. J Clin Endocrinol Metab 1993;76:1439–1445.
19. Friedman AJ, Daly M, Juneau-Norcross M, et al. Long-term medical therapy for leiomyomata uteri: a prospective, randomized study of leuprolide acetate depot plus either oestrogen-progestin or progestin "add-back" for 2 years. Hum Reprod 1994;9:1618–1625.
20. Laufer LR, Erlik Y, Meldrum DR, Judd HL. Effect of clonidine on hot flashes in postmenopausal women. Obstet Gynecol 1982;60:583–586.
21. Lebherz TB, French L. Nonhormonal treatment of the menopausal syndrome. A double-blind evaluation of an autonomic system stabilizer. Obstet Gynecol 1969;33:795–799.
22. Storm T, Thamsborg G, Steiniche T, et al. Effect of intermittent cyclical etidronate therapy on bone mass and fracture rate in women with postmenopausal osteoporosis. N Engl J Med 1990;322:1265–1271.

23. Watts NB, Hauis ST, Genant HK, et al. Intermittent cyclical etidronate treatment of postmenopausal osteoporosis. N Engl J Med 1990;323:73–79.
24. Surrey ES, Fournet N, Voigt B, Judd HL. Effects of sodium etidronate in combination with low-dose norethindrone in patients administered a long-acting GnRH agonist: a preliminary report. Obstet Gynecol 1993;81: 581–586.
25. Surrey ES, Voigt B, Fournet N, Judd HL. Prolonged gonadotropin-releasing hormone agonist treatment of symptomatic endometriosis: the role of cyclic sodium etidronate and low-dose norethindrone "add-back" therapy. Fertil Steril 1995;63:747–755.
26. Karpf DB, Shapiro DR, Seeman E, et al. Prevention of nonvertebral fractures by alendronate. A meta-analysis. JAMA 1997;277:1159–1164.
27. Finkelstein JS, Klibanski A, Schaefer EH, et al. Parathyroid hormone for the prevention of bone loss induced by estrogen deficiency. N Engl J Med 1994;331:1618–1623.
28. Overgaard K, Hansen MA, Nielsen VAH, et al. Discontinuous calcitonin treatment of established osteoporosis—effects of withdrawal of treatment. Am J Med 1990;89:1–6.
29. Buclin T, Randin JP, Jacquet AE, et al. The effect of rectal and nasal administration of salmon calcitonin in normal subjects. Calcif Tissue Int 1987;41: 252–258.

CHAPTER

14

Morbidity Associated with Myomectomy

Richard E. Leach
Michael P. Diamond

The reported complications associated with myomectomy and their occurrence vary widely. While some investigators have reported no complications in a combined series of 119 patients (1–3), others have reported complications in over 50% of patients who underwent myomectomy (4–8) (Table 14.1). The more common complications include febrile morbidity, ranging from 0% to 38%, and hemorrhage, requiring transfusion ranging from 0% to 52%. It is suggested by one author that the variable rate of complications associated with myomectomy supports the opinion that experience and surgical technique may play an important role (4). This chapter reviews the risks of complications associated with myomectomy and discusses possible techniques to reduce them.

EARLY COMPLICATIONS

Hemorrhage

Hemorrhage remains a significant potential complication when myomectomy is performed.

Preoperative adjuvant therapy has been proposed as a method to significantly reduce intraoperative blood loss. However, some contro-

TABLE 14.1

Reported complications associated with abdominal myomectomy

COMPLICATION	LAMORTE ET AL, 1993 (4) N = 128 (%)	GOLAN ET AL, 1993 (5) N = 21 (%)	KILTZ ET AL, 1994 (6) N = 28 (%)	HUTCHINS, 1992 (7) N = 67 (%)	FRIEDMAN ET AL, 1989 (8) N = 18 (%)
Fever	15 (12)	8 (38)	NA	7 (10)	9 (50)
Transfusion	26 (20)	11 (52)	6 (21)	2 (3)	4 (22)
EBL > 1000 mL	6 (5)	NA	NA	NA	0
Hysterectomy	1 (1)	0	0	1 (1)	0
Postoperative complication	3 (2) 1 DVT 1 wound infection 1 ileus	1 (5) 1 wound infection	NA	2 (2) 1 ileus 1 pelvic thrombophlebitis	0
Total	51 (40)	20 (95)	6 (21)	11 (16)	13 (72)

NA, not available (not evaluated); EBL, estimated blood loss; DVT, deep venous thrombosis.

versy remains as to whether gonadotropin-releasing hormone agonist (GnRHag) therapy will significantly reduce intraoperative blood loss in all situations (Table 14.2). Friedman et al (8) showed no significant difference in estimated blood loss (EBL) in women who underwent myomectomy between leuprolide acetate–treated patients (n = 9) preoperatively and control untreated patients (n = 9), with EBLs of 242 mL and 189 mL, respectively. Further, no change occurred in the preoperative versus postoperative hematocrit, measured 4 weeks later, at 1.3% and 1.4%, respectively. Two patients in each group required blood transfusion. When the patients were stratified according to their preoperative uterine volume, in those women with uterine volume greater than 600 mL (n = 5), GnRHag treatment resulted in a significant

TABLE 14.2

Estimated blood loss and number of transfusions after myomectomy with and without GnRHag pretreatment

AUTHOR	GROUP (N)	EBL (ML)	Δ HCT	TRANSFUSIONS
Friedman et al (8)	Treated (9)	242	−1.30%	2
	Control (9)	189	−1.40%	2
Hutchins (7)	Treated (48)	300	NA	2
	Control (19)	257	NA	0
Golan et al (5)	Treated (12)	320	NA	6
	Control (9)	476	NA	4
Kiltz et al (6)	Treated (19)	700*	−12%	3
	Control (9)	700*	−10%	3

EBL, estimated blood loss; Hct, hematocrit; NA, not available (not evaluated).
*Extrapolated from bar graph.

reduction in blood loss when compared to those with pretreatment uterine volume of less than 600 mL (n = 4). The authors recommended GnRHag therapy as having potential use in patients with large preoperative uteri (>16 wk) and anemia. Hutchins (7) found no significant difference in the EBL between control or leuprolide acetate–treated patients and two of the treated patients required transfusion. The results from this study are difficult to interpret since the treated patients had significantly larger uterine volume preoperatively than the control untreated group. Golan et al (5) found a significant difference in the EBL in the treated versus the control group, 320 mL versus 476 mL, respectively. However, six patients in the treated group and four in the control group required transfusion. Kiltz et al (6) tested the effect of two doses of leuprolide acetate, 3.75 mg and 7.5 mg, versus control and showed no significant difference in EBL between both doses of treatment and control group. Three patients in the treated and three in the control group required transfusion. The clinical significance of the differences in EBL in the studies cited remains to be determined; however, there appears to be no difference in the number of transfusions whether or not patients have had presurgical GnRHag treatment. Hemorrhage, and its treatment by transfusion, is especially important in the current era of hepatitis C and human immunodeficiency virus (HIV). Many patients are extremely concerned about the risk of these and other infectious diseases.

GnRHag therapy has been reported to induce hypoestrogenism, amenorrhea, and significant reduction in uterine volume in women with leiomyomata uteri (8). Despite these effects some women will continue to bleed after continued therapy. The occurrence of significant vaginal hemorrhage with GnRHag therapy has been reported in three women (9). In all three cases, the estradiol level was less than 20 pg/mL at the time of hemorrhage. After the patients were stabilized, they underwent emergent myomectomies after receiving four units of packed red blood cells (RBCs) in each case. In all three patients histopathologic analysis revealed hyaline degeneration with focal necrosis and hemorrhage. It is possible that rapid involution of the submucous fibroids found in each case is responsible for the hemorrhage. These authors had a similar experience with three different premenopausal women who were being treated for leiomyomas with GnRHag and profuse vaginal bleeding 7 to 11 weeks after initiation of treatment (10). GnRH therapy was discontinued and each patient was treated with combination oral contraceptives (OCP) and ferrous sulfate. The profuse vaginal bleeding stopped within 48 hours of the initiation of OCP treatment and the hemoglobin returned to normal. Subsequently, each patient underwent definitive surgical treatment within 4 to 6 weeks without need for blood transfusion. Submucous myomas were also identified in these patients.

Controlling intraoperative loss by mechanical interruption of the uterine and ovarian vessels has been proposed to be the simplest method to control uterine incision bleeding. These surgical tenets of Victor Bonney, who promoted the advantages of myomectomy in the early 1930s, remain the basis by which myomectomies are performed today. Bonney (11) introduced a clamp, named after himself, that not only occludes the uterine vessels in the lower uterine segment but also provides a means of uterine elevation. Rubin (12) described the technique of using a tourniquet method by incising the broad ligament bilaterally and introducing a rubber drain around the lower uterine segment, compressing the uterine arteries and clamping the tourniquet in the cul-de-sac. Lastly, a rubber shod bulldog clamp placed over the infundibulopelvic ligament bilaterally can help to control bleeding (13). Intermittent release of any of these vascular occluding techniques is important in preventing undue necrosis secondary to ischemia. The application of the Bonney clamp or the tourniquet technique described by Rubin may be difficult to apply in patients with large cervical and broad ligament leiomyomas. Care must be taken not to evulse tissue grasped by the clamps while performing the myomectomy (13). It should be recognized that while these mechanical techniques are widely utilized, their use has not undergone rigorous examination. Similarly, the effect of these techniques on postoperative adhesion development remains to be determined.

Another technique utilized to minimize blood loss is the uterine injection of vasopressin, first described by Dillon in 1962 (14). The doses used have ranged from two units diluted in 5 mL to 20 mL lactated Ringer's solution. The solution is injected into the serosa overlying the myoma in the region of the intended incision and also into the base of the fibroid, with a resultant characteristic blanching. The strategy for the location of the incision should consider several factors: First, the placement of an incision is made to accommodate the removal of as many myomas through that incision as possible (15). Secondly, placement of an anterior uterine incision is preferred to minimize the risk of adhesion formation to the adnexa, which is not uncommon with posterior incisions. Third, avoiding the cornual region will prevent inadvertent intramural tubal damage and possible occlusion with the suture intended to close the myometrial defect.

After the myoma is identified and the initial incision is made, traction on the myoma with a towel clamp or a large-caliber suture delineates the adherent myometrial fibers and associated blood vessels. The use of unipolar cautery in a blended coagulation-cutting mode or laser can adequately coagulate and cut the tissue that has been exposed using either hemostats or a Teflon-tipped probe. As this process is performed circumferentially, the myoma becomes enucleated. Rarely are bleeding vessels identified within the remaining myometrium; rather, typically a generalized ooze is seen. Proper closure of the incision site includes complete reapproximation of the denuded myometrium, usually in several layers, with nonreactive absorbable sutures of 2.0 or 3.0 caliber. With large defects, a continuous, intermittently interlocking, spiral pattern of suturing will accomplish a symmetric closure of the spherical defect, more closely approximating the shape of the uterus. The serosa is typically closed with 4.0 nonreactive absorbable sutures in a running continuous stitch in order to seal the incision from the venous ooze that is usually present.

A case of disseminated intravascular coagulation (DIC) has been described following myomectomy after 52 myomas were removed from a uterus that measured 36 cm above the pubic symphysis (16). The exact cause for the DIC is not known and may include myometrial tissue damage that resulted both in the consumption of coagulation factors needed to maintain hemostasis in the multiple myomectomy sites and the possible dissemination of tissue thromboplastin systemically from the myometrium. The authors went on to conclude that patients with extremely large myomatous uteri should be counseled about the risk of coagulopathy associated with extensive myometrial dissection (16).

Febrile Morbidity

Occurrence of febrile morbidity associated with myomectomy is varied, ranging from 0% to 50% (see Table 14.1). This is due in part to the differences in the definition of febrile morbidity. LaMorte et al (4) defined febrile morbidity as a temperature of 100.4°F or greater after the first 24 postoperative hours. Friedman et al (8) defined febrile morbidity as a temperature greater than 100.4°F or greater on two occasions, 6 hours apart. None of the other authors define febrile morbidity in their manuscripts. LaMorte et al found that 70% of the myomectomy cases were treated with antibiotics prophylactically, presumably in an attempt to lower postoperative infection.

Unintended Total Abdominal Hysterectomy

The possibility of an unintended abdominal hysterectomy is a complication that should be discussed with the patient preoperatively and included in the surgical consent form. Although the occurrence is reportedly small, around 1% (see Table 14.1), the possibility is increased in cases of large uteri, multiple fibroids, and those fibroids that are positioned laterally near or that involve the vasculature of the uterus. Those large fibroids located in the lower uterine segment are in a more ominous position, where careful dissection is more difficult due to the proximity of ureter, major vessels, and bladder.

LATE COMPLICATIONS

Adhesion Formation

In general, postoperative adhesion formation after gynecologic surgery occurs 60% to 80% of the time, with potential long-term sequelae, including pelvic pain, infertility, and small-bowel obstruction (17). Myomectomy appears to be a very adhesiogenic surgery, with adhesions found to occur in 90% to 95% of cases at the time of second laparoscopy (18) (Table 14.3).

Contributing factors to the formation of adhesions after myomectomy include posterior uterine incisions, incomplete hemostasis, thermal tissue necrosis, and ischemic incision closures. Despite the use of compulsive surgical technique, including hemostasis control, irrigation of tissues, and atraumatic tissue handling, adhesion formation remains prob-

TABLE 14.3

The occurrence of postoperative adhesions after abdominal myomectomy

AUTHOR	ADHESIONS PRESENT (%)
Tulandi et al, 1993 (17)	15/16 (94)
Myomectomy Adhesion Multicenter Study Group, 1995 (18)	25/27 (92)
Total	40/43 (93)

lematic. Recently, the application of polytetrafluoroethylene barrier (Gore-Tex Surgical Membrane; W.L. Gore and Associates, Flagstaff, AZ), evaluated by the Myomectomy Adhesion Study Group, revealed a significant reduction in the adhesion score and the percentage of patients who were free of adhesions to the uterus at the time of second-look laparoscopy (18) (Table 14.4).

There is some evidence in animal models that GnRHag therapy may reduce postoperative adhesion formation (19,20). Wright and Sharrpe-Timms (19), in a rat model, showed significant reduction in adhesion scores using both an adhesion and endometriosis model in GnRHag-treated animals when compared to controls (Table 14.5). This effect was also found in a primate model when GnRHag-treated animals showed reduction in adhesion scores with a significant correlation to serum estradiol levels (20). Human studies are needed to confirm this intriguing suggestion.

Small-bowel obstruction remains a serious complication from postoperative adhesion formation. Its occurrence as a result of gynecologic surgery is not well documented. Insight is gained by a retrospective review of women with a discharge diagnosis of intestinal obstruction from 1988 to 1991 at the Columbia Presbyterian Medical Center in New York (21). The cause of intestinal obstruction was found to be

TABLE 14.4

The reduction of postoperative adhesion formation with Gore-Tex application at myomectomy

SITE	GORE-TEX	CONTROL
Adhesion free	15/27 (56%)	2/27 (7%)
Adhesion score	1.9/11	7.6/11

Source: Myomectomy Adhesion Multicenter Study Group. An expanded polytetrafluoroethylene barrier (Gore-Tex Surgical Membrane) reduces postmyomectomy adhesion formation. Fertil Steril 1995;63:491.

TABLE 14.5

The reduction of postoperative adhesion scores with GnRHag pretreatment in the rat

Drug Treatment	Endometriosis Model	Endometriosis Sham	Adhesion Model	Adhesion Sham
GnRHag	1.1 ± 0.2	1.1 ± 0.2	0.3 ± 0.1	0.0 ± 0.0
Diluent	2.2 ± 0.2	1.1 ± 0.2	0.6 ± 0.1	0.0 ± 0.0

Source: Wright J, Sharrpe-Timms K. Gonadotropin-releasing hormone agonist therapy reduces postoperative adhesion formation and reformation after adhesiolysis in rat models for adhesion formation and endometriosis. Fertil Steril 1995;63:1094.

postoperative adhesion formation in 60% of the patients. In these women, the most common gynecologic procedure performed was a total abdominal hysterectomy with or without bilateral salpingo-oophorectomy. Interestingly, myomectomy was the only preceding surgery in 11% of the cases identified. This figure is compared to the overall performance of myomectomy, which only accounted for 1% of the gynecologic procedures performed in the United States in 1990 (21). Thus prior myomectomy is a cause for intestinal obstruction more than would be expected from the low numbers of myomectomies that are being performed. As myomectomy becomes an increasingly popular conservative procedure, the problem with adhesion formation remains a significant complication.

Uterine Rupture

The catastrophic event of uterine rupture occurs in one in 1500 deliveries. Myomectomy precedes 1 in 50 cases of uterine rupture (22). Most instances of uterine rupture occur in the third trimester or in labor and are sometimes associated with invasive placentation. Golan et al (23) reported a rare case of spontaneous uterine rupture at 20 weeks' gestation following myomectomy. The placenta penetrated the uterine wall at the site of the previous myomectomy incision (23). Harris (24) described a case of uterine dehiscence following laparoscopic myomectomy. A 3 cm × 2 cm fibroid was excised from the posterior surface of the uterus using electrocautery to maintain a homeostasis. Only the uterine serosa was reapproximated with 4-0 polyglycolic sutures. A uterine dehiscence occurred at 34 weeks' gestation. Uterine rupture was thought to be due to incomplete healing secondary to excessive coagulation during dissection, lack of tissue approximation, and infection. The instillation of indigo carmine into the uterus preoperatively by a pediatric Foley catheter will stain the endometrium to facilitate identification of the endometrial cavity. In a series of 158 women who had undergone laparoscopic myomectomy, 6 were found to have fistulas between the endometrial cavity and the parietal peritoneum (25). This complication is thought to be due to lack of myometrial closure at the time of laparoscopy. This has led the authors to modify their technique to a laparoscopic assisted myomectomy in which the myomectomy is closed completely through a minilaparotomy incision (26). In general, vaginal delivery is recommended after myomectomy if the uterus has been properly closed.

Malignant Change

The risk of leiomyosarcoma increases with increasing age. It should be suspected with rapid uterine growth. Additionally, the lack of uterine volume reduction after GnRHag treatment should lead the surgeon to suspect leiomyosarcoma. A case of unsuspected leiomyosarcoma treated with GnRHag has been reported (27). The definitive diagnosis of leiomyosarcoma could not be made intraoperatively and the patient's strong desire for preservation of her uterus required a second exploratory laparotomy after a permanent pathologic diagnosis was made. Two additional cases of unsuspected leiomyosarcoma after GnRHag therapy were reported (28,29). The rare occurrence of leiomyosarcoma treated with GnRHag therapy and its incumbent delay in diagnosis should be discussed with each patient before therapy.

The effect of GnRHag preoperative treatment on the histopathologic changes of myomas after GnRHag therapy has been investigated (30–32) (Table 14.6). The results from three studies remain controversial regarding the effect of GnRHag on myoma cellularity and hyaliniza-

TABLE 14.6

Effect of GnRHag on histopathologic characteristics of myomas when compared to untreated controls

AUTHOR	CELLULARITY	HYALINIZATION	MITOTIC ACTIVITY
Upadhyaya et al, 1990 (30)	Reduced	Not done	No difference
Cohen et al, 1994 (31)	Increased	Increased	No difference
Gutmann et al, 1994 (32)	No difference	No difference	No difference

tion. However, there is agreement that GnRHag exposure does not affect the mitotic activity in myomas. Therefore, mitotic cellular changes identified at the time of surgery cannot be attributed to GnRHag therapy.

Recurrence of Myomas

Before myomectomy the patient should be informed of the recurrence rate, which is both myoma number and time dependent (33). Solitary myomas have a recurrence rate of 27%, compared to 59% in women undergoing multiple myomectomies. The recurrence rate is time dependent with an increase from 19% at 2 years to 31% at 5 years. There appears to be no difference in recurrence rates in women who have received GnRHag when compared to controls.

CONCLUSION

Uterine myomas are the most commonly occurring tumors of the female pelvis, being symptomatic in 30% to 50% of cases. They may be responsible for menstrual irregularity, pelvic pain and pressure, infertility, and repetitive pregnancy loss. Myomectomy offers conservative therapy for women with these indications during reproductive age. Significant early complications including fever and hemorrhage are associated with abdominal myomectomy. The late complication of postoperative adhesion formation is generally considered to be responsible for postoperative pain and infertility, the very indication in some instances for the myomectomy. In those patients in whom future fertility is not a concern, the remaining risk of small-bowel obstruction should be weighed against any potential benefits. Each of the complications presented should be considered when the benefits of myomectomy are weighed against the possible risks.

REFERENCES

1. Smith DC, Uhlir JK. Myomectomy as a reproductive procedure. Am J Obstet Gynecol 1990;162:1476.
2. Starks G. CO_2 laser myomectomy in an infertile population. J Reprod Med 1988;33:184.
3. Rosenfeld DK. Abdominal myomectomy for otherwise unexplained infertility. Fertil Steril 1986;4:328.
4. LaMorte Al, Lalwani S, Diamond MP. Morbidity associated with abdominal myomectomy. Obstet Gynecol 1993;82:897.
5. Golan A, Bukovsky L, Pansky M, et al. Preoperative gonadotropin-releasing hormone agonist treatment in surgery for uterine leiomyomata, Hum Reprod 1993;8:450.
6. Kiltz R, Rutgers J, Philips J, et al. Absence of a dose response effect of leuprolide acetate on leiomyomata uterine size. Fertil Steril 1994;61: 1021–1026.
7. Hutchins FL Jr. Myomectomy after selective preoperative treatment with a gonadotropin releasing hormone analog. J Reprod Med 1992;37: 699.
8. Friedman AJ, Rein MS, Harrison-Atlas D, et al. A randomized, placebo-controlled, double-blind study evaluating leuprolide acetate depot treatment before myomectomy. Fertil Steril 1989;52:728–733.
9. Friedman AJ. Vaginal hemorrhage associated with degenerating submucous leiomyomata during leuprolide acetate treatment. Fertil Steril 1989;52: 152.

10. Friedman AJ. Combined oestrogen-progestin treatment of vaginal haemorrhage following gonadotropin-releasing hormone agonist therapy of uterine myomas. Hum Reprod 1993;8:540–542.
11. Bonney V. The techniques and results of myomectomy. Lancet 1931; 220:171–177.
12. Rubin I. Progress in myomectomy. Am J Obstet Gynecol 1942;44:196–212.
13. Verkauf B. Myomectomy for fertility enhancement and preservation. Fertil Steril 1992;58:1–15.
14. Dillon T. Control of blood loss during gynecologic surgery. Obstet Gynecol 1962;19:428–435.
15. Buttram VC, Reiter RC. Uterine leiomyomata: etiology, symptomatology and management. Fertil Steril 1981;36:433.
16. Sacks P, Hoyne P. Disseminated intravascular coagulation, hemolytic anemia, and acute renal failure associated with extensive myomectomy. J Reprod Med 1992;79:835–838.
17. Tulandi T, Murry C, Guralnick M. Adhesion formation and reproductive outcome after myomectomy and second-look laparoscopy. J Reprod Med 1993;82:213.
18. Myomectomy Adhesion Multicenter Study Group. An expanded polytetrafluoroethylene barrier (Gore-Tex Surgical Membrane) reduces postmyomectomy adhesion formation. Fertil Steril 1995;63:491.
19. Wright J, Sharrpe-Timms K. Gonadotropin-releasing hormone agonist therapy reduces postoperative adhesion formation and reformation after adhesiolysis in rat models for adhesion formation and endometriosis. Fertil Steril 1995;63:1094.
20. Grow DR, Coddington CC, Seltman H, Hodgen GD. Role of hypoestrogenism or antiestrogens in adhesion formation after myometrial surgery in primates. Proceedings of the 50th Annual Meeting of the American Fertility Society, O-002, S1, 1994.
21. Stricker B, Blanco J, Fox H. The gynecologic contribution to intestinal obstruction. J Am Coll Surg 1994;178:617–620.
22. Shrinsky D, Benson R. Rupture of the pregnant uterus: a review. Obstet Gynecol Surg 1978;33:217.
23. Golan D, Aharoni A, Gonen R, et al. Early spontaneous rupture of the post myomectomy gravid uterus. Int J Gynecol Obstet 1990;31:167–170.
24. Harris W. Uterine dehiscence following laparoscopic myomectomy. Obstet Gynecol 1992;80:5445.

25. Nezhat C, Nezhat F, Silfen SL, et al. Laparoscopic myomectomy. Int J Fertil 1991;3;275.
26. Nezhat C, Nezhat F, Bess O, et al. Laparoscopically assisted myomectomy: a report of a new technique in 57 cases. Int J Fertil 1994;39:39.
27. Meyer W, William R, Mayer A, et al. Unsuspected leiomyosarcoma: treatment with gonadotropin releasing hormone analogue. Obstet Gynecol 1990;75:529–531.
28. Hitti I, Glasberg S, McKenzie C, Meltzer B. Uterine leiomyosarcoma with massive necrosis diagnosed during GnRH: a therapy for presumed uterine fibroids. Fertil Steril 1991;56:778–780
29. Loong E, Wong F. Uterine leiomyosarcoma diagnosed during treatment with gonadotropin releasing hormone analogue for presumed uterine fibroids. Fertil Steril 1990;54:530–531.
30. Upadhyaya N, Doody M, Googe P. Histopathological changes in leimyomata treated with leuprolide acetate. Fertil Steril 1990;54:811.
31. Cohen D, Mazur MT, Jozefczyk MA, Badawy SZA. Hyalinization and cellular changes in uterine leiomyomata after gonadotropin releasing hormone agonist therapy. J Reprod Med 1994;39:377.
32. Gutmann J, Thornton K, Diamond M, Carcangiu M. Evaluation of leuprolide acetate treatment on histopathology of uterine myomata. Fertil Steril. 1994;61:622.
33. Malone LJ. Myomectomy: recurrence after removal of solitary and multiple myomas. Obstet Gynecol 1969;34:200.

CHAPTER

15

Myoma Coagulation

Michael S. Baggish
Marvin D. Almquist
Jenn-Ming Yang

Uterine myomas characteristically occur in three locations: submucous, subserous, and intramural. The principal reason for treating these tumors is bleeding, which is usually cyclic, prolonged, and heavy (1). Secondary indications include pressure on neighboring structures, pain, rapid growth, and infertility.

A characteristic of myomas that makes coagulation a reasonable alternative to excision in selected cases is their altered blood supply. This is evidenced by the fact that hyaline (coagulation) necrosis is observed in most myomas (60%). Forssman (2), using xenon 133 during laparotomy, has shown not only a decreased blood supply within myomas compared to surrounding myometrium, but also a diminished uterine blood supply to myomatous uteri as compared to normal uteri (3,4). Kurjak et al (5), employing transvaginal color-flow Doppler, compared uterine blood flow impedance in 101 patients with palpable myomas and 60 women without myomas. Decreased resistance to flow was observed in the women with myomas. Weiner et al (6) found that blood vessels detected in uterine myomas had elevated resistance indices with color-flow Doppler. Sapozhnikov (7) noted a two- to four-time decrease in the volume of microvessels in the central areas of myomas, whereas peripheral areas of the myomas had higher specific volumes of blood microcirculatory beds. Clearly, uterine leiomyomas are highly susceptible to the coagulating effects of lasers or electrosurgical devices (8).

PREPARATION

A variety of drugs can be utilized to 1) reduce the size of the myoma, 2) decrease the vascularity, and 3) render the operation easier to perform.

For submucous myomas, danazol, 400 g twice a day, and megestrol acetate (Megace), 40 mg four times a day, have been utilized by the authors. More recently, gonadotropin-releasing hormone (GnRH) agonists leuprolide acetate (Lupron) or goserelin acetate (Zoladex) have been selectively used because of convenience and better patient compliance. Since 3.75 mg Lupron or 3.60 mg Zoladex is injected only once a month, the dependency on patient motivation is largely eliminated. The maximal reduction in myoma size or vascularity regardless of location is seen after 3 consecutive months of drug administration.

Another class of drugs utilized intraoperatively are vasoconstrictors. Although epinephrine or phenylephrine (Neo-Synephrine) can be selected, the most effective peripheral agent is vasopressin. Since vasopressin can *cause* systemic effects, for example, hypertension, bradycardia, and arrhythmia, it must be diluted. For the most effective vasoconstriction with the least risk to the patient, a 1:200 dilution is recommended. A 1 mL vial of vasopressin containing 20 units per milliliter is diluted with 199 mL sterile water for injection. Each milliliter will contain 0.1 unit of vasopressin. Generally, 25 to 30 mL of this solution can be injected into the myoma with a 23-gauge needle. The myoma typically will blanch white after injection. Vasopressin will significantly (>50%) reduce the amount of intraoperative bleeding.

ENERGY DEVICES

Myoma coagulation is performed via two major energy methods, neodymium (Nd):YAG laser and bipolar electrosurgery. Interestingly, the common end point is identical for the two categories: *thermal action.*

The neodymium:YAG light energy is transmitted at 1065 nm via quartz or silicon fibers that range in diameter from 600 to 1200 μ. The newest fibers are sculpted in order to fit different clinical applications. The laser penetration into tissue by sculpted versus plain fibers is vastly different. The latter emits parallel unfocused light that has greater penetrating power. The Nd:YAG laser is a front scatter device that traverses liquid or air, exerting a maximal effect beneath the tissue surface. It is principally a coagulating laser, the heating action of which spreads in a fashion analogous to that of an isodose curve and proportional to the time on tissue (9). Larger volumes of tissue will be coagulated by lower laser wattage (20–30 W) kept on tissue for a longer time. In contrast, less tissue injury will be observed with high-power input coupled with a shorter dwelling time.

Bipolar electrosurgical devices offer significantly better safety than do monopolar delivery systems. With bipolar, no grounding pad (neutral electrode) is needed because the system conducts current through one insulated electrode (active) and returns it to the generator through a second insulated electrode (return). The thermal action coagulates tissue between the electrodes. Surrounding tissue is affected only by heat conduction rather than by electron flow. This system produces tissue actions that are very similar to laser effects but is even safer in actual practice since forward penetration injuries are virtually eliminated. If the bipolar delivery is coupled to a sophisticated electrosurgical unit (ESU) equipped with automatic bipolar, then the system represents the best modality for inducing controlled tissue coagulation for the following reasons: lowered tissue resistance, lower power requirements, pure sine wave output (lower peak to peak voltage), and automatic cutoff when tissue temperature reaches 100°C (Fig. 15.1).

Monopolar electrosurgery is not well suited to interior myoma coagulation surgery and is a poor second choice from the standpoint of safety when compared to bipolar particularly for laparoscopic techniques. The reasons for this are: 1) Monopolar electric current flows through higher resistance, necessitating higher power; 2) electrons flow through the patient and require a ground plate (neutral electrodes); 3) open circuits create even higher voltage and dangerous induced direct current; 4) front penetration injuries can and do occur; and 5) capacitive

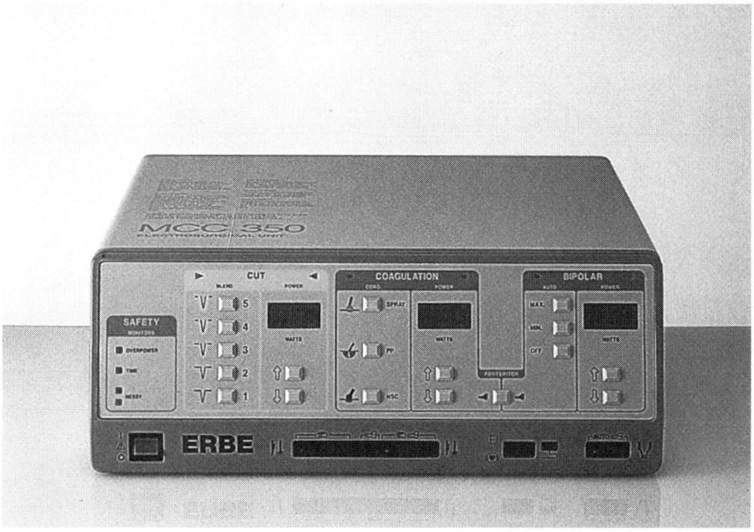

FIG. 15.1.

ERBE electrosurgical generator (Tubingen, Germany) is equipped for automatic bipolar coagulation. The ICC 350 model also has true bipolar cut mode.

coupling, direct coupling, and insulation failure injuries constitute serious potential patient risks.

HYSTEROSCOPIC TECHNIQUES

The operating hysteroscope utilized consists of a multichannel sheath that measures 8 mm in diameter. Separate channels are dedicated for the 4-mm telescope, distention medium, and 3-mm operating instruments. The sheath is constructed of an internal fluid delivery and an outside fluid collecting system; therefore, the uterus is continuously flushed (Fig. 15.2).

The authors prefer a 0-degree telescope in order to allow precise viewing of instruments in either close-up or in the extended panoramic position. A 2.8-mm bipolar electrode with ½- to 1-cm needle tips measures 50 cm in length and slides through the 3-mm operating channel.

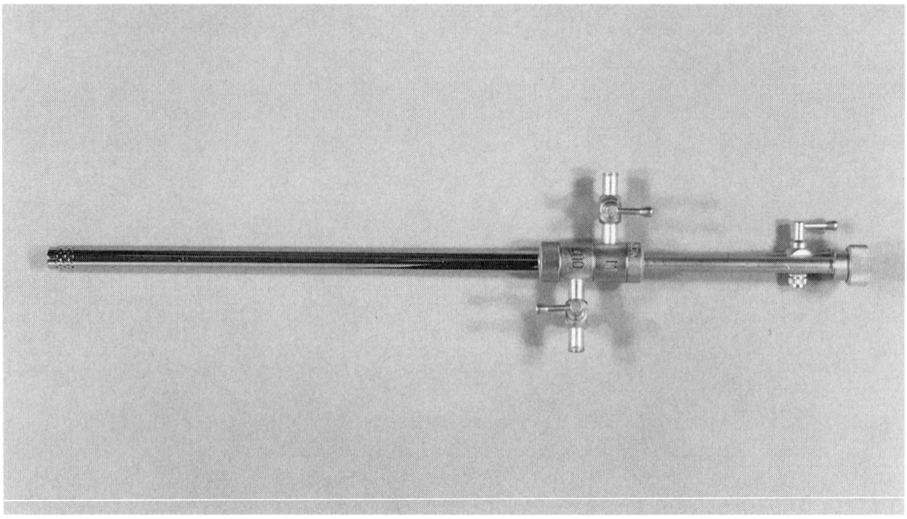

FIG. 15.2.

Isolated-channel and continuous-flow hysteroscope, 8.3-mm diameter (Bryan Corp, Woburn, MA).

Alternatively, a 1.0-mm silicon-quartz Nd:YAG laser fiber can traverse the 3-mm operating channel. A No. 9 French polyethylene aspirating cannula (Cook OB/GYN, Bloomington, IN) is attached to an intravenous extension tube and then to a 60-mL syringe. This can be inserted through the operating channel to clear the uterus of debris.

Myoma coagulation surgery can be performed with the safest distending medium, that is, normal (0.9%) saline. This medium can be used since bipolar and Nd:YAG laser surgery are best performed through electrolytic (saline, lactated Ringer's solution) rather than nonelectrolytic (glycine, sorbitol, water, mannitol) media.

TECHNIQUES

Several methods for coagulating submucous myomas have been utilized by the authors. The method selected depends on the size and location of the mass.

Myomas that are 1 cm or less can be ablated to the level of the surrounding endometrium by means of the Nd:YAG laser at 40 to 50 W of power. For fundal or cornual myomas of this size, power should be reduced to 30 W. The fiber is simply dragged across the myoma until it is obliterated. If the lesion is studded with large vessels, a hysteroscopic injection needle (23–25 gauge) can be passed into the myoma and 3 to 5 mL of 1:200 vasopressin injected before ablation. Operative time approximates 15 to 20 minutes.

Bipolar needles are used for intermediate-sized myomas ranging from 2 to 4 cm. The myoma is first injected with 5 mL of 1:200 vasopressin (Fig. 15.3). The bipolar needles are multiply thrust into the substance of the lesion (20–40 punctures) and current is activated using automatic bipolar. The ESU is set at 30 to 40 W power. This operation is very simple and can be completed in 15 minutes. Large myomas, that is, greater than 4 cm, are treated with the Nd:YAG laser by multiple sec-

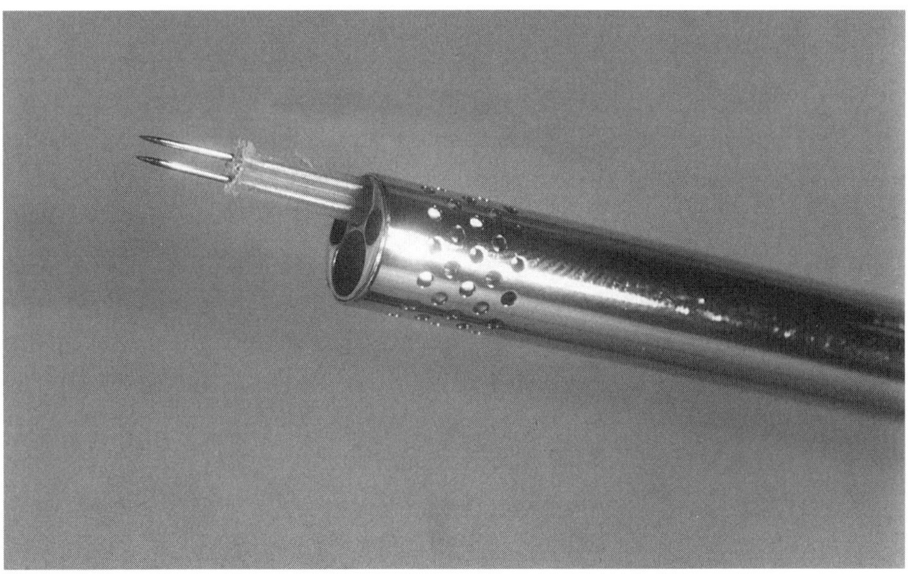

FIG. 15.3.

Hysteroscopic bipolar electrode extends out from the large (3 mm) operating channel. The openings on either side are medium inflow ports. The outer sheath (multiple puncture holes) is the medium outflow channel.

tioning. The laser fiber is drawn across the surface of the myoma slowly allowing the laser to cut deep swaths into the myoma. Several sections are cut in this manner ending up with a result akin to a sectioned orange. The thermal injury created to the myomatous mass is extensive depending on the size of the myoma. The operation will take approximately 30 minutes to complete. Donnez et al (10) have described a two-step procedure combining partial excision and multiple jabs into the remainder of the myoma with the Nd:YAG laser (11).

RESULTS

Coagulation of submucous myomas creates minimal trauma to surrounding tissue and is associated with minimal blood loss. The end result of coagulation is the production of a shrunken, white, avascular shell of the former myoma. Of 80 women on whom the authors have performed hysteroscopic myomectomy, 51 were treated by Nd:YAG laser or bipolar needle coagulation. Six patients required either secondary procedures (2) or underwent hysterectomy (4). The hypermenorrhea and menorrhagia were eliminated in 46 cases (90%). Both of the women who had repeat hysteroscopy had multiple myomas. In 1 case, the patient had repeat hysteroscopy, with resultant return to normal menstrual pattern and elimination of all myoma-related bleeding. The second patient subsequently underwent hysterectomy.

Histologic examination of the interior of a coagulated myoma reveals extensive thermal necrosis. The degree of microscopic injury is proportional to the number of penetrations and the time on tissue of the energy-emitting device (see Plate 10).

COMPLICATIONS

No serious complications have been reported in association with coagulating techniques. Among 233 cases, Donnez et al (11) reported no major complications. This was also true in Dubuisson's and our own series (12). Conversely, complications that have been reported in association with excisional surgery include perforation, hemorrhage, infections, and media reaction (pulmonary edema, hyponatremia). Delayed expulsion of all or a portion of the myoma has followed coagulation injury and subsequent devascularization.

FOLLOW-UP THERAPY

Patients for whom fertility is not a concern are continued on suppressive medication for 4 to 6 weeks postoperatively. The goal of this regimen is to ensure maximal scar formation and to prevent regrowth of any portion of the myoma by inhibiting neovascularization. The suppression of the endometrium additionally will enhance scar formation within the cavity in and around the deteriorating myoma.

Women in whom the myomectomy was performed to improve their chances of childbearing or those who wish to maintain the option for future fertility are treated by the administration of estrogen, 2.5 mg/day for 30 days postoperatively. Although there is a risk of myoma regrowth, this is superseded by the need to stimulate rapid endometrial growth to prevent intrauterine adhesions.

Although several reports have been published about the risk of uterine rupture following hysteroscopic myomectomy, the chances of uterine rupture after uncomplicated myoma coagulation appear to be remote. None have been reported to date; however, only a relatively small number of cases have as yet been performed using this technique.

LAPAROSCOPIC TECHNIQUES

Both the Nd:YAG laser and bipolar needles have been employed for the treatment of subserous and intramural myomas via operative laparoscopy. The laser fiber can be delivered either through the instrument channel of the operating laparoscope or via a second puncture trocar/sleeve. The

A

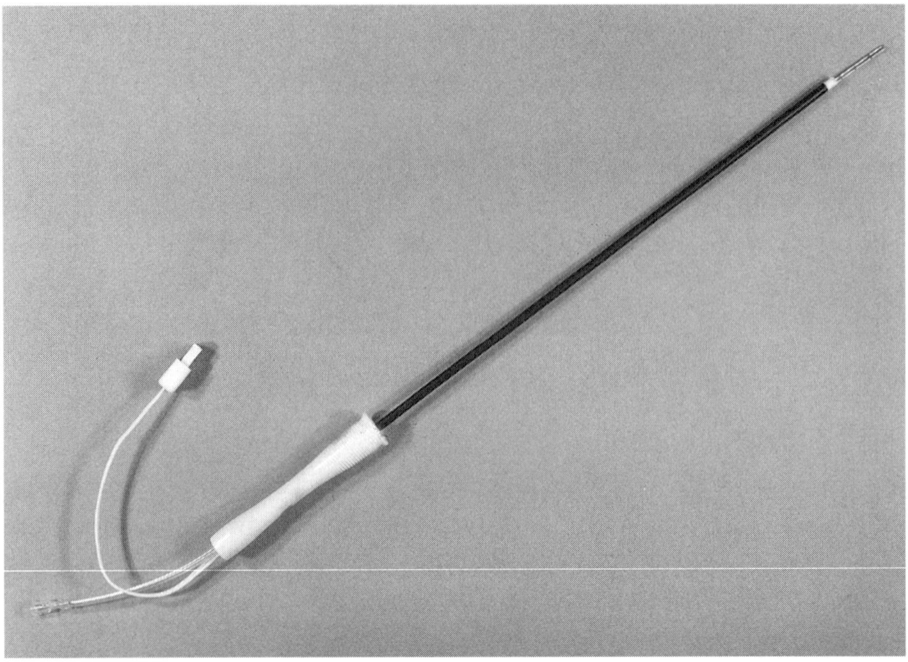

B

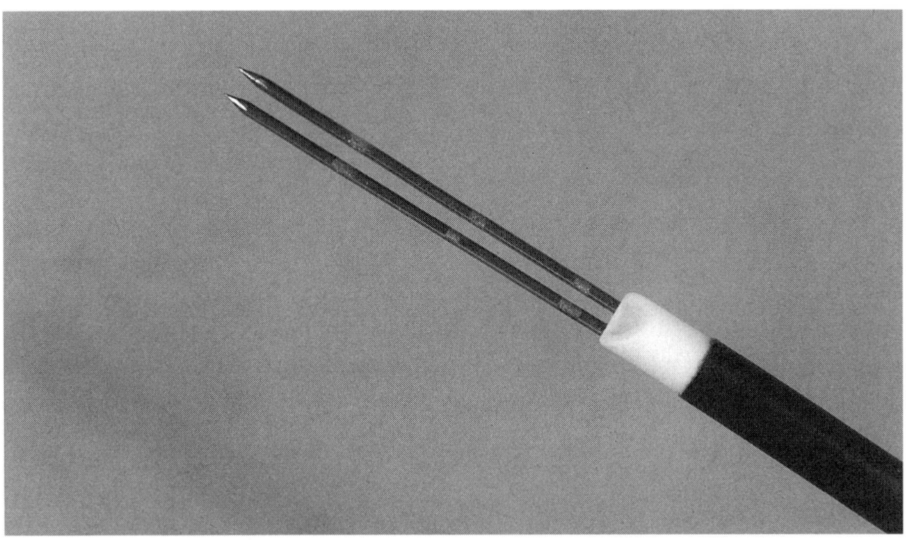

FIG. 15.4.

A. Bipolar laparoscopic myolysis needles (Everest Medical, Minneapolis, MN), panoramic view. The needles are delivered into the abdomen via a 5-mm sleeve. B. Close-up of the bipolar needles. Note the irrigating port located at the base of the needle.

bipolar needles are usually delivered through a second puncture entry site (Fig. 15.4).

Although myomectomy by open techniques (laparotomy) is an established procedure, the same operation by laparoscopic approach is still questionable. Laparoscopic excision of intramural and subserous myomas has been reported by several investigators. The difficulties encountered with the procedure, particularly related to intramural myomas of greater than 5 cm, include closure of the uterine defect, extraction of the myomatous mass, adhesion formation, and control of bleeding (12–14).

Goldfarb (15) and Nisolle et al (16) have reported Nd:YAG laser myoma coagulation. A bare 600-μ fiber penetrates the myoma and the laser is fired utilizing powers in the range of 50 to 80 W. The technique advocates 10 punctures per centimeter of estimated myoma diameter. Tumors up to 10 cm in diameter have been treated, with subsequent reduction of mass averaging greater than 50%. No serious complications were reported and blood loss was negligible in this combined series that numbered 123 patients. In 7 patients who accepted second-look laparoscopy at 6 months postoperatively, dense fibrous adhesions were observed between the myoma(s) and the small intestine. The myoma(s) itself was white and devoid of vasculature.

The use of bipolar needles is advantageous from several standpoints. The procedure is safe, requires relatively low wattage, and permits known depth of penetration. Additionally, protective glasses or shutters are unnecessary. The myoma is thoroughly irrigated with normal saline in order to enhance the bipolar coagulation. The foot pedal is activated just as the needles come into contact with the serosa and is continuously depressed as the needles enter the myomatous mass. When coagulation is complete, the needles are withdrawn and then the operator disengages the foot pedal. Utilization of a generator equipped with automatic bipolar facilitates the operation. Goldfarb (17) has performed this operation in 110 women for myomas that ranged in size from 2 to 10 cm with reductions of myoma mass averaging 75% to 80% (Fig. 15.5; see also Plate 11).

The authors have performed this operation in 20 women with intramural myomas that ranged from 5 to 7 cm in diameter. The

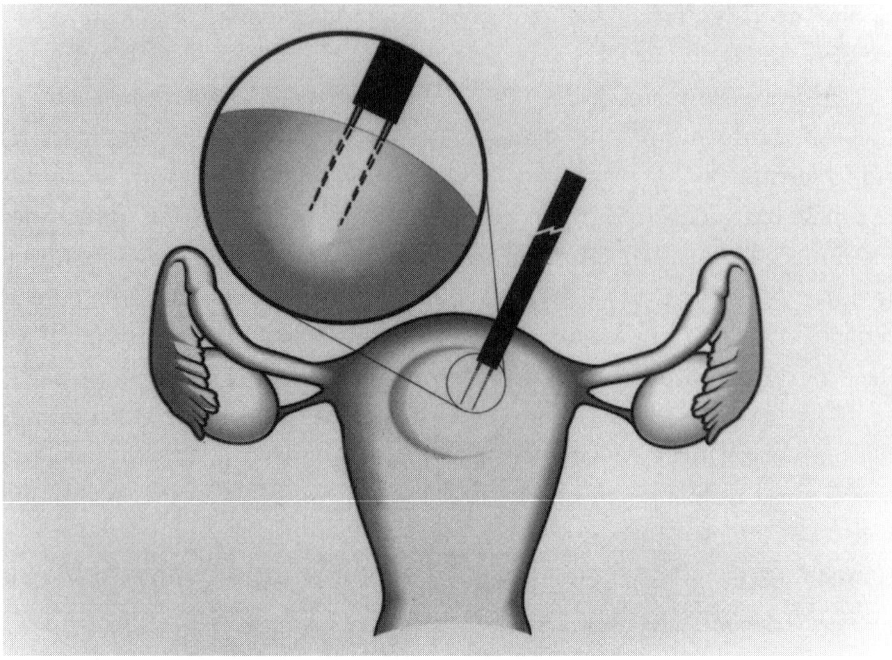

FIG. 15.5.

Schematic drawing showing bipolar needles penetrating a posterior intramural myoma. The major destruction of myometrium occurs between the two needles. Some heat is conducted radially from the needles. Automatic bipolar ESUs reduce the volume of conduction injury. (By permission of M.S. Baggish, MD.)

maximal reduction in mass averaged 60%. Second-look laparoscopy revealed white avascular remnants associated with adhesions in 50% (6) of the cases surveyed. The number of punctures ranged from 40 to 70. Power was set at 40 W. The mean time to complete the operation was 50 minutes. The patients were discharged on the day of surgery. Average estimated blood loss was less than 100 mL. No complications were observed.

Myoma coagulation is an easy operation that is ideally suited for the laparoscopic approach. The most serious negative aspect of the technique is the high percentage of adhesion formation observed in cases in which second-look laparoscopy was performed. Unfortunately, none of the series has reported the use of adhesion prevention adjuvants such as absorbable oxidized regenerated cellulose (Interceed, Johnson & Johnson, New Brunswick, NJ) following myoma coagulation. Clearly the use of such adjuvants should be studied particularly for posterior and fundal lesions.

FOLLOW-UP THERAPY

Women who undergo laparoscopic myoma coagulation are uniformly continued on suppressive medication for 8 weeks following surgery. The authors administer two doses of goserelin acetate, 3.60 mg subcutaneously at monthly intervals. We believe that this regimen enhances the subsequent degeneration of the myoma. The once per month injection of GnRH agonist and the consistency of reduced vascularity in the myoma are superior to the results obtained with currently available oral drugs. However, a recent article reported excellent results with gestrinone administered orally in a dose of 5 mg three times a week (18). We have not used this drug since it is not available in the United States at this time.

CONCLUSIONS

Myoma coagulation is a rapid, safe, and effective alternative to excision and is well suited to endoscopic surgery. The technique is easily taught and does not require a protracted learning curve to master. The recent resurgence of bipolar technology coupled with new delivery systems and electrosurgical generators undoubtedly will result in more surgeons performing this type of operation. Finally, coagulation techniques are attractive and cheap alternatives to hysterectomy for women who wish to preserve their uterus. More data are required to ascertain the true efficacy of the technique.

REFERENCES

1. Baggish MS, Sze EHM, Rosenzweig BA, et al. Direct hysteroscopic observation to document the reasons for abnormal bleeding secondary to submucous myoma. J Gynecol Surg 1989;5:149–154.
2. Forssman L. Distribution of blood flow in myomatous uteri as measured by locally injected xenon. Acta Obstet Gynecol Scand 1976;55:101.
3. Farrer-Brown G, Beilby JOW, McPath DM, et al. Microvasculature of the uterus. Obstet Gynecol 1970;35:21.
4. Forssman L. Blood flow in myomatous uteri as measured by intraarterial xenon. Acta Obstet Gynecol Scand 1976;55:21.
5. Kurjak A, Kupesic-Urek S, Miric D. The assessment of benign uterine tumor vascularization by transvaginal color Doppler. Ultrasound Med Biol 1992;18:645–649.
6. Weiner Z, Beck D, Rottem S, et al. Uterine artery flow velocity waveforms and color imaging in women with peri-menopausal and postmenopausal bleeding. Acta Obstet Gynecol Scand 1993;72:162–166.
7. Sapozhnikov AG. Structure of the blood microcirculatory bed in intramural uterine myomas. Vopr Onkol 1987;33:43–48.
8. Verkauf BS. Myomectomy for fertility enhancement and preservation. Fertil Steril 1992;58:1–15.
9. Cornier E. Traitement hysterofibroscopique ambulatoire des metrorragies rebelles par laser Nd-YAG. J Gynecol Obstet Biol Reprod 1986;15: 661.
10. Donnez J, Gillerot S, Bourgonjon D. Neodymium-YAG laser hysteroscopy in large submucous fibroids. Fertil Steril 1990;54:999–1003.
11. Donnez J, Nisolle F, Clerckx F, et al. Advanced endoscopic techniques used in dysfunctional bleeding, fibroids and endometriosis, and the role of gonadotrophin-releasing hormone agonist treatment. Br J Obstet Gynaecol 1994;101:2–9.
12. Dubuisson JB, Lecuru F, Herve F, et al. Myomectomy by laparoscopy: a preliminary report of 43 cases. Fertil Steril 1991;56:827–830.
13. Ginsburg ES, Benson CB, Garfield JM, et al. The effect of operative technique and uterine size on blood loss during myomectomy: a prospective randomized study. Fertil Steril 1993;60:956–962.
14. Nezhat C, Nezhat F, Nezhat C. Operative laparoscopy: state of the art. J Gynecol Surg 1992;8:111–141.

15. Goldfarb HA. Nd-YAG laser laparoscopic coagulation of symptomatic myomas. J Reprod Med 1992;37:636–638.
16. Nisolle M, Smets M, Malvaux V, et al. Laparoscopic myolysis with the Nd-YAG laser. J Gynecol Surg 1993;9:95–99.
17. Goldfarb HA. Removing uterine fibroids laparoscopically. Contemp OB/GYN 1994;39:50–72.
18. Coutinho EM. Treatment of large fibroids with high doses of gestrinone. Gynecol Obstet Invest 1990;30;44–47.

CHAPTER

16

Laparoscopic Myomectomy

Howard C. Topel

Uterine leiomyomas will occur in approximately 25% of women and commonly develop during the third and fourth decades of reproductive life. Most fibroids remain small, produce few symptoms, and result in little clinical significance. However, about one third of women with myomas will experience significant morbidity that will affect their well-being and require treatment. The most common symptoms produced by myomas are abnormal uterine bleeding and lower-abdominal or pelvic pain. Large-sized fibroids can cause pressure on the bladder and bowel, resulting in complaints of urinary frequency, incontinence, and constipation. The severity and frequency of problems created by leiomyomas are often dependent on the size, number, and location within the uterus. However, it is not uncommon for a large uterus filled with multiple fibroids to produce only minimal symptoms.

At the present time, medical treatment for uterine leiomyomas is incomplete with only temporary relief of symptoms and reduction in myoma size and number. Surgery remains the only definitive treatment for symptomatic leiomyomas. Conservative surgical management such as myomectomy has been traditionally reserved for those patients who desire future reproduction. For many gynecologists, hysterectomy is the preferred treatment when future reproduction is no longer a concern. This is substantiated by the fact that the most common indication for hysterectomy in the United States is uterine fibroids. However, a greater number of older women, often not interested in future fertility but desirous of preserving the uterus, are seeking a more conservative alternative to hysterectomy. For many in this selected group, myomectomy is a reasonable therapeutic choice.

The standard operative technique for myomectomy has been an open laparotomy approach. However, operative laparoscopy, employing a minimally invasive technique, may offer significant advantages, such as reduced morbidity, shorter hospitalization, faster recovery, and improved incisional cosmetics. At the present time, however, laparoscopic myomectomy remains a controversial technique. Critics cite issues such as prolonged operative time, difficulty with myoma removal, inadequate uterine reconstruction, and excessive thermal injury with poor tissue healing. Proponents, however, believe that in properly selected patients, myomectomy can be skillfully performed with a laparoscopic microsurgical technique and less intraoperative blood loss. Skillful endosuturing can restore normal uterine anatomy, and preserve uterine function with no compromise in patient well-being. Critical to successful laparoscopic myomectomy are two key elements: careful patient selection and the correct operative technique.

Though proper patient selection is crucial for most laparoscopic operations, it is absolutely essential for the successful performance of laparoscopic myomectomy. Surgical indications for performing a laparoscopic myomectomy remain consistent as with open myomectomy. However, many significant variables influence patient selection for a laparoscopic approach. These variables are myoma size, location within the uterine wall, number of fibroids, endometrial involvement, the patient's desire for future fertility, and the skill level of the laparoscopic surgeon. Each of these variables must be thoroughly evaluated and considered before the patient enters the operating room. Laparoscopic myomectomy may not be appropriate for every patient, and not every surgeon will be inclined to perform such a complex operation.

Vaginal ultrasound is routinely employed to determine the size, location, and often the number of myomas present within the uterus. All patients who are considered for laparoscopic myomectomy will have a vaginal ultrasound to assess, preoperatively, the feasibility of a minimally invasive approach. Only with complex or poorly defined uterine pathology is a computed tomographic (CT) scan or magnetic resonance imaging (MRI) needed to assess the extent of uterine leiomyomas or to identify adenomyosis. Careful attention should be directed to determine the depth of the myoma penetration into the myometrium, and to assess its relationship with the endometrial canal (Fig. 16.1). Although this can occasionally be accomplished with vaginal ultrasound, other techniques, such as hysterosalpingography, office hysteroscopy, or saline sonohysterography, will be needed to evaluate involvement of the uterine cavity.

Saline sonohysterography is a simplified office technique for the assessment of endometrial pathology that employs saline distention of the uterine cavity with simultaneous vaginal ultrasound observation. A small plastic insemination catheter is placed into the uterine cavity and 10 to 15 mL sterile saline is injected into the endometrial canal. The sub-

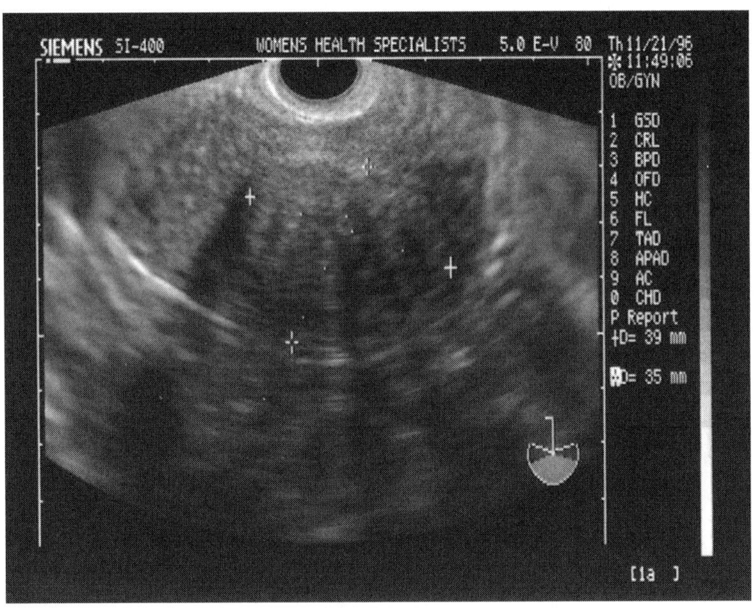

FIG. 16.1.

Localization and depth of penetration of posterior myoma with vaginal ultrasound.

sequent cavity distention creates a separation of the anterior and posterior uterine walls. The internal uterine contour can be easily visualized by performing, at the time of saline distention, a vaginal ultrasound. This simple and fast office technique permits easy identification of uterine pathology such as polyps or fibroids that enter into, or lie in close proximity to, the endometrial cavity (see Plate 12). A saline ultrasound hysterogram can easily identify the submucosal component of a large intramural fibroid. Endometrial involvement may represent a relative contraindication to performing a laparoscopic myomectomy and may influence the surgeon to choose an open technique. This is an important consideration when the patient desires future pregnancy, or if the surgeon's endosuturing skills are inadequate to close a large uterine defect.

A thorough preoperative evaluation permits the laparoscopic surgeon to properly select those patients who will maximally experience all the benefits of a minimally invasive operation, and achieve an excellent surgical end result, with no compromise in uterine function or in patient well-being. General guidelines for laparoscopic technique are the following: solitary myoma size smaller than 10 cm, depth of penetration 50% or less, five myomas or less with the largest myoma not to exceed 6 cm, and no precarious myoma location such as under the bladder, parametrial, or deep posterior. Careful preoperative patient selection for laparoscopic myomectomy is essential if the laparoscopic surgeon is to enjoy a high level of success, and to minimize surgical complications and patient morbidity.

In order to help facilitate laparoscopic removal of a large leiomyoma, a long-acting gonadotropin-releasing hormone (GnRH) agonist can be administered preoperatively. When prescribed, leuprolide acetate depot (Lupron), 3.75 mg IM per month, is given for 3 months before surgery in an effort to decrease myoma size, reduce myometrial vascularity, or correct anemia secondary to heavy uterine bleeding. At present, myomas greater than 6 cm in size on vaginal ultrasound, or those located in a posterior or interligamentous lateral location, are considered for preoperative treatment. When employed, serial ultrasounds are performed every 6 weeks to evaluate any reduction in myoma size. The GnRH hypoestrogenic induced anovulation is reported to produce a 30% to

50% decrease in uterine volume, and to inhibit further myoma growth. Patient response to GnRH treatment, however, is often inconsistent and variable with almost 50% demonstrating little reduction in myoma size. This variability must be carefully considered and explained to the patient since the medication is costly and the hypoestrogenic side effects can be uncomfortable. Severely anemic patients can be treated with oral iron during this medically induced amenorrhea. At times, because of work or social demands, a patient will need to delay treatment. GnRH treatment can be given to control symptoms or slow myoma growth while awaiting surgery. Many believe that a myoma, after GnRH treatment, is more difficult to remove from the myometrium due to poorer recognition of the pseudocapsular tissue plane. I have found this concern to be quite variable, and it may merely reflect myomas that have existed for a long time and have undergone extensive degeneration.

Laparoscopic myomectomy should be performed in either the later follicular or early luteal phases of the menstrual cycle. Frequently, those patients pretreated with a GnRH agonist will have surgery 3 to 4 weeks following the last treatment. In addition to the standard preoperative laboratory testing, a coagulation profile is routinely obtained. In those patients who request or have borderline blood counts, autologous or donor blood will be available at the time of surgery. A Fleet enema is commonly given the night before surgery to empty and decompress the lower colon. Before a laparoscopic myomectomy is performed, patients are informed of all available treatment options. A detailed discussion of the operative technique, potential complications, indications for conversion to laparotomy, and postoperative patient expectations follows.

TECHNIQUE

With the patient in the lithotomy position, a Foley catheter is placed in the bladder for the duration of the procedure. The uterus is sounded and a uterine manipulator is inserted into the entire length of the endometrial cavity. It is important to use a strong manipulator that will support the increased uterine weight and permit movement of the uterus from anterior to posterior and from side to side. In addition, the manipulator must be able to rotate the uterus along its long axis. This rotational movement provides a torquing effect that maximizes exposure to all surfaces of an irregularly shaped leiomyoma, which is essential for identifying the correct dissection planes for myoma enucleation.

Trocar placement for laparoscopic myomectomy consists of a 10-mm trocar positioned at the umbilicus. A 10-mm 0° laparoscope with an attached video camera is placed through the umbilical port. Ancillary trocars will vary in size and location depending on the total uterine size, as well as the location, size, and number of individual myomas. In general, three 10- to 12-mm trocars are placed along the suprapubic area and adjusted, as the pathology dictates, to either more superior or lateral positions. Large trocars with reducer caps are used to maximize the flexibility and variety of instrumentation at each trocar site. Trocar location must be carefully determined in order to provide multiple working angles, and to maximize the optimal mechanical advantage when this complex operation is performed. Attention to this important technical detail of trocar placement can often determine the success or failure of this operation, and the avoidance of serious intraoperative complications.

Following trocar insertion, the entire abdominal cavity and pelvis should be inspected and the uterine pathology evaluated. At this time, one must determine if the operation is feasible with laparoscopic technique, or whether the patient will be best served with a laparotomy approach.

Laparoscopic myomectomy consists of four technical steps:

1. Enucleation of the myoma
2. Hemostasis of the myometrial bed
3. Suture reconstruction to normal anatomy
4. Specimen removal from the abdominal cavity

Enucleation of the Myoma

The first operative step, myoma enucleation, begins with injection of a dilute (10–20 units in 100 mL saline) solution of vasopressin into the uterine serosa. With the uterus elevated, a long 6-in. 18-gauge needle with a 20-mL syringe is inserted through the anterior abdominal wall under direct vision (see Plate 13). Multiple sites are injected around the circumference of the myoma base. Usually 10 to 15 mL is sufficient to create an intense vasoconstriction of the uterine serosa and myometrium (see Plate 14). Proper precautions are observed to avoid direct intravascular injection, and the anesthesiologist should be informed when vasopressin is administered.

The uterine serosal layer is incised with a laparoscopic endoknife or microscissors. This initial serosal incision can be made in either a vertical or horizontal direction, depending on the location of the myoma. In general, most serosal incisions are vertical, except when the myoma is located anterior near the bladder or posterior near the corpocervical junction. The incision is slowly made into the uterus until the glistening white fibroid surface is located and the pseudocapsular plane is identified (see Plate 15). Great care should be exercised to precisely locate this plane, and to avoid cutting too deep into the fibroid or remaining too high in the myometrium or serosa. It is critical to dissect and perform this initial myoma enucleation step within the avascular pseudocapsular plane, in order to minimize bleeding and to prevent excessive tissue damage. Video magnification greatly facilitates the identification and helps to localize the dissection within this tissue plane.

Often all three ancillary trocar sites are employed to complete the myoma dissection. This requires frequent movement of graspers and energy sources from the various ports in order to gain maximal exposure to the correct tissue plane, and to avoid dissection into the myometrium or inadvertent entry into the endometrium.

Enucleation of a leiomyoma from the myometrium can be accomplished with a variety of laparoscopic energy sources. Electrocautery, laser, harmonic scalpel, argon beam, endocoagulation, and scissors dissection have all been employed in performing laparoscopic myomectomy with varying degrees of success. However, depending on the size, location, and consistency of the myoma, a combination of several energy sources will frequently be used for enucleation. Thus, it is important to be skillful with a variety of energy sources and to understand their particular advantages, tissue effects, and limitations.

An ideal energy source for laparoscopic myomectomy should provide for precise dissection through the capsular plane while at the same time allowing adequate coagulation to the deeper vascular myometrial bed. One must be careful not to create excessive thermal injury within the myometrium, which could result in poor tissue healing and compromise future uterine function. My personal preference is to initially develop and dissect this important pseudocapsular plane with a Semm blunt endocoagulation probe set at 130°F (see Plate 16).

With deeper dissection into the myometrium, large heavy fibroids will become difficult to control and stabilize. A large, 10-mm corkscrew instrument or an endoscopic tenaculum can be placed into the center of the fibroid. The fibroid tissue can now be effectively controlled and manipulated for better exposure. The highly vascular myoma bed can be precisely dissected with bipolar scissors and simultaneously coagulated with bipolar cautery. Great care must be taken to work close to the myoma and not to extend the dissection into the peripheral myometrial wall. Any break in this technique will cause increased bleeding and excessive cauterization of the myometrium. As a consequence the extensive tissue necrosis and inadequate hemostasis create the potential for poor wound healing and subsequent complications. Dissection of the deeper vascular tissue planes must be slowly developed and all vessels precisely secured in order to prevent delayed postoperative bleeding. Exposure to this deeper plane is possible with lateral traction on one side of the uterine wall, while the fibroid is elevated and pulled to the opposite side (see Plate 17). Instruments are then rotated through all three ancillary trocar ports to gain adequate exposure to the entire vascular bed. In contrast to the open technique, strict adherence to identifying and meticulously dissecting within this pseudocapsular plane will result in surprisingly little blood loss and will limit the potential for myometrial injury.

Hemostasis of the Myometrial Bed

The second step in laparoscopic myomectomy is establishment of excellent hemostasis within both the deep and superficial layers of the myometrium and serosa. If the enucleation technique is followed as described, only a small amount of capillary bleeding will be present, which can be gently controlled with endocoagulation or bipolar cautery (see Plate 18). Heavy central bleeding must be selectively secured with either more aggressive electrocautery or placement of a suture. The use of monopolar cautery is strongly discouraged in the performance of a laparoscopic myomectomy. Excessive thermal injury to the myometrium secondary to monopolar cautery use may be the cause of reported fistula formation, uterine dehiscence, and extensive postoperative adhesions.

Suture Reconstruction to Normal Anatomy

Uterine reconstruction back to normal anatomy should only be initiated after hemostasis has been established. In general, I employ endosuturing techniques for anatomic reconstruction, but not to control bleeding. A variety of endosuturing techniques, both extra- and intracorporeal, can be utilized to close the uterine defect. A good guideline to follow is to suture those uterine defects that would normally be closed when an open myomectomy is performed. A large myometrial incision can be approximated in several layers with an intracorporeal curved-needle endosuturing technique. Precise alignment of the deeper myometrium is only possible with a curved suture needle and the rotational motion needed to pass the suture needle through deeper tissue (see Plate 19). I prefer polyglactin (Vicryl) suture on a CT-2 or CT-3 needle for laparoscopic suturing because of its strength, limited memory, and ease of handling.

A simplified intracorporeal twist knot-tying technique is demonstrated in Plate 20. One end of the suture is grasped and then twisted around the shaft of the instrument. After three or four twists, the suture tail is removed from the instrument as the other end of the suture is grasped and pulled through. This twist knot-tying technique greatly facilitates the formation of square "surgeon" knots with no slippage of the suture of separation of the incision edges. Since a large uterine defect can be under a great amount of tension, it is essential that the first suture be secured with minimal slippage. In addition, this curved-needle and knot-tying technique permits a deep suture to be reliably placed into the myometrium in order to obliterate the dead space and to provide the necessary tight approximation of the sidewalls deep within the myometrium.

Uterine reconstruction can also be accomplished with a continuous endosuturing technique. An interrupted tension suture of 2-0 Vicryl must first be placed along the midportion of the incision, and a double square knot tied to reduce tension on the opposing sidewalls. An absorbable polydioxanone (PDS) laparo-tye clip attached to the end of a 3-0 Vicryl suture will serve to anchor the continuous suture line. After the needle is passed into the apex of the incision, the suture is pulled through as the PDS clip becomes locked and buried within the myometrium. A continuous locking suture can be placed along the serosal surface. When the suture line is completed, it is anchored and secured with a second PDS clip (see Plate 21).

The goal of every laparoscopic myomectomy is to reconstruct the myometrial defect with good hemostasis and with an excellent anatomic approximation. Advanced endosuturing skills are essential to the successful performance of laparoscopic myomectomy, and should be a prerequisite for performing this operation. With proper techniques and reconstructive skills, acceptable standards of care can be maintained and well-established surgical principles need not be compromised (see Plate 22).

Specimen Removal from the Abdominal Cavity

The last technical step in laparoscopic myomectomy, specimen removal, is often the most tedious and time consuming. Care must be taken during fibroid removal to avoid patient injury, as one's patience and fatigue level are often challenged. Small fibroids can be removed with a 10-mm morcellating instrument. The myoma must be soft and pliable in order to be removed with this technique. This instrument, however, is ineffective with large or calcified fibroids.

A second technique for removal is to place an endoknife into the abdominal cavity, and to sharply dissect the fibroid into smaller pieces. The fibroid is grasped and stabilized through both lateral ports, while an endoknife is placed down the central midline port. The knife must be visualized and controlled at all times to avoid injury to the patient (see Plate 23). A large 10-mm scissors can also be used to morcellate a fibroid into smaller pieces. A harmonic scalpel is an effective dissector and can safely divide large amounts of fibrous tissue in a reasonable amount of time. The smaller morcellated pieces can be removed from the abdominal cavity through a trocar site. When needed, a large segment of fibroid can be brought up through the trocar site and partially exteriorized. Morcellation can now take place outside the abdominal cavity.

With the appropriate patient, the posterior vaginal fornix provides a fast and readily accessible pathway for fibroid removal. A sponge stick can be placed into the posterior fornix, and a laparoscopic colpotomy incision is made with a scissors or needle-tip cautery. It is important to identify the rectum before making the colpotomy incision. The pneumoperitoneum is rarely lost, as the small vaginal incision is tamponaded when the fibroid is placed into the cul-de-sac. The fibroid is grasped through the vagina and gently removed from the abdominal cavity. The opening in the posterior fornix is sutured closed from the vaginal side. Posterior colpotomy removal is ideal for hard myomas that are resistant to morcellation, or for very large fibroids that are difficult and often time-consuming to debulk. The pelvis is irrigated with 200 mL fluid and the patient is given a single dose of antibiotic. Contrary to previous impressions, we have encountered no increased morbidity in 43 patients with colpotomy removal of uterine fibroids.

For many surgeons, difficulty with endosuturing and tedious specimen removal are the two critical causes that prevent widespread acceptance of laparoscopic myomectomy. A new technique called gasless laparoscopy may provide the solution to improving laparoscopic techniques for myomectomy. A small doughnut-shaped balloon is positioned under the abdominal wall and then attached to an external mechanical elevation arm. The anterior abdominal wall can be gently elevated with creation of a large internal space, which provides excellent visualization and sufficient room for performing a myomectomy (see Plate 24). Since a pneumoperitoneum has been eliminated, standard laparotomy instrumentation can be introduced through small valveless rubber ports. A videoendoscopic operation can now be performed using conventional laparotomy graspers, scalpels, scissors, and needle holders. Uterine reconstruction is now achieved with standard needle drivers and large curved needles (see Plate 25).

The techniques of endosuturing and knot tying are made significantly easier with conventional instrumentation and a gasless technique. In addition, myoma morcellation is rapidly performed with a large scalpel and removal of larger-sized pieces through the abdominal wall (see Plate 26). As a long-time proponent of gasless surgery, I believe that this technique affords many advantages over carbon dioxide laparoscopy, and that it will become the preferred technique for performing a laparoscopic myomectomy.

CONCLUSION

At the present time, a limited number of studies have been published on laparoscopic myomectomy. Reports of intraoperative or delayed bleeding, fistula formation, adhesion formation, and uterine rupture have contributed to a sense of skepticism toward this technique. This procedure is a complex operation that places great demands on the operator's skill, judgment, and patience. However, experienced endoscopists, who routinely perform laparoscopic myomectomy, eagerly attest to the technical feasibility and low morbidity associated with this operation. In my personal series of 173 laparoscopic myomectomies, we have experienced no pelvic infections, no postoperative ileus, no delayed bleeding, no reoperations, two readmissions for unrelated problems, and a return to normal activities in 97% of patients within 2 weeks after surgery.

With careful patient selection, preoperative assessment, strict adherence to operative technique, good hemostasis, and suture reconstruction, many additional patients with symptomatic fibroids can now be afforded the significant benefits of endoscopic surgery. Laparoscopic myomectomy can be safely performed with restoration of normal anatomy and preservation of uterine function (see Plate 27).

BIBLIOGRAPHY

Chin A, et al. Mechanical peritoneal retraction as a replacement for carbon dioxide pneumoperitoneum. J Am Assoc Gynecol Laparoscopists 1993; 1:62.

Dubuisson J-B, et al. Myomectomy by laparoscopy: a preliminary report of 43 cases. Fertil Steril 1991;1:827.

Dubuisson J-B, et al. Gonadotrophin-releasing hormone agonist and laparoscopic myomectomy. Clin Ther 1992;14:51–56.

Dubuisson J-B, Chapron C. Laparoscopic myomectomy: operative procedure and results. Ann NY Acad Sci 1994;734:450.

Harris WJ. Uterine dehiscence following laparoscopic myomectomy. Obstet Gynecol 1992;80:545.

Hasson HM, et al. Instruments and methods. Obstet Gynecol 1992;80:884.

Nezhat C, et al. Laparoscopically assisted myomectomy: a report of a new technique in 57 cases. Int Fertil 1994;39:39.

Turner RT, et al. Improved demonstration of endometrial polyps and submucous myomas using saline-enhanced vaginal sonohysterography. J Am Assoc Gynecol Laparoscopists 1995;2:421.

Verkauf BS. Myomectomy for fertility enhancement and preservation. Mod Trends 1992;58:1.

Verkauf BS. Changing trends in treatment of leiomyomata uteri. Curr Opinion Obstet Gynecol 1993;5:301.

Index

Note: Numbers followed by f indicate figures; those followed by t indicate tables.